# Medical Imaging and Radiotherapy Research

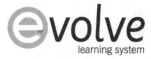

evolve
learning system

Evolve Learning Resources for Students and Lecturers.
See the instructions on the inside cover for
access to the web site.

**Think outside the book**. . .**evolve**

*Commissioning Editor:* Claire Wilson
*Development Editor:* Catherine Jackson
*Project Manager:* Annie Victor
*Designer:* Stewart Larking
*Illustration Manager:* Bruce Hogarth
*Illustrator:* Gillian Richards

# Medical Imaging and Radiotherapy Research

## Skills and Strategies

Edited by

## Aarthi Ramlaul MA(UK) BTechRad NDipRad(SA)

Senior Lecturer, Department of Radiography, University of Hertfordshire, Hatfield, Herts

Foreword by

## Professor Peter Hogg

Professor of Radiography and Diagnostic Imaging Research Lead, University of Salford, Salford

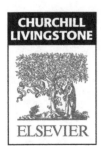

Edinburgh  London  New York  Oxford  Philadelphia  St Louis  Sydney  Toronto  2010

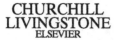

© 2010 Elsevier Ltd. All rights reserved.

ISBN 978 0 7020 3104 5

**British Library Cataloguing in Publication Data**
A catalogue record for this book is available from the British Library

**Library of Congress Cataloging in Publication Data**
A catalog record for this book is available from the Library of Congress

your source for books,
journals and multimedia
in the health sciences
**www.elsevierhealth.com**

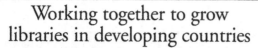

The
Publisher's
policy is to use
paper manufactured
from sustainable forests

Printed in China

# Contents

# Foreword

Radiography, as a profession, has progressed significantly since its inception in the early 20<sup>th</sup> century. In its initial phases the profession rightly placed a major emphasis on practice-based and patient-related activities within what might be described as traditional therapeutic and diagnostic roles. However by the late 1980s and early 1990s, various opportunities presented themselves to further enhance the clinical impact of the profession and the notion of advanced clinical practice was born. Supporting this development, in the early 1990s, the profession became graduate entry and the majority of post-basic clinical competencies became embodied within a postgraduate framework. Graduate and higher graduate education and training therefore provided a firm foundation on which practice would evolve

It is important that we recognise the importance of such university-based education, because without this the service offered to patients would be limited due to the potential lack of appreciation of the value of research in clinical practice. As clinical standards evolved the requirement to use good quality evidence to inform practice has become paramount. In line with this the radiographic profession has been required to use, and where necessary generate, quality evidence on which to base clinical practice. Within the UK, and other countries too, the need for skills in research therefore became an essential component of basic and advanced radiographic competencies.

*Medical Imaging and Radiotherapy Research* is the first book of its kind, bringing together and contextualising important research-related matters that are of relevance to the radiographic profession. This book outlines key reasons as to why research is important in healthcare, making clear why practitioners need a firm comprehension of research processes across a broad range of professional roles and levels. In support of this argument, the book concerns itself with a variety of relevant research paradigms, thereby making it a valuable resource for practitioners, postgraduate and undergraduate students and those whose job role is more focused to research per se.

For those new to research this book will serve to provide a useful framework - not least because it explains particularly well some of the fundamental concepts and terms. It also provides good practical tips from experienced researchers in the field of radiography. As radiography is unusual given the close interface it has between caring for patients and using high technology, the inclusion of a broad but pertinent range of methodologies in this book is important.

My final comment is in regard of the chapter authors and the book editor. If you were to examine radiographic literature over the past 10-15 years you would realise immediately that the contributors are people who are well known in the radiographic profession - they are active participants in our research community. Their individual and collective conference work and journal publications presents as an impressive record of their contribution to our professional knowledge base. Consequently it is right to congratulate the editor on the selection of the chapter authors. On reading this book you will see that their collective knowledge and experience provides us with an excellent research compendium that has direct relevance to the radiographic profession.

Peter Hogg
*Professor of Radiography*
*University of Salford*

The Health Professions Council and the Society of Radiographers requires *inter-alia* practitioners to use evidence from research to inform their everyday practice. Higher education institutions are simultaneously providing training that encourages an interest in research activities among their students.

It is hoped that as a profession, we increase the amount of research that we undertake and prioritize research activities as fundamental to changing practice. In so doing, we become active learners who are committed to improving our profession by embracing lifelong learning. These endeavours contribute to enhancing practice and providing quality care that is uncompromised and benefits the patient, who is at the heart of all considerations.

Radiography has emerged as a discrete profession, which has been demanding because ongoing research is essential and as such, research is a new and challenging area with which we must engage. This text has been written to enable you to develop research skills by the experience gained 'doing it yourself', and aims to take you through the process in the hope of exploring new territories or challenging old ones. In doing so I am sure that you will feel apprehensive at times, but this is all a normal part of discovery.

This text is directed primarily towards those undertaking research studies in radiography for the first time, i.e. undergraduate and postgraduate students. However, the information contained herein would also benefit qualified medical imaging and radiotherapy practitioners who are undertaking research studies for the first time, as well as allied health professionals such as physiotherapists, sports therapists, nurses, dieticians, etc., who have research interests in aspects of radiography. Hence, the text supports inter-professional working, learning and development.

Students can feel overwhelmed by the number of textbooks on their reading lists; in particular, those dealing with research that are not directed specifically to meeting their needs as medical imaging and radiotherapy practitioners. The aim of this textbook is to provide the necessary guidance, support and direction for the novice radiography researcher. The tools provided will help develop the skills needed to generate, develop and undertake research in a methodical and reliable manner.

It is not the intention of the book to present the chapters as stages within the research process, as prescribed steps to follow. Rather it is intended that opportunities for skills development and useful strategies be provided so that each individual can find a style relevant to his or her own work. The research process is dynamic. Often the direction the study takes is dictated by constraints experienced due to the nature of the study. You will find practical examples of the recommended steps to follow; use these as guide in finding your own balance with your study.

This text starts off with background information on the history of research and its context within radiography. Generic aspects of the research process, from literature searching and information management to research governance and ethical considerations, are described. Although generic in concept, the context within which this is set relates to medical imaging and radiotherapy practice. It is intended that this style of presenting these concepts will aid your understanding.

The main types of information or data gathered from research studies are explained and tools for collecting, testing and interpreting data are provided. The quantitative analysis chapter is supported by an interactive demonstration of the statistics tests described within the chapter. This resource is accessible online through *Evolve*, and allows students to work their way through the case examples provided.

The chapter on health technology assessment is a vital tool in our profession today as it enables high quality information on the costs and implications for use of the various technologies to be assessed. By evaluating technologies, we are using the evidence to improve patient outcomes and make efficient and effective use of healthcare resources.

The inclusion of chapters on research outcome measures, reflective practice, dosimetry, quality assurance and clinical audit provides the reader with a comprehensive package of core aspects of our profession.

Novice researchers should benefit from the guidance in structuring, writing, publishing and presenting research findings. Writing up assignments seems to be a somewhat daunting experience for students, whether it is a simple 1000 word essay or a 10 000 word dissertation. These chapters provide you with straightforward guidance on how to structure and present your writing. Guidance on cohesion of information and referencing techniques is given. Using these tools should enable you become a confident writer and publisher.

For those considering applying for research grants, there is a chapter on applying for research funding which provides guidance on the application process, and lastly, some good practice tips to bear in mind throughout the research process as well as pitfalls to avoid. This chapter has been written particularly with the undergraduate student in mind; however, it is aimed equally at all practitioners who need guidance in this skilled technique.

In addition, a glossary of terms can be found on pages 273–275 for clarifying terminology. Where relevant, authors have also added suggested reading material which you will find useful.

You will notice that links have been drawn between chapters and there is repetition of information. Repetition in this context is good as it reinforces understanding and fosters a deep approach to learning.

Where reference to 'radiography' is made, this is generically applicable to both diagnostic and therapeutic practice. Where reference to 'practitioner' is made, this is applicable to radiographers in diagnostic and therapeutic practice and radiologic technologists, as well as allied health professionals.

The overall strength of the text lies in the unique way that concepts are related to examples from medical imaging and radiotherapy practice. Although practices within both these disciplines incorporate somewhat different interaction frameworks between practitioner and patient, care has been taken to present examples from practice that should enable students from both disciplines to connect with the concepts discussed.

As we embark on another era in radiography development and discovery, it is my pleasure to offer this text to enhance and maintain our valuable profession. I hope that the experiences you are about to gain from your research studies encourage and motivate you to continue the process of enquiry throughout your careers.

Aarthi Ramlaul
Spring 2010

# Acknowledgements

I would like to take this opportunity to thank a few key persons without whom this project would not have been possible.

- Class of radiography (2003/4 and 2004/5 - UH) for their feedback and suggestions for the chapter inclusions.
- Dr Richard Price, for his guidance and encouragement throughout the project.
- Martin Vosper, for his advice on various aspects of the text and for developing the online material.

- Professor Gill Marshall who kindly read the drafts and provided guidance on the overall structure of the text.
- Rachel Harris (Professional Research Officer for the Society of Radiographers) for her support and advice.
- All the contributors, who have been patient with me during the editing process and have made this text possible.
- Last, but not least, my family for their unwavering support and encouragement.

# Contributors

**David Allen** BA HDCR
Senior Lecturer, Division of Radiography, Birmingham City University, Birmingham

**Lisa Booth** BSc PhD
Senior Lecturer, School of Medical Imaging Sciences, University of Cumbria, Lancaster

**Stephen Brealey** BSc PhD
Research Fellow, Department of Health Sciences, University of York, York

**Paul Brown** PhD MSc TDCR HDCR(T) DCR(T) FHEA
Deputy Director, Department of Radiography, School of Healthcare Studies, Cardiff University, Cardiff

**Alan Castle** BEd MA PhD TDCR
Principal Lecturer, Radiography, University of Portsmouth, Portsmouth

**Susan Cutler** HDCR MSc PGCE
Senior Lecturer, School of Health and Social Care, University of Teeside, Cleveland, Teeside

**David M Flinton** MSc BSc(Hons) DCR(T) PGCE
Senior Lecturer, Department of Radiography, City University, London

**Julie Hall** DCR(T) PgDip
Senior Lecturer in Radiotherapy, Birmingham City University, Birmingham

**Leon Jonker** BSc(Hons) MSc PhD
Senior Research Fellow, Faculty of Health, Medical Sciences and Social Care, University of Cumbria, Lancaster

**Karen Knapp** BSc(Hons) PgC PhD
Senior Lecturer, University of Exeter, Exeter, Devon

**Jagdeep Kudhail** DCR(T) MSc
Superintendent Radiographer/Quality Manager, Radiotherapy Department, Mount Vernon Hospital, Northwood, Middlesex

**Gill Marshall** MA MSc SFHEA HDCR TDCR
Professor of Medical Imaging Education, Faculty of Health, Medical Science and Social Care, University of Cumbria, Lancaster

**Fiona Mellor** BSc(Hons)
Research Radiographer, Institute for Musculoskeletal Imaging and Clinical Implementation, Anglo-European College of Chiropractic, Bournemouth, Dorset

**Elizabeth Miles** MPhil BSc(Hons) DCR(T)
Co-ordinator, National Trials QA Team, Radiotherapy Physics, Mount Vernon Hospital, Northwood, Middlesex

**Andrew Owens** BSc(Hons) DCR(R) DRI PGCert FETC
Lecturer in Nuclear Medicine, Department of Radiography, City University, London

**Richard Price** PhD MSc FCR
Head of School of Health and Emergency Professions, University of Hertfordshire, Hatfield, Herts

**Heidi Probst** PhD MA BSc(Hons) DCR(T)
Senior Lecturer, Faculty of Health and Wellbeing, Department of Allied Health Professions, Sheffield Hallam University, Sheffield

**Aarthi Ramlaul** MA(UK) BTechRad NDipRad(SA)
Senior Lecturer, Department of Radiography, University of Hertfordshire, Hatfield, Herts

**Pauline Reeves** MSc PhD PgDip PgCert TDCR
Superintendent Radiographer, Radiology Department, Arrowe Park Hospital, Wirral, Cheshire

**Andrew Scally** DCR(R) BSc(Hons) MSc
Senior Lecturer, School of Health Studies, University of Bradford, Bradford

**Martin Vosper** MSc PgDip HDCR
Senior Lecturer, Division of Diagnostic Radiography, University of Hertfordshire, Hatfield, Herts

**Barbara Wilford** MA PgC DCR
Teaching Fellow/Principal Lecturer Medical Imaging, School of Health & Social Care, Teesside University, Middlesbrough, Tees Valley

**Peter Williams** BEd(Hons) MA MSc
Research Fellow, University College London, London

# List of abbreviations and acronyms

| | |
|---|---|
| AAPM | American Association of Physicists in Medicine |
| ABPI | Association of British Pharmaceutical Industry |
| ALARA | As Low As Reasonably Achievable |
| ALARP | As Low As Reasonably Practicable |
| ANOVA | Analysis Of Variance |
| AP | Antero-posterior |
| ARR | Absolute Risk Reduction |
| ARSAC | Administration of Radioactive Substances Advisory Committee (UK) |
| AUC | Area Under the Curve |
| BMA | British Medical Association |
| BPA | British Paediatric Association |
| BSc | Bachelor of Science (degree) |
| CCTV | Closed Circuit Television |
| CI | Confidence Interval |
| CIT | Critical Incident Technique |
| CLD | Central Lung Depth |
| COIN | Royal College of Radiologists Clinical Oncology Information Network |
| CPD | Continuing Professional Development |
| CR | Computed Radiography |
| CT | Computed Tomography |
| CTDI | Computed Tomography Dose Index |
| CHART | Continuous Hyperfractionated Accelerated Radiotherapy Trial |
| CHI | Commission for Health Improvement |
| DAP | Dose Area Product |
| DMC | Data Monitoring Committee |
| DMPA | Depot Medroxyprogesterone Acetate |
| DoH | Department of Health |
| DR | Digital Radiography |
| DXA | Dual Energy X-ray Absorptionmetry |
| EBP | Evidence Based Practice |
| EER | Experiment Event Rate |
| EORTC | European Organisation for Research and Treatment of Cancer |
| EPID | Electronic Portal Imaging Device |
| ESD | Entrance Surface Dose |
| ESTRO | European Society for Therapeutic Radiology and Oncology |

| | |
|---|---|
| GCP | Good Clinical Practice |
| GP | General Practitioner |
| FSD | Focus to Skin Distance |
| Gy | Gray |
| HCC | Health Care Commission |
| HEI | Higher Education Institution |
| HPC | Health Professions Council |
| HTA | Health Technology Assessment |
| ICH | International Conference on Harmonization |
| IGRT | Image Guided Radiotherapy |
| IMRT | Intensity Modulated Radiotherapy |
| IPEM | Institute of Physics in Engineering in Medicine |
| IR(ME)R | Ionising Radiation Medical Exposure Regulations |
| IRAS | Integrated Research Application System |
| IRR | Ionising Radiation Regulations |
| ISO | International Standards Organization |
| ITT | Intention To Treat |
| IVE | Immersive Visualization Environment |
| KSF | Knowledge and Skills Framework |
| kVp | Kilovoltage peak |
| LINAC | Linear Accelerator |
| mAs | Milliampere seconds |
| MCID | Minimally Clinically Important Difference |
| MLC | Multi-leaf Collimator |
| MRA | Magnetic Resonance Angiography |
| MRC | Medical Research Council |
| MRI | Magnetic Resonance Imaging |
| MSc | Master of Science (degree) |
| MU | Monitor Unit |
| NHS | National Health Service |
| NICE | National Institute for Health and Clinical Excellence |
| NIHR | National Institute for Health Research |
| NNT | Number Needed to Treat |
| NPSA | National Patient Safety Agency |
| NRES | National Research Ethics Service |
| NSF | National Service Framework |
| OBI | On Board Imaging |

| | |
|---|---|
| PA | Postero-anterior |
| PACS | Picture Archive and Communication System |
| PICO | Population/Participant Intervention Comparison Outcome |
| PIS | Participant Information Sheet |
| PROMS | Patient Reported Outcome Measures |
| PTV | Planning Target Volume |
| PhD | Doctor of Philosophy (degree) |
| QA | Quality Assurance |
| QALYs | Quality Adjusted Life Years |
| QART | Quality Assurance in Radiotherapy |
| QC | Quality Control |
| QMS | Quality Management System |
| QUADAS | Quality Assessment for Diagnostic Accuracy Studies |
| QUOROM | Quality Of Reporting Of Meta-analysis Statement |
| QUS | Quantitative Ultrasound |
| R&D | Research & Development |
| RBE | Relative Biological Effectiveness |
| RCT | Randomized Controlled Trial |
| REC | Research Ethics Committee |
| RISRAS | Radiation Induced Skin Reaction Assessment Scale |
| ROC | Receiver Operating Characteristic |
| RTOG | Radiotherapy and Oncology Group |
| SCoR | Society and College of Radiographers |
| SHA | Strategic Health Authority |
| SIGN | Scotland Intercollegiate Guidelines Network |
| STARD | Standards for Reporting Diagnostic Accuracy Studies |
| STROBE | Strengthening the Reporting of Observational Studies in Epidemiology |
| Sv | Sievert |
| TLD | Thermoluminescent Dosimeter |
| UICC TNM | International Union against Cancer Tumour-Node-Metastases |
| VAS | Visual Analogue Scale |
| WHO | World Health Organization |

# Section 1

## Getting started with research

# History of research

David Allen   Julie Hall

## CHAPTER POINTS

- Modern clinical practice must be developed using evidence from research.
- The research process allows practitioners both to confirm existing knowledge and to acquire new knowledge.
- Different approaches to research will be required to address different issues. Researchers must choose appropriate methodologies and be transparent in acknowledging the assumptions which underpin their choices.
- Whatever paradigm is chosen the research process itself should remain rigorous and systematic.
- Research may be primary, in which data is gathered first hand, or secondary, where use is made of other sources and acknowledged as such.
- The research community requires that the results of work are shared and are open to retesting and peer review.

This chapter draws on the origins of research, lending a historical perspective on the application of its theories to modern day practice.

## Research and radiography

Unless they have taken on a specialist role, medical imaging and radiotherapy practitioners do not appear to be directly involved in research on a daily basis. Although the ethos is changing, this could explain why research is often not recognized as an integral part of the role of the practitioner and why many students of radiography, both undergraduate and post graduate, have questioned the inclusion of research and statistics material in their courses. However, practitioners rarely, if ever, dispute the need to develop clinical practice upon a sound evidence base, and research is required to obtain this foundation.

Research is about the spirit of enquiry. It can lead almost anywhere you choose. In the medical world it provides evidence which can be used to justify your practice, or to challenge existing dogma. In both the imaging and treatment aspects of the profession, there is a responsibility on the individual to maintain their skills in line with an ever-changing knowledge and evidence base. The radiographic role may vary around the world, with a scope of practice ranging from practitioner to autonomous consultant practitioner, but this responsibility remains constant. It requires a work ethic which embraces continued professional development and life-long learning to ensure the radiographic work force is well informed and effective.

Practitioners therefore require research skills for the following purposes:

- to allow participation in studies contributing to the discipline of radiography
- to address specific problems that may arise in clinical practice
- to develop practice.

It is important to consider how our underpinning knowledge base is formed and the extent to which we are open to new information. This consideration leads directly to the fundamental question, 'What is knowledge?' As researchers, it is important that we understand the philosophy of knowledge and its emerging paradigms as we need to apply these concepts to our daily practice.

# What is knowledge?

Epistemology is the name given to the study of the nature of knowledge; it is essentially a philosophical issue. We not only use information to survive, we also speculate on the nature of that information and our place in relation to it. This is far from being a new preoccupation, as ancient Greece is traditionally identified as the home of the first philosophers. For example, we can easily recognize a modern outlook emerging in Aristotle's (384–322 BC) close observations of the natural world and his application of logic to attempt an explanation of what he saw. It is then not a difficult step to recognize that it is possible, and probably necessary, to distinguish between the world as it is and the world as we perceive it.[1] Knowledge therefore poses certain problems which research must acknowledge in its attempts to separate so-called 'fact' from belief.

Moving briskly forward almost 2000 years, this problem was taken up by a Cambridge-educated English philosopher, Francis Bacon (1561–1626). Bacon believed in the need for a new learning, free from the 'idols' of superstition, prejudice and the preconceptions of the human mind.[2] He was a strong admirer of Aristotle but differed in his insistence that observations should drive the logical process rather than vice versa. Thus, an inductive process of building up a logical structure rooted in observation was established as being a more reliable method than starting with the logic and then applying it to experience in a deductive, top-down fashion. This philosophy gave rise to a systematic method of enquiry which, for the first time, could be termed 'scientific'.

It would probably be contentious to try and fix a date when the scientific process truly came of age. Certainly Isaac Newton set a dramatic and definitive new standard in bringing together observations of the natural world with the theoretical model purporting to explain it. The eighteenth century in Europe, dubbed 'the Enlightenment', recognized this and was characterized by an insistence that belief and observation should be mutually consistent. Its philosophers prized intellectual progress, and perceived this as a measure of the advance of reason over superstition.[3] Indeed, the scientific method has been so successful that it can be argued (and often is) that it has become a dogmatic system in its own right. The strength of the challenge it offers to existing dogmas was clearly seen in the reaction provoked at the time of Darwin's publication of *On the Origin of Species*. Interestingly, over a century later there is still fierce debate between those who believe in creationism and intelligent design, and those who believe in the scientific theory of evolution through natural selection.

Clearly the definition of knowledge and its relation to belief are not separable from social pressures, and so in looking at the pursuit of knowledge it is necessary to be transparent in taking these pressures into consideration.

# Social context of research: paradigms and the pursuit of knowledge

Once a topic of enquiry has been conceived, an appropriate method of investigation has to be applied to it. Immediately, this requires the researcher to consider the beliefs and assumptions they may already hold which could limit or distort their approach. Thomas Kuhn[4] identified that research will inevitably take place within a dominant paradigm – an overarching theoretical context or set of expectations which is socially agreed, perhaps unconscious in its effect, and rooted in culture and history. For this reason, the most significant advances in knowledge and understanding are experienced as revolutionary – so called paradigm shifts. This view was strongly endorsed by Paul Feyerabend,[5] who argued that 'Science is essentially an anarchic enterprise' and that new insights are likely to meet strong resistance, citing Galileo's difficulties with the Catholic Church at that time by way of illustration. However, this contextual basis of research need not be a problem so long as it is recognized as such. Indeed, that being the case, the structure offered by research paradigms can then serve an essential function in supporting the generation of knowledge.[6] In recognizing that a particular enquiry falls within a particular paradigm, the researcher is more likely to produce a credible outcome. Simply put, the method of enquiry must be consistent with the nature of the research question being addressed, and both are likely to be derived within a particular paradigm. It is necessary therefore to identify some common paradigms, and three main contenders can be described: *positivism*, *interpretivism*, and *critical theoretical*.

# Positivism

As noted above, the scientific version of knowledge has become increasingly dominant in modern times, and this dominance is associated in the public mind with a belief that the information that science yields is true and reliable. This popular perception is drawn from a particular paradigm which is defined as positivistic. The assertion that a belief must be testable in observed experience is clearly a powerful driving force, and the fact that this is just an assertion can easily be forgotten. The positivist outlook tends to support this belief and rests on an assumption that an objective and measurable reality exists. It would simply remain then for the researcher to devise a way of measuring the right thing as accurately as possible. This is exactly what seems to have happened. Practical experimentation and observation have been pursued with increasingly subtle ingenuity and investment in advanced technology, and society can see the material fruits of this in everyday life. We can split the atom, put a man on the moon, and decode genetic structures. Clearly, in a practical sense, this sort of science works. So long as there is a quantity to be measured and an objective observer to measure it, positivists believe that eventually the truth will be revealed. From a philosophical point of view this is something of an oversimplification, but it does provide methodologies by which certain sorts of theory can be tested. This is because the positivistic notion of a separate reality allows for the manipulation and control of that reality with no consequent loss of validity. Thus an experimenter can manipulate an independent variable and control confounding variables, and be reasonably confident that the dependent variable will yield a reliable and valid outcome.

For example: using a diagnostic radiographic phantom it is possible to vary the kilovoltage peak (kVp) for a given exposure and measure the consequent effect on image contrast, resolution and density. In radiotherapy the dose on a linear accelerator may be varied when imaging a phantom on a treatment set. In both examples the expectation is that the researcher has control over all identifiable variables, and in particular can isolate and measure the effect of varying a specific parameter.

In medicine this method forms the basis of randomized controlled clinical trials. A typical example would be where a sample of volunteers is randomly allocated to one of two groups, one of which receives a placebo drug or treatment and the other of which receives a new version, with all other factors being the same for both groups. An attempt is thus made to eliminate systematic bias and minimize chance variability in the expectation that any subsequent difference experienced by the two groups will therefore arise as a consequence of the new intervention. The logic is sound, the outcome is measurable, and the system works pretty well. However, there are many other situations in medicine which also require firm evidence but which are not amenable to this sort of approach. It is often necessary therefore to recognize the limits of the positivist outlook and adopt a more appropriate paradigm.

# Interpretivism

People and their circumstances are not easy to control or measure. It may be a simple matter to check an individual's blood pressure or record their weight, but this tells us nothing about what they are thinking or feeling. It is necessary therefore to recognize that in certain areas there is a problem of measurement and equally so of the role of the person doing the measuring. The appropriate paradigm for this sort of enquiry is defined as interpretivist and it differs from the positivist outlook in fundamental ways. The interpretivist paradigm works on the principle that reality is socially constructed, and so emphasizes subjectivity rather than objectivity and regards the observer as essentially inseparable from the phenomena under observation. It is more likely therefore that the sort of data gathered will reflect the *quality* of an experience rather than its *quantity*, and will tend to be concerned with theory building rather than theory testing.

For example: in both diagnostic and radiotherapy settings a researcher may wish to use a questionnaire to conduct a survey into the participants' experience of their illness or treatment. Researchers would then need to be alert to the extent to which their own expectations could influence the choice of questions put to the participants, and also to a possible similar bias in the subsequent analysis of the responses.

Historically, we have seen how science fought to establish itself against dogma as a reliable source of information and have noted its subsequent increasing dominance. Perhaps it was inevitable that at some point it would reach the limits of its applicability, and risk becoming a dogma in its own right.

A good example of this is the progress of behaviourism as a psychological model. At the start of the 20th century Wilhelm Wundt suggested that the subject matter of psychology should be consciousness, and the method of enquiry introspection. However, John Watson and B. F. Skinner later insisted that the only observable phenomenon is outward behaviour and that it was not possible therefore to comment directly on possible mental events. This idea took hold and by the latter half of the 20th century psychology was largely given over to a biological and operant conditioning model of learning. Society moved on, and it was felt that in ditching consciousness 'the baby had been thrown out with the bathwater'. Eventually a variety of humanistic models reasserted the central importance of inner experience, with methodologies to suit.[7] So, for example, a positivistic view of learning as a change in behaviour can be compared with an interpretivist version: 'learning occurs when individuals ... respond, or try to respond, meaningfully to what they experience and then seek to ... integrate the outcomes into their own biographies'.[8]

In order to capture the lived quality of an individual's experience, an interpretivist paradigm must be embraced. This brings with it the need for a methodology which can deal with subjectivity but which is nevertheless rigorous and systematic, and in that sense scientific and credible. Within the interpretivist paradigm it is possible to identify several distinct approaches and these need to be briefly described.

## Phenomenology and hermeneutics

Typically an interpretivist approach will involve recording someone's own account of something they have experienced. The problem is to do it in such a way that the person's words are captured and used to present a credible insight which is faithful to that experience. Phenomenology aims to achieve this. Edmund Husserl (1859–1932), usually regarded as the founder of phenomenology, believed that it was possible to delineate an individual's conscious experience by a process of 'bracketing'. This involves the deliberate attempt to identify and set aside the researcher's own preconceptions, so that one is left with a complete yet unadorned description of the phenomenon in the respondent's own terms.[9] Clearly, however, there may be difficulty in achieving the desired level of objectivity when immersed in essentially subjective material. Furthermore it may be questioned whether such a description would be

meaningful anyway, since the respondent's own terms are themselves a product of that individual's circumstances. This latter point rests at the heart of hermeneutics, a phenomenological approach developed by German philosopher Martin Heidegger (1889–1976), in which bracketing is dismissed and the researcher aims to capture individual meaning through subjective dialogue with the material.[10]

For example: diagnostic imaging and therapy practitioners both come into contact with people who present with serious illness and may wish to understand their patients' condition more thoroughly. In this example it would be appropriate to talk with willing participants and allow them to describe and discuss their personal experience in some depth. A suitable methodology here may be to conduct an extended interview, gathering as much spoken and non-verbal communication as possible, and then transcribe it faithfully. Researchers would need to immerse themselves in such material and try to make sense of it while setting aside their own biases and opinions.

This is clearly a far cry from the positivist approach, which tends to ignore individuals and their social context.

## Symbolic interactionism, grounded theory and ethnomethodology

The impact of social context and the roles that we derive from it form the subject matter of symbolic interactionism. The sense of self is here regarded as arising out of the interplay between members of a social group in which we communicate by means of words, gestures and display. The clothes we wear, the words we choose and the mannerisms we adopt all contribute to a social consensus within which our own identity is established with reference to other people. At the level of large groups of people or populations this process is addressed through ethnomethodology, which focuses on socially agreed customs. Within the same sociological tradition, Glaser and Strauss[11] pioneered the approach known as grounded theory, which acknowledges that individuals constantly change, and so does research.

For example: a suitable application of grounded theory could be to explore the student practitioner's experience of clinical placement. Students could be asked to maintain a journal while on placement in which they record their thoughts, feelings and behaviour. The researcher could then look for themes in these written accounts, perhaps meet with the participants, and suggest a possible analysis of the main factors which the students themselves regarded as significant to their learning. Having developed such an analysis the researcher would need to meet again with the students to confirm the extent to which the researcher's version 'rang true'. In the light of the new participant response the researcher would need to revisit their explanatory model, iterating this consultative process until consensus is reached that the model is credible.

The method is inductive, aiming to build theory from the 'bottom up' using participants' reports, and revisiting those people to check that the result is in accordance with their experience. The process of data collection and analysis is therefore iterative and ongoing, with constant elaboration and refinement in an attempt to establish a consensus.

Thus, interpretivism seeks to understand the world, while positivism expects to predict it. The third paradigm, the critical theoretical, aims to change it.

## Critical theoretical

Both paradigms discussed so far incorporate an ethos that the process of research is in some way separable from the area being researched. The positivist approach takes this as axiomatic and interpretivism, although it addresses individuals' experiences within their social context, still proceeds as if that context is well defined. In contrast, the critical theoretical paradigm starts with the premise that not only is research embedded in its social context, it is actually part of it. Furthermore, because society itself is neither fixed nor well defined, the validity of the product of research is therefore called into question. Thus research is faced with both a challenge of credibility and an opportunity to be an agent of change. Action research, for example, specifically sets out to evaluate and possibly recommend change in a system at the very same time that it is gathering data on the system. This requires a team approach and potentially offers emancipatory power to the participants, but brings problems of its own, to do with a need for flexibility and a possible challenge to existing power relationships. In this respect, it is not difficult to see the same concerns at the heart of the standpoints on research of feminists and black people. The former approach points to the failure of traditional research to address topics of particular relevance to women and places women firmly in the role of researcher and women's issues at the focus of enquiry. Likewise the latter approach is a response to the need for culturally sensitive and competent research with an emphasis on the impact of ethnicity and culture on life and life chances. These differing standpoints share the concern that in order to be meaningful, research must be transparent in recognizing personal and societal agendas. In order to achieve this, the researcher must adopt a postmodern awareness of the complexity of how the world presents to us, and how we in turn choose to perceive it. This requires the researcher to look for the 'truth behind the truth' by deconstructing existing social terms and forms of representation.

For example: role extension provides a possible example within radiography of where the status quo might be questioned or even challenged by critical theoretical research. The practitioner's role can be defined on a spectrum ranging from protocol driven, technical tasks to autonomous patient management at consultant level. The latter end of this spectrum particularly needs to be supported by a credible evidence base, and in acquiring such a base the issue of professional boundaries would need to be addressed. The terms, conditions and scope of the research and the researcher's own agenda cannot now be regarded as separate from the underpinning research aim. Existing power relationships will come into play and the researcher must recognize these, allow them to inform his or her work, and so deal with them.

Language is thus crucial to any line of enquiry. Discourse analysis, for example, looks beyond the text that is supplied by a research participant, and investigates the beliefs which their words belie.[12] In addition, language is not regarded as a passive vehicle for fixed propositions, but as an active component in their establishment and propagation. Van Dijk,[13] for example, draws attention to the multilevelled nature of discourse, the strategies we employ in comprehending it, and the consequent encoding of social structures and power relationships in the very words that people use. Thus all players in the research process have agendas and it is necessary to identify and declare these. Within the critical theorist paradigm, not only is knowledge provisional but also, in the words of Habermas,[14] there is a 'singular interlocking of knowledge and interest'.

Clearly the type of knowledge being sought and the methods used to seek it are interdependent, and Box 1.1 attempts to summarize this relationship.

## Box 1.1

### Summary of research terms

#### Epistemology

The study of the nature of knowledge or what is out there to know in the world around us.

#### Paradigms

The assumptions we make about the world which influence our expectations of what it is possible to know and how we go about knowing it.

Examples: positivism, interpretivism, critical theoretical.

#### Methodologies

These are the general approaches to research found within each paradigm.

For example: an experimental approach is an appropriate methodology within the positivist paradigm.

#### Methods

These are the particular ways of carrying out a given methodology.

Using the experiment as an example of a general approach, a particular way of conducting the experiment could be a randomized controlled trial.

The divisions in Box 1.1 do not necessarily indicate the order in which a researcher works. It is not wrong to start with a methodology or even a method. Often we start with a question in mind, develop a method that seems appropriate, and only then appreciate how the paradigm can inform or constrain our research design.

It can also be convenient to divide research into quantitative and qualitative approaches. Quantitative approaches are often associated with the positivistic paradigm and qualitative approaches are often similarly associated with the interpretivist paradigm. However, this can be an oversimplification and it may therefore be safer simply to use the terms 'quantitative' and 'qualitative' as descriptions of the methods that we use, the data that we collect and how we analyse it. For example, consider a study designed to explore the feelings of a patient undergoing a diagnostic examination or a course of radiotherapy treatment. We may assume that the approach being taken is a qualitative one because we are trying to capture the nature of their experience and the data collected would be in the form of words requiring interpretation. However, the distinction would become slightly blurred if our analysis then involved counting the number of times that a

particular feeling was expressed, because these numbers would make our approach more quantitative. The researcher may perhaps be forgiven for wondering how useful the distinction really is; however, the important thing to get right is to choose a methodology which allows you to answer your research question.

In summary, therefore, it is necessary to recognize that any particular piece of research will be limited in what it can achieve, and these limits are set by the world view or paradigm within which the researcher is operating. We have identified three different paradigms, but whichever approach is adopted there is a common requirement that the process of enquiry itself should be rigorous and systematic, and it is to this that we turn next.

## Evidence-based medicine: a systematic approach to knowledge

We have thoroughly explored the proposition that knowledge does not arise in a vacuum. In fact, putting philosophy to one side, there is nowadays an expectation that research will lead to useful applications – not least in the field of health care. It is this expectation that underpins the practice of evidence-based medicine, whereby current clinical activity is constantly reviewed in the light of new research. It is accepted therefore that knowledge is only ever provisional, and with that caveat in place the research process must be robust enough to offer a definitive version of the latest 'best practice'. Improving clinical practice must place the patient's well-being at the heart of our endeavours. To do this we must consider both the objective and physiological together with the subjective and emotional aspects of the patient experience. This demands that the researcher adopt whichever approach is most appropriate for the topic being pursued, but in all cases to still aspire to a credible outcome which is open to peer review. In practice this is achieved by following a common systematic approach, by breaking up a rather large project into bite-sized chunks and allowing yourself to work through this in an organized manner (see Chapter 7).

Thus an organized process is used to connect with existing knowledge and yield a result which is communicable and, if necessary, open to retesting. Possibly the most difficult of these is the very first question, namely 'what do you want to do?' Clarity of focus is crucial since it will determine the nature of the methods you use, and a clear focus does not have to be a narrow one.

## Secondary research

So far the assumption has been that research is all about discovering, assessing and comparing new data. Practice can also be informed by revisiting the research carried out by others.

This can be done by combining a number of studies in order to answer a specific research question (or to summarize the findings) and usually takes the form of a systematic review. A systematic review involves the painstaking collection of all relevant studies, whether they have been published or not. A good quality systematic review applies the same rigour in the review of research evidence as should have been applied in the original production of that evidence and presents the collated evidence in an impartial and balanced way. Meta-analysis is used to combine the statistical data from these combined studies in a meaningful way as it takes into account the relative sizes of the studies included in the systematic review. A good literature source for recommendation would be the Cochrane Collaboration,[15] which is a global network that provides systematic reviews on healthcare interventions. Interventions for relieving the pain and discomfort of screening mammography and exercise for women receiving adjuvant therapy for breast cancer are just two examples of reviews that can be accessed.

## Secondary data

Another approach to research is to use secondary data. Secondary data are data previously collected by someone else, possibly for some other purpose. However, care must be exercised when defining what constitutes secondary data. For example, if you compiled a new data set unique to your study from existing survey material you would be considered to be doing primary research, but if you used existing summary results or results compiled by other researchers this would be considered secondary data and so your research would also be considered as secondary.

# Conclusion

As practitioners we are professional people, and as such we have an obligation to maintain our clinical practice to the highest standards. We act as the interface between high technology and the patient; and our duty to the patient is matched by a responsibility to pull our weight within the medical team. Modern medicine proceeds on the basis of clinical evidence and the way to acquire this is through research. We have argued that research should be a systematic and rigorous process of collecting, analysing and sharing data, and that this work must be done in a way which transparently acknowledges its social context. We may wish to predict, interpret or even change the world we live in and we should recognize that the knowledge we acquire is likely to be influenced by our own interests. All the more reason, therefore, for a firm knowledge base, derived using an appropriate methodology. We can build theories from qualitative interpretation or test them by making quantitative measurements, but the fundamental principle to observe in all cases is to develop a clear focus for the research question and allow this to inform our actions.

# References

[1] Harré R. The Philosophies of Science. London: Oxford University Press; 1972.

[2] Peltonen, Markku, editor. The Cambridge Companion to Bacon. Cambridge: Cambridge University Press; 1996.

[3] Cassirer E. The Philosophy of the Enlightenment. Princeton: Princeton University Press; 1968.

[4] Kuhn TS. The Structure of Scientific Revolutions. 2nd ed. Chicago: The University of Chicago Press; 1970.

[5] Feyerabend P. Against Method. 3rd ed. London: New Left Books; 1975.

[6] Ernest P. An Introduction to Research Methodology and Paradigms. Exeter: Research Support Unit, School of Education, University of Exeter; 1994.

[7] Roth I, editor. Introduction to Psychology Vol 1. London: The Open University; 1990.

[8] Jarvis P, Holford J, Griffin C. The Theory and Practice of Learning. 2nd ed. London: Kogan Page; 2003.

[9] Parahoo K. Nursing Research: Principles, Process and Issues. London: Macmillan; 1997.

[10] Miller S. Analysis of phenomenological data generated with children as research participants. Nurse Researcher 2003;10:70–3.

[11] Glaser B, Strauss AL. The Discovery of Grounded Theory.

London: Weidenfeld & Nicolson; 1967.

[12] Abbott P, Sapsford R. Research Methods for Nurses and the Caring Professions. 2nd ed. Maidenhead: Open University Press; 1998.

[13] Van Dijk TA, Kintsch W. Strategies of Discourse Comprehension. London: Academic Press; 1983.

[14] Habermas J. Knowledge and Human Interests. London: Heinemann; 1972. p. 209.

[15] Cochrane Collaboration. Available online: http://www.cochrane.org/reviews/index.htm (accessed 10 December 2008).

# Finding and formulating a research question

## 2

Martin Vosper

## CHAPTER POINTS

- Research questions should be clear, specific and focused to the purpose of study.
- Time and resources are the main constraints which affect the feasibility of studies.
- For an undergraduate project, keep to a maximum of about three aims, and use this as a guide to build up to a postgraduate project, e.g. at Master's level, or develop significantly for a project at Doctoral level.
- Qualitative and quantitative methods of enquiry form the two main avenues of research.

This chapter takes you through the various steps involved in finding a suitable research idea or topic and formulating it into a workable question to answer.

## Step one: identifying a question

Why is it important to have a question when starting out in medical imaging or radiotherapy research? Well, having a clear and specific question permits the following things:

- it provides a focus
- it identifies a gap in existing knowledge, or a set of circumstances which need to be explained
- it prevents us from becoming 'side-tracked' into irrelevant enquiries
- it reminds us of the purpose of our research
- it enables us to find answers and make conclusions
- it helps others to decide whether our work is of interest to them.

The lack of an obvious research question is one of the main reasons why research proposals are rejected, be

it by academic tutors, health ethics committees or funding bodies. At this point the frustrated and disappointed researcher might well ask the question 'Why on earth am I doing this?' This is a very good question to ask.

There are of course many reasons why people do research: perhaps to get a diploma or degree, to advance their careers, to benefit their patients within the healthcare system, or even to expand the boundaries of human knowledge. Their expectations will vary in line with these goals, from modest to ambitious. Very few of us will do truly revolutionary research in our lifetimes, such as splitting the atom, discovering X-rays or developing the ultimate cure for cancer. It is not often that research questions are completely ground-breaking and original. But a question does not have to be 100% novel to be of value. There are always questions that others have asked already, but in different circumstances. For example, we might explore whether the radiation doses to our patients are different this year from last, or the same at hospital A and hospital B. Surveys of stress are nothing new, but it could be that no one has ever done a stress survey of patients receiving a particular type of palliative radiotherapy or diagnostic X-ray examination at your workplace. To be worthwhile, a research question does not have to be new, but it *does* have to be *worth asking*.

To be worth asking, a research question should try to avoid producing what I could call the 'so what?' response from other people. This consists of a mix of negative feelings, including:

- 'So what is the purpose of this research?' (there isn't one?)

- 'So what new understanding or information will this research give us?' (none?)
- 'So what benefit could this research bring to imaging or radiotherapy?' (none?)
- 'So who cares?' (so what?)

Medical imaging and radiotherapy research is most likely to succeed when it has a clear purpose, is capable of increasing understanding and likely to benefit patients. For undergraduate research leading to an academic award these principles could perhaps be relaxed slightly, as 'new understanding' might include a student's improved awareness of the research process. But the three principles of purpose, understanding and benefit still apply.

This might sound daunting, but it really is not. Finding a suitable research question is within everyone's reach. In fact there are questions which present themselves every day, both in clinical practice and at university or college. There are too many to be answered in a lifetime, with new questions constantly arising as clinical practice changes and new technologies emerge. All we need to do is lift our eyes up from the coal face of our routine work and be observant – ask questions and keep notes on a daily basis.

What types of questions can we ask? There are too many possibilities to list fully, but the following may provide some suggestions:

- Are there variations between practices, workplaces or people?
- What is happening nationally in this type of clinical practice?
- Is A performing better or worse than B? (this could apply to procedures, environments, information, or education systems)
- What has changed since date X?
- What are people's feelings, knowledge, attitudes or opinions? (patients, staff, students, tutors or the general public)
- What are the effects of this particular technology, or service? (benefits and risks for patients, diagnosis, treatment, costs, waiting times, technical quality, training, education)
- What happens if we alter this? (technique, procedure, parameter)
- What is the size or extent of this?
- Why did things go wrong or right in this situation?
- What is the current 'state of the art' (knowledge or advancement) in this topic area?

If we are completely stuck and cannot think of any research questions, it is often a good idea to look through published journal articles in medical imaging and radiotherapy for sources of inspiration. Reading them can highlight topic areas that we would not otherwise have considered. Also the authors may list recommendations for further research at the end of their articles – research that we might be in a position to do.

Whatever question is chosen, the researcher needs to feel *interested* in it and also that the question is of interest to others. Having a love (or at least a liking) for a topic helps a researcher get through the long hours of data collection and writing up that will follow. Sometimes a research question is chosen for weak reasons, because it seems easy to answer or will not need ethics approval. Although this is understandable, the result can be a first taste of research which is boring and dissatisfying. Having completed the project and got the qualification, the student closes the book on research and vows never to open it again!

It is important to ask a research question, no matter whether we are doing a piece of primary research (gathering fresh material) or secondary research (reviewing published material). Finding a fresh question is vital if a review of existing literature is to be of interest. Since there may already be published reviews in the topic area, it is best if a different angle on the material is chosen, or different inclusion criteria are used. Also if there has been some time since the last review, it may be possible to ask an existing question but with the benefit of new articles.

## Step two: is my question feasible?

There are many questions to ask, but not all of them can be answered, or certainly not within the time or resources available. Research into cancer survival rates following treatment is valuable but will probably need a period of years to undertake, rather than the 6–8 months of a student project. Likewise it would be interesting to survey whether the dose from a diagnostic X-ray procedure causes an increase in cancer rates, but as the radiation dose will be small and induced cancers few, we would need a huge sample of patients to test our question. Questions such as these can indeed be answered, but perhaps only within the wider framework of a Doctoral thesis or a large funded project.

The following points should be considered by anyone starting out on a piece of research:

- Is this research question answerable?
- How big a sample will I need to have a good chance of providing an answer?
- How much time have I got?
- What resources do I have (especially money and skills)?
- Has the question already been answered, to such an extent that there is nothing new to say in this topic area?

An example of an unanswerable question might be one which depends on historical data. Let us suppose that we want to ask whether the performance of a radiography procedure has improved over time. Past hospital or patient records might be missing or incomplete, meaning that no comparison can be made with the present day – the situation is essentially unknowable. This is often a problem with *retrospective studies*. Another unanswerable question might be 'What are the true causes of adverse patient reactions to this radiological contrast agent at our hospital?' Although reaction types and rates might be recordable, the real nature of the physiological changes taking place would only be knowable after thorough tests on each patient.

More is said about sample sizes in Chapters 7 and 10. But we can note here that in any research study we need enough data to be able to reach valid conclusions. It would be silly, for example, to make assumptions about the national views of clinical practitioners after getting questionnaires back from only 10 people. When writing a research question we need to consider how feasible it will be to gather data. If we are part of a big student cohort, it should be fairly straightforward to gather plenty of student attitude information, assuming that people are available when we need them and prepared to take part. But if the research topic is, for example, based on a fairly unusual clinical condition or procedure, we might not be able to gather many cases during the research time we have available.

Time available to us as researchers is a real issue, and clearly more can be achieved when we have 3 years to do the work, rather than 6 months. Long-term projects can be more ambitious and more thorough. But in reality most research, whether it be for a university degree or an external funding body, is driven by tight deadlines. After deciding on a research question, time is needed to explore the previously published literature on the topic, gather data

and then write up the work. Each of these stages can take longer than expected and it is important to map out a target timetable, paying attention to what are the key aims and objectives for each stage. In this respect I would argue that it is better to answer a simple question well rather than a complex question inadequately, especially when time is short. It is important to ask 'What is my key question?' when doing research, rather than becoming sidetracked into other minor queries, no matter how interesting they might appear to be. 'Fuzziness' or lack of focus is one of the most frequent reasons why research projects under-perform in assessment.

When considering the resources available to us, one key factor is money (or lack of it). The costs of doing research might include:

- postage, paper and envelopes
- travel
- reimbursing participants
- photocopying and printing
- ordering journal articles
- setting up an online survey
- software packages and computer hardware
- paying research assistants or statisticians (in funded projects)
- paying for use of clinical facilities, such as scanner time (in funded projects).

Some of these things might possibly be available on a 'no charge' basis to students, but it is wise to be realistic, for example when proposing to undertake a national survey involving all hospitals.

Resources also include our own special talents and abilities. Someone who is especially good at statistics might be drawn to a project which involves a lot of complex data analysis, while a person who is a good communicator might be more suited to doing an interview survey. Although statistical help is often available at colleges and hospitals, many people become so scared of statistics that they try to avoid them altogether. This is not normally a good idea as it can restrict the analysis of research findings. But of course it is not true that *every* piece of research must make use of statistical tests. Some numerical findings can be reported perfectly well descriptively, using tables and charts, while analysis of interviews would not usually require statistics at all. I would recommend using a statistical test when it adds something useful to the research findings, but not merely for the sake of trying to 'show off' when there is little justification for the test's inclusion.

There are some research questions which have already been answered so completely that there can be little scope for fresh discoveries in the topic. As an example, it is well known that giving a caudal beam angulation for postero-anterior (PA) chest radiography can slightly reduce the dose to the patient's thyroid gland. Published dose data were available for this many decades ago, but the question is still a popular choice for undergraduate research proposals in radiography. There can be little real justification for proposals of this type, although the measurements involved might form a useful exercise within an undergraduate science course. If the answer to a research question is already well known from standard textbooks on the subject, there is little point in asking it again, unless a new approach can be used.

## Step three: types of questions

People can ask research questions for different reasons in radiography; for example:

- *To test a theory or idea*. This is often the case in experimental research. An experiment sounds rather lab-based but can be much broader than this, including social science, not just physics. Testing the effects of two radiotherapy regimes in clinical practice or bringing in a new patient information leaflet could be considered to be experimental studies, as could dosimetry research using a phantom. We might also be making observations and trying to create a theory to explain what we see.
- *To measure a position or situation*. This could take place in surveys – for example to determine the state of current practice in digital imaging at hospital sites or practitioner attitudes to a Government policy.
- *To improve clinical practice*. Asking questions about what we do as clinical practitioners, making use of research findings and altering our procedures accordingly, is known as 'evidence-based practice' or 'evidence-informed practice'. Such questioning also forms a part of the process of reflection (see Chapter 5, Reflective practice).
- *To explore feelings, viewpoints and attitudes*. These might include the anxieties of patients receiving a clinical procedure, or the factors which influence job satisfaction among staff.

The types of questions we can ask could be categorized as being directed towards:

- explaining (e.g. testing theories and idea*s)*
- *describing* (e.g. measuring positions and situations, making observations)
- exploring (e.g. looking at feelings and attitudes)
- controlling (e.g. implementing change, improving quality).

These types of questions can be found within the two main avenues of research, that is, quantitative and qualitative. More will be said about these avenues in Chapters 7 and 8 but quantitative research is more likely to be based on numerical data and seeks to ask questions such as 'What?' or 'How much?', while qualitative research is more likely to be based on attitudes and opinions and asks the question 'Why?'. Questions which fall within the 'exploring' category are usually associated with qualitative research. The research tradition in medical imaging and radiotherapy has mostly been quantitative, linked to measuring the statistical performance of diagnostic tests, cancer therapies and associated equipment. However, qualitative work has a vital and perhaps neglected role to play in exploring the attitudes, beliefs and opinions of patients and staff. Research can often bring together both approaches, gathering statistical data and also insights into the underlying reasons as to why things are as they are. An example might be a study of quality performance in radiography which looks at numerical trends and also staff attitudes.

When doing a piece of research, we may be faced with the dilemma of asking just a single key question, or asking several. In addition, we may ask ourselves, 'Should we stay fixed and focused on a single issue or should we be responsive to the findings that we make during the research process?' Researchers' views on this will generally differ according to their research background. Quantitative research tends to address a single question (or perhaps several closely related questions), while qualitative research is much more free in its philosophy and would regard a single research question as an unhelpful restraint. Qualitative research needs to be free to find and develop new research questions as people's verbal comments are explored. Putting these differences aside for a moment, however, I would advise anyone who is submitting a research proposal for a degree project or external funding to opt for a single principal question initially, for the reasons I gave at the start of this chapter.

## Does research have to have a hypothesis?

The answer is no, not always. A hypothesis is a research question which aims to test out a theory. Traditionally we mean 'scientific' theory here, which is based on experimental observations and attempts to make sense of the world by explaining these in terms of proposed theories. The term 'hypothesis' could be used in research which asks 'explaining' questions, but not in that which uses 'describing' or 'exploring' questions. It would not generally be found in qualitative research. As an example, it would be quite normal to have a hypothesis when doing a physics experiment in the X-ray lab, but not when exploring the belief systems of student practitioners.

People often get confused when the terms 'null hypothesis' and 'alternative hypothesis' appear. Hypotheses generally test theories about whether relationships between measurable things (*variables*) are real or not. There are two possibilities: either one variable will influence another, or it will not. For example, we could propose a theory that the size of the X-radiation dose to living tissues is a factor influencing an irradiated person's health. Rather confusingly, this relationship would be termed the 'alternative hypothesis', which is given the symbol $H_1$. A proposal that there is no relationship at all between X-ray dose and health would be called the 'null hypothesis'. A null hypothesis is given the symbol $H_0$.

If there are two possible relationships between variables, for example where one variable might vary inversely or directly with another, we can have two alternative hypotheses. The first alternative hypothesis, symbol $H_1$, could here describe the more likely inverse relationship between radiation dose and health (as dose increases, health decreases), while the second alternative hypothesis, symbol $H_2$, could describe a less likely direct relationship (as radiation dose increases, health increases). These days we all accept that increased X-ray doses may reduce health and would thus reject hypothesis $H_2$, but this was not at all obvious to the early radiation pioneers. Indeed a theory called radiation hormesis, in which small doses of radiation might actually be beneficial in some respects, has been proposed (but is not accepted by the majority of scientists).

## Step four: answering our question

Once we have decided upon a research question, we need to take the work forward by developing a structure for the project. It is important to create aims and objectives – indeed these are normally an expected part of a research project proposal.

It is very common for students to get the terms 'aims' and 'objectives' mixed up. An aim is a defined goal or aspiration for the research and is much easier to write if we have a clear research question. In general there should not be too many aims, or else the project is at risk of becoming confused in its intentions, over-ambitious, cumbersome and not feasible. I would recommend that there should not be more than about three aims at most for an undergraduate research project, and using this as a guide to build upon for a postgraduate project. Objectives are step-by-step targets for the research process, often arranged within a timeline, setting out the practical means by which the project aims will be achieved. There will normally be more objectives than aims.

Let us consider an example of a survey project which is asking the question 'Does the general public know less about radiography than about physiotherapy or nursing?' Possible aims for a project like this might be:

- to determine the general public's awareness of radiography, physiotherapy and nursing
- to survey a representative sample of the general public
- to undertake a questionnaire survey.

Possible objectives for this project might include:

- to search the available published literature covering public awareness of the health professions
- to explore possible means of targeting the general public
- to decide survey limits and sample size
- to submit a research proposal
- to produce a draft questionnaire
- to obtain ethics approval
- to pilot the questionnaire
- to rework the questionnaire as necessary
- to distribute the questionnaires
- to analyse the questionnaire data
- project write-up
- submission
- possible publication.

# Further reading

Crombie IK, Davies HTO. Research in Health Care: Design, Conduct and Interpretation of Health Services Research. Chichester: Wiley; 1996.

Polit DF, Beck CT. Essentials of Nursing Research: Methods, Appraisal and Utilization. Philadelphia: Lippincott, Williams and Wilkins; 2006.

Sim J, Wright C. Research in Health Care: Concepts, Designs and Methods. Cheltenham: Nelson Thornes; 2000.

# Literature searching

# 3

## Martin Vosper

## CHAPTER POINTS

- Conducting a good literature search enables you to take a broad view and to interpret your research findings in light of existing knowledge.
- There are a number of ways in which you can search for information, the most popular being the online search engines.
- It is good practice to develop a literature search strategy or method so that this plan can guide you through your searches and keep you focused on the aims and objectives of your study.
- Most literature reviews will need you to submit an indication of the search strategies or methods used. This forms the methodology of the literature review and would include the main inclusion and exclusion criteria for literature searching.

This chapter describes the need for searching literature sources of information and provides guidance on how to conduct a search, how to extract information and how to manage this information.

## Why search the literature?

Searching the published literature within our chosen research topic is vital, both in primary research (for example a *new* experiment or survey) and in secondary research (a review of existing findings). Literature searches can be used in many ways, to give:

- a supporting background to help justify a research proposal
- a source of ideas for new research
- guidance on pitfalls and problems in the topic area, drawing upon the experiences of previous researchers
- a check on what has already been done (or not done) in the topic
- an update of current evidence to inform best clinical practice
- a chapter on previous published findings within a primary research project
- the content material for a systematic review
- evidence to support what we say in essays, guidance documents and policies.

So it can be seen that everyone, from a first year diagnostic imaging or radiotherapy student to the head of the National Health Service, has reasons to search the literature. Literature searching is not a tool that can be packed away at the end of an undergraduate degree and never used again.

The research that we do may be weak and ill-informed if we are unaware of the findings of others in the field. There may then be a tendency to promote our own pet theories. Of course, even top scientists like to push their personal viewpoints, but they run the risk of having narrow discussions and reaching biased conclusions if they ignore alternative evidence. This applies to us as novice researchers too. Doing a good literature search enables us to take a broad view and to interpret our own research results fully in the light of existing knowledge. It also gives us more to say within the analysis of our findings, as we can compare our own data with those previously gathered by others elsewhere.

# How wide a literature search do we need to do?

Well, this very much depends on the task in hand. Some suggestions are given in Table 3.1.

Suggestions for the numbers of references in Table 3.1 apply to typical student work at undergraduate degree level. For postgraduate or funded research, the expectations would be greater. But there are always some topics, perhaps very recent, specialist or obscure, in which little published research is available. In these cases it would be accepted that fewer references might be used – *provided that the researcher really has done a thorough literature search.* It is quite common for students to report, rather despondently, that they 'can't find anything on the subject', when a subsequent online search brings up several journal articles which they have missed. It is important to search widely when looking for literature and to use the right tools for the job. These issues are discussed below.

Researching in an area where little previous work is available can restrict the literature review section of a project, but it can be a positive advantage too.

There is probably more chance that the research findings will be novel and original. It may also help with publication, provided that the topic is not so obscure that it is of no interest to others.

*How recent should literature references be?* The pace of technological change in medical imaging and radiotherapy means that older clinical references may be outdated and no longer relevant to current practice. As a guide, I would recommend only using literature sources from within the last 5 years (normally) in any topic area which is experiencing rapid change. Examples might include computed tomography and intensity modulated radiotherapy. Even in subjects like these, there may be earlier research which should be included because it is key to understanding in the subject or contains evidence which was, and still is, of vital importance. It is sometimes suggested that research from countries which have technically advanced health care systems (the USA is often quoted in this regard) may be slightly ahead of its time and that this should be taken account of too when thinking of a 5-year cut-off point for useful sources.

As mentioned above, secondary research consisting of a literature review makes the most extensive

**Table 3.1  The number of literature references typically needed within common research tasks at undergraduate level**

| Research task | Suggested number of references | Reasons for the literature search |
|---|---|---|
| 1. Writing a research proposal | About 10 should suffice. These should be recent key references in the topic area | To set the background<br>To show awareness of the topic<br>To justify the proposed research<br>To identify issues and opportunities |
| 2. Doing a literature review chapter within a primary research project | The number depends upon how many references are available in the topic. However, fewer than about 30–40 would be disappointing to most tutors | To set the background<br>To identify other relevant work in the topic<br>To provide comparisons with our own findings<br>To inform our method, discussion and conclusions |
| 3. Doing secondary research (a systematic review of literature) | All recent relevant research in the topic should be included<br>*But* limitations will include language of publication (if other than English), type of publication, personal resources<br>The number depends upon how many references are available in the topic, but it should be larger than in (2) above<br>About 80+ would typically be expected for an undergraduate review in a topic where ample literature is available | To provide a rigorous overview of recent available research in the topic area, without major omissions<br>To portray the current state of knowledge and/or clinical practice in the topic area<br>To synthesize the available research evidence and reach informed conclusions regarding current issues, trends and practice |

use of literature searching. A 'systematic review' is the term used for a really thorough appraisal of all available research evidence in a topic. True systematic reviews are normally the work of funded agencies or a chapter within a Doctoral research project, and would not be expected within an undergraduate degree. Most undergraduate researchers will not have the time, money or language skills to assemble and translate every possible piece of literature on their chosen topic published worldwide. But a reasonably complete overview of recent published evidence (in English) is achievable within a timeframe of about 6–9 months for an undergraduate review.

## Literature sources

So where should we start looking for evidence? The sources of available research literature have expanded over the years and now include:

- journal articles (in traditional paper journals and e-journals)
- systematic reviews (such as Cochrane Reviews)
- textbooks
- so-called 'grey literature' (unpublished material such as theses and conference proceedings)
- media articles (newspapers, magazines)
- internet sites.

In fact there is such a wide array of available material these days that it can appear bewildering. Accessing evidence electronically, via web-based and library search engines has never been easier, but is important to have the right tools for the job and to screen out stuff that is not relevant to our needs.

The majority of medical imaging and radiotherapy researchers would regard journal articles as the most important source, as they tend (usually) to be reliable, of good quality and widely read by clinical practitioners. This is where new research gets published, although the key content may have been reported earlier at conferences. Useful journals in medical imaging and radiotherapy include: *Academic Radiology*, the *British Journal of Radiology (BJR)*, *Clinical Imaging*, *Clinical Radiology*, the *European Journal of Radiology*, the *Journal of Diagnostic Radiography and Imaging*, the *Journal of Radiotherapy in Practice*, the *International Journal of Radiation Oncology, Biology and Physics*, *Radiology*, *Radiography*, *Radiotherapy and Oncology*. There are many others.

Systematic reviews, such as those produced by the Cochrane Collaboration in the United Kingdom

(see Systematic reviews and meta-analysis in Chapter 12) are very useful as they provide a thorough overview of published work in a clinical topic area at the date of publication, with reporting of overall trends. They are not available for every speciality, however – there are more reviews for therapies than diagnostic tests. Textbook content tends to lag slightly behind new developments as a result of unavoidable delays in writing and publication, but may provide a useful overview of a subject area. There are also certain key textbooks which contain important theories and principles, written by their original advocates. It is often important to refer to these, especially in subjects such as research methods, psychology and social studies. Media articles from internet news sites and newspapers are useful for providing interesting 'scene-setting' and quotations for research projects, but should not be relied on too heavily for factual accuracy.

Although internet sites can be used as references in some circumstances, journal articles should form the main part of a good literature search. This is because the material found on most personal, special interest and corporate internet sites is not subject to the same process of academic peer review and quality assessment that takes place before publication in journals. It is thus more likely to be of a variable standard and may be subject to personal bias. However, there are many reputable peer-reviewed electronic journals available on the web which can normally be relied on.

I need to mention again that web-based search engines such as MEDLINE (PubMed) are very valuable as a tool for finding journal articles and that their use is highly recommended – in fact essential. In years gone by a literature search would be a very slow and expensive task and would often result in a great pile of photocopied articles sitting on the researcher's desk. Nowadays it is possible to find a wide range of articles quickly and to download them onto a convenient memory stick for electronic storage.

Medical imaging and radiotherapy research is not only about physics, biology and technology. It is also concerned with people – patients, clients, the general public and staff. As a result, researchers may need to think laterally, also considering sources within general health, psychology, social sciences and even economics. 'Search widely' is good advice. It is important to look at research in other fields such as nursing, physiotherapy and general industry if we are exploring topics such as manual handling, job satisfaction or anxiety (for example), which have a huge literature but not much that is specifically about radiography. In such situations useful comparisons can be made between experiences in radiography and other professions. Of course, if we are doing research in a very 'radiographic' area such as radiation doses, it is unlikely that we will find much relevant material outside the radiological and medical physics literature, but even in this case it may be worth looking at sources in medical health, oncology, molecular biology, epidemiology and immunology, to name just a few.

A literature source is the *original* published article, book or conference proceedings. Although people sometimes find and use abstracts (which are short summaries) of published articles, because it is quicker and easier to do so, this is never a good idea. A 200–300 word abstract can never convey the full findings of a journal article, and although there are usually some summary results, many important details, complexities and angles will be missed. Similarly, it is best to look for an author's views within their original book or article, rather than relying on secondary quotations in other sources. Other people may be selective when quoting an author's words, in order to support their own arguments.

# Writing a literature search method

Although the term 'method' is associated in many people's minds with a survey or an experiment in the laboratory, methodology is a vitally important (and sometimes forgotten) part of a literature search too. A good literature review will include details of the search strategies used, in the same way that a primary research project will have a methods chapter. Components of the method should include:

- approaches used to access the literature (such as 'hand searching' and the names of electronic databases used)
- database search terms (key words, which should hopefully allow related articles of interest to us to be found electronically)
- inclusion and exclusion criteria (justifiable reasons for leaving literature in or out of the review)
- data extraction (details of the types of information that we want to get from the literature).

Literature searching needs to be planned and methodical, just like other aspects of research. In fact it can be regarded as being similar to an observational

study in terms of what it sets out to achieve (see Chapters 4 and 9 for the types of research studies). It needs to ask clear questions, gather necessary information and report findings.

## Approaches used in the search

Nowadays the most important approach for finding research literature is to use a computerized database, which will be available at libraries and hospitals. This has hugely improved the search process and electronic copies of articles can be readily downloaded for storage, provided that the institution subscribes to the journal in question or the article is free of charge. There are a number of information databases available online in health and related subjects, including:

- Academic Search Complete, multidisciplinary full-text journal articles
- CancerNET UK, a good resource for oncology, from the National Cancer Institute
- CINAHL, which includes nursing and allied health
- EMBASE, the *Excerpta Medica* Database, produced by Elsevier
- International Cancer Research Portfolio (ICRP), a collaborative indexing of cancer research
- MEDLINE (PubMed), the most widely known, covering most aspects of medical and health literature and produced by the US National Library of Medicine
- Open SIGLE (System for Information on Grey Literature in Europe), which covers unpublished ('grey') literature, categorized by country and subject area
- PsycINFO, covering psychological literature
- the Cochrane Library, a valuable source for health interventions and therapies, especially 'controlled trials' (see Chapter 4), as well as systematic reviews in health care. It contains several individual databases, such as:
  - ○ CDSR (the Cochrane Database of Systematic Reviews)
  - ○ DARE (the Database of Abstracts of Reviews of Effectiveness)
  - ○ CENTRAL (the Cochrane Central Register of Controlled Trials).

The large number available seems a bit overwhelming, and many people just end up using a single database, such as MEDLINE. But it is important to know that each database will bring up articles that might be missing on the others and that no single database covers everything (that includes MEDLINE). Sometimes in libraries it is possible to do a combined search using more than one database, but beware that this may give duplicate 'hits' for the same article via different databases, giving a very long list of references. The Embase.com site, produced by Elsevier, usefully combines the MEDLINE and EMBASE resources.

There are other databases which can be used on the web to find research articles, including those from the journal publishers, such as:

- Blackwell Synergy
- Ingenta Connect
- Link-Springer Journals
- Sage Journals Online
- Science Direct, from Elsevier
- Wiley Interscience.

The content of these depends of course on each publisher's range of journal titles, but they are a useful extra source in many cases. The web search engine Google Scholar can also bring up useful journal articles and other material such as electronic book extracts.

Table 3.2 gives an indication of the amount of material available via the various web-based search tools and gives some indication of their potential usefulness to diagnostic imaging and radiotherapy.

A database search will not bring up every article that we are looking for, because:

1. no database can include all published articles ever written, and
2. the key search words and phrases we use might not take us to some articles.

Indeed at a lot of unrelated material can be brought up by a simple search term such as 'radiotherapy'. Often articles will not contain our search words in their title/abstract or the database will not recognize our search words. In these cases it may be necessary to do a 'hand search' which might mean sitting down in a library with a stack of journals such as *Radiography* that we think should be a promising resource and looking through back issues, volume by volume. Nowadays we are lucky, as the electronic archives of most journals are conveniently available online and there are usually search facilities within them. Even so, looking through article titles by eye on the computer screen, using contents pages, can still yield useful stuff that we would otherwise have missed. Realistically, a hand search (either manual or electronic) is more likely to be done by a student who is writing a systematic review rather than one who is writing a literature review chapter for a

**Table 3.2  Numbers of hits for the search word 'radiotherapy' using some well known electronic databases and journals**

| Database, web search engine or electronic journal | Number of hits | Comments |
|---|---|---|
| MEDLINE (PubMed) | 202 000 | This database contains over 18 million citations, dating back to the 1950s |
| CINAHL Plus | 10 600 | Articles from over 3200 journals |
| PsycINFO | 430 | Consists of several parallel databases covering different date ranges |
| Allied and Complementary Medicine Database (AMED) | 660 | Contains articles relating to alternative and complementary therapies |
| International Cancer Research Portfolio | 580 | Search for the period 2007–2008 |
| Cochrane Library | 5400 | For the Cochrane Database of Systematic Reviews |
| Science Direct (from Elsevier) | 25 700 | Articles from over 1000 journals |
| *Radiology* | 2000 | The journal *Radiology* |
| *British Journal of Radiology* (BJR) | 820 | For a search within abstracts of articles in the journal BJR |

primary research project. But I would still recommend a hand search to anyone who wants to be thorough in searching for literature on a topic.

Additional search approaches include visiting a specialist library, such as that of the British Institute of Radiology in London, which contains student projects and subject-specific literature. It is worth contacting the librarian of such a centre before the visit, in order to check whether there are likely to be any materials there which are relevant to your research, especially if a long trip is involved. Major national libraries, such as the British Library, contain journals that might not be available locally, but do remember that electronic copies of articles can be ordered, often free of charge to university students or hospital staff.

Not all original research gets published and a thorough literature search may also include unpublished material (often referred to as 'grey literature') such as Masters or Doctoral theses and dissertations, reports of meetings and conference proceedings. This is often to be found in university libraries and repositories such as the British Institute of Radiology Library.

The search approaches used should all be listed in the literature review methodology.

## Database search terms

In the literature search methodology we need to list the search terms which we have used when hunting for articles via electronic databases. Search terms are words and phrases which we hope will score hits by bringing up relevant articles which are of interest to us. The terms are entered in a search box within the database. The precise choice of words and phrases will very much affect the number and type of hits that we get – the results can be a bit surprising. The database will usually look for matches between our search terms and key words contained in the title, abstract and text of journal articles. Sometimes, even when we know for sure that there are articles available in a topic area, a database will not retrieve them for us and this can be frustrating. Possible reasons for this include:

1. the database we are using does not include these articles (no database contains everything ever written)
2. the database does contain the articles but the search terms we are using are not recognized or are not precise enough.

The search phrase 'X-ray' might well be a useful one to include, but just entering it on its own might bring up a huge number of hits from non-radiographic fields, such as X-ray astronomy, X-ray crystallography, general physics and so on (depending on the type of database we are using). More advice is given on issues such as this later in this chapter.

## Inclusion and exclusion criteria

We need to have some standard in our methodology for deciding whether each piece of published research should be included in our written literature review, or excluded from it. Every researcher needs to produce his or her own standard and there is no universal guidance for this. This is because each research topic is unique and so rules which are set in tablets of stone would not work. But generally we are likely to leave out articles which are:

- inapplicable
- out of date
- unreliable.

Inapplicable evidence is evidence which is not relevant to our research; examples might be research from other countries (where the healthcare system is very different from our own), or studies of diagnostic imaging in children when we are researching radiography of adults.

Research from many years ago might have become irrelevant if there have been rapid changes in clinical practice since then. Each researcher needs to decide a cut-off point for inclusion, after which date research is still applicable today and before which it is not. The date chosen will very much depend on the topic area – for example, human anatomy does not change over the years but chemotherapy does.

Deciding whether research evidence is reliable is often the hardest decision to make when considering whether or not to include it. More is said about literature appraisal in Chapter 4, but it is best to exclude articles which we feel are of poor quality. Poor quality research articles (as seen by us as reviewers) might be ones with small sample sizes, flawed methods, obvious bias, weak statistics and analysis, and so on. A randomized controlled trial (see Chapter 12) is usually regarded as the best quality clinical research evidence, but such trials are rare in medical imaging (although there are more in cancer therapies). Thus a researcher writing a review in radiology might need to compromise a bit when considering articles for inclusion (or risk having none).

When writing a literature review it may be wise to pay more attention to the findings of research which compares the effectiveness of one diagnostic test (or cancer therapy) with another on the same set of patients. Most research will only look at a single intervention, however.

To give an example of a set of inclusion and exclusion criteria for a literature review, let us suppose that are doing a systematic review examining the usefulness of magnetic resonance imaging (MRI) in diagnosing suspected adult brain tumours.

Inclusion criteria in this example might consist of articles which:

- are written in English
- have been published within the last 5 years
- are original primary research
- use commonly available MRI technologies
- have symptomatic adults as their sample group
- involve first presentation of disease or symptoms
- use a sample size of at least 25 clinical cases
- are felt to be reliable and of good quality.

Exclusion criteria would mostly follow on from this and might be articles which:

- are in languages other than English (unless we have language skills)
- are older than 5 years
- are reviews of other work
- involve MRI technologies not generally available elsewhere
- include asymptomatic adults (such as volunteers and health screening cases)
- involve recurrence of disease or symptoms
- have a sample group of less than 25 clinical cases
- are felt to be unreliable as evidence, due to poor quality.

## The data extraction process

One very valuable – but often omitted – part of a literature search method is the data extraction form. This lists the key information which the researcher is aiming to extract from the literature. I would recommend filling in the form for every research article, as this gives a valuable summary of major findings and also acts as a reminder about what information was found where. Otherwise we might be left later on with a pile of paper articles and no clue about which one contained that important finding.

**Table 3.3 Example of a data extraction form**

| Key data categories | Entries |
|---|---|
| Title of article | |
| Authors | |
| Year of publication | |
| Country of publication | |
| Type of MRI scanner | |
| Field strength of MRI scanner | |
| Type of research study (randomized trial, observational study, review, etc.) | |
| Is MRI compared with any other test and if so with what? | |
| Is a 'gold standard' test used? | |
| Number of patients in the study | |
| Are sensitivity and specificity data included? If so state the values | |
| Are cost data included? | |
| Is there any mention of patient outcome measures, such as survival, quality of life, alteration of treatment or diagnosis, satisfaction, etc.? | |

An example of a data extraction form is included in Table 3.3, for the previously mentioned review of MRI in diagnosing adult brain tumours. Again this is not a rigid template, just an example – every literature review will be different.

## Tips and tactics for doing the literature search

Doing a literature review can either proceed smoothly, or be very frustrating. The following tips and tactics may help you:

- Consider all of the possible words and phrases that might commonly be used by authors when they are writing articles in your chosen topic area. Using these words as search terms should help you find related articles. It is often a good idea to see which words are used in the reference lists of the first articles that you find. Be broad minded in your choice of search terms.

- When using a database, look for search terms in the abstract and body of articles, not just in their titles. Many authors use rather odd or catchy phrases as article titles, which do not connect well with the actual subject area. It would be easy to miss these articles if you only searched for words in their titles.

- When using the MEDLINE database, an initial search can often bring up loads of articles that are not connected with your subject area. Get round this problem by using the Medical Subject Headings (MeSH) tool to see what key words and phrases MEDLINE recognizes in your topic. A repeat search using these recognized words usually gives more hits.

- Do not just rely on MEDLINE as a search engine. You may find that other databases such as Science Direct or Google Scholar give you more returns. No database covers all of the available literature and each will have good coverage in some specialist areas.

- If you find that an author (or team of authors) research quite frequently in your topic area, try doing a search using that author's name.

- Always click on the 'related articles' that appear when you do a search using a database such as MEDLINE. These in turn will lead you to other related articles in the subject area.

- If you find that articles from your topic area often appear in the same published journal, try doing a search, volume by volume, through all of its content for the last few years. This can be done electronically or manually if your library has hard copies. You will often find that you come across other relevant articles, editorials and correspondence that you would otherwise have missed.

- It may seem a bit obvious, but do look through the reference lists of those journal articles which you have already got saved to your computer or printed off. Sometimes authors will quote references which do not appear in your database searches.

## Problems with literature searches

We do not want to dwell on negatives, but it is best to be pre-warned about possible pitfalls. It can be difficult sometimes to find all of the relevant research

that has been written in our chosen topic area, even with the help of electronic databases such as MEDLINE. Having a thorough search method will increase our chances of success.

But is the published material an accurate picture of research in medical imaging and radiotherapy? The answer is 'Well, yes, sometimes – but not necessarily'. Often there is a tendency for research which shows positive benefits from treatments or diagnostic tests to get published, while negative findings may end up filed in a drawer. Also, definite or statistically significant results (whether positive or negative) may be more attractive to a publisher than findings which are null or equivocal. Although journals are not like newspapers, there may still be pressure to print material which is likely to excite the readership. This tendency is called 'publication bias' and it is present in many areas of health research, including funded work. This bias can skew clinicians' perceptions of the usefulness of treatments and there have been situations where the effectiveness of certain therapies (for example, certain chemotherapies) have been over-exaggerated. Since most clinical staff get their updates from journal articles and conferences, this is hard to avoid.

Definite or positive findings are not only more likely to be published, they are also more likely to be published quickly. This means that the first rush of publications in a developing clinical technique may tend to give a rosy picture, while delayed reports may be more cautious. This is called 'time lag' bias.

A student searching the literature will often find several articles in a topic which are from the same group of authors. This may sometimes be essentially one piece of research, written up in slightly different ways and presented in several journals, and can lead to 'multiple publication' bias. Multiple publication can be attractive to researchers since producing more 'outputs' not only increases their street credibility but can also bring promotion and other rewards. Of course if the articles are from widely different years, it is more likely that each is a separate piece of research, and some authors are very prolific in producing original work, even within a single year. No one would accuse authors of cheating where multiple publications of the same findings takes place, but a student doing a literature review should record the findings as *one piece of research evidence*, not several.

In technology-driven fields such as medical imaging and radiotherapy, there can also be another effect, which I will call 'one-upmanship' bias. This means that hospital centres with the most 'whizzy' new scanners or linear accelerators may be more likely to get their research published. It is true that cutting-edge work is more likely to be done using the newest equipment, and active clinical researchers are attracted to the best funded centres, hence the greater number of publications from these sites. But someone doing a literature review should reflect that these advanced technologies may be unavailable at most hospitals, and thus this research may not reflect the real world situation in the major part of the health service.

The biases mentioned above will be present in the research literature, and the available evidence will be influenced to some degree. Researchers cannot escape this fact, *but they can be aware of possible biases and reflect accordingly*.

What if we are doing historical research, for example, looking at the development of radiography during the period from the 1920s to the 1960s? Most journal articles are only available electronically in full text form over the last 10–15 years and this can cause a problem. In these cases it may be necessary to visit a national collection such as the British Institute of Radiology library, and do a hand search. The same problem also applies to older and out-of-print books. Museum and Public Record Office collections may be a good resource, if we can get access to them. A researcher living in a large city such as London is more conveniently placed to visit specialist science and medical libraries. The limited availability of older

sources is not normally a problem in medical imaging and radiotherapy research, since most (but not all) older publications are no longer relevant to current clinical practice.

To access a wide range of literature we need to go via an institutional library and there can be a problem if our institution does not pay to subscribe to the electronic full text version of the key journals we need. In such cases it will be necessary to order copies of articles from elsewhere. This is always possible but may have cost and time implications. The library may hold paper copies of journals, but sometimes these are missing, misfiled or have pages ripped out (sad but true). It is a good idea to check the library's holdings of full text journals as soon as possible, not in the last few weeks before a review has to be submitted. Remember that databases such as MEDLINE will help us to find the title and location (journal, year, volume, page number) of articles we need, but will not normally link to the full text unless it is available free to non-subscribers. Abstracts are usually available via MEDLINE, but *do not* rely on these alone.

Searching the literature can be an exciting quest, as it always gives fresh insight to the person doing it themselves for the first time. No matter that hundreds of other people have done the job previously – since new things are constantly being published, each search is unique. Literature searching can be frustrating too, but use of the right tools and the right method eases the journey.

## Further reading

Greenhalgh T. How to Read a Paper. London: BMJ Books; 2001.

Hart C. Doing a Literature Search. London: Sage; 2001.

Mayer D. Essential Evidence-Based Medicine. Cambridge: Cambridge University Press; 2004.

Straus S, Richardson WS, Glasziou P, et al. Evidence-Based Medicine:

How to Practice and Teach EBM. Edinburgh: Churchill Livingstone; 2005.

# Literature evaluation and critique

**4**

Andy Scally    Stephen Brealey

## CHAPTER POINTS

- All health professionals are expected to be able to identify and critically evaluate research evidence relevant to their practice.
- In order that they can do this, an understanding of the different study designs is essential, as is an appreciation of the circumstances in which each can be appropriately used.
- The inherent limitations of the different study designs need to be understood and an awareness is needed of recommended standards in the design and conduct of each study type.
- A critical appraisal requires a systematic approach, relevant to the specific study design employed. Methodological standards and critical appraisal tools have been developed and are widely available to assist in this task.

This chapter looks at methods of evaluating and critiquing literature, including examples of how to go about this. There are good practice guidelines that have been recommended as well as useful web resources that you may wish to refer to.

## Introduction

In the global modern healthcare environment, there is an expectation that you as a healthcare professional should base your practice upon the best available research evidence. Given that new 'evidence' continues to emerge at a rapid rate, all health professionals must be able to evaluate findings that are relevant to their clinical practice and judge whether to incorporate change when this is necessary.

This ability to critically appraise claims from research that are published in the literature, and independently evaluate the strength of such claims, is vital to diagnostic imaging and radiotherapy.

Although the idea of evidence-based medicine, or more generally evidence-based healthcare practice, has been traced back to the 19th century, the quality of health research has improved steadily. Unfortunately, this does not mean that nowadays all research is conducted in a way that ensures the robustness of the conclusions. Established best practice is not always followed by researchers, and even where it is there is still the potential for hidden biases to be present in the research that cannot easily be identified, eliminated or controlled for.

Standards for best practice in healthcare research have been published within recent years and these publications are an extremely valuable resource, both for students and for qualified practitioners, in helping them make informed judgements on the quality and relevance of published research. Several organizations have also developed critical appraisal tools which enable you critically to appraise research papers in a systematic way that involves the consistent application of the same relevant key questions for a given research design (see Appendix 4.1 – Resources for critical appraisal – for web addresses).

## Hierarchies of evidence

A natural hierarchy of research evidence quality has emerged which is informed by the ease with which potential biases can be avoided or controlled. This is covered in useful texts by Sackett and colleagues and

**Table 4.1 The traditional hierarchies of evidence**

| Rank | Study design | Comment |
| --- | --- | --- |
| 1 | Systematic review | Ideally of well designed homogeneous RCTs. May or may not include a meta-analysis. Status in hierarchy may be relegated if RCTs are heterogeneous or if the review is of observational studies |
| 2 | Randomized controlled trial | Judgement required of the size and quality of the study and whether the results are definitive |
| 3 | Cohort study | Large, well designed study may be more persuasive than a weak RCT, but cohort study more prone to bias |
| 4 | Case-control study | Causal inference more difficult to establish and more prone to bias than a cohort study |
| 5 | Cross-sectional study (survey) | Causal inferences cannot be made. Provides information at a single instance of time |
| 6 | Ecological study | An observational study that uses aggregate level data, in the absence of an assessment of individual exposures |
| 7 | Case reports | Lack generalizability due to very limited sample size and their selective nature |

by Greenalgh.[1-4] Although there are variations on the precise structure of this hierarchy, in particular to take account of qualitative research,[5] it is broadly as outlined in Table 4.1.

The highest level of evidence is widely considered to be a systematic review of well designed randomized controlled clinical trials (RCTs), all of which aim to answer the same research question. However, the quality of a systematic review is necessarily constrained by the quality of the individual trials of which it is composed and not all systematic reviews are reviews of clinical trials. Also, it is worth bearing in mind that published randomized controlled trials may be relatively uncommon in diagnostic imaging and radiotherapy. It is perfectly reasonable to perform a systematic review of observational studies when there is little or no evidence from RCTs in a particular area of interest. The second level in the standard hierarchy, a large, well designed RCT, is therefore considered by some to represent the strongest kind of evidence. The third level of evidence is an observational cohort study, the fourth and fifth are observational case-control studies and cross-sectional studies (surveys), while the sixth is an observational ecological study (where individual-level patient exposure data is lacking, but aggregate, population-level data are available). Ecological studies are not common in medical imaging or radiotherapy, but are conducted occasionally. The lowest level of evidence is considered to be individual case reports, owing to their usual lack of generalizability.

Although this hierarchy reflects the reliability of the different study designs in terms of researchers' ability to eliminate or control biases within them, it should not be assumed that an observational study is always inferior to an RCT. Randomized controlled trials have their own potential problems and may not always be the most appropriate design for diagnostic imaging studies. They are not even ethical or appropriate in many situations, for example when studying the health effects due to exposure to toxic agents, such as ionizing radiation or chemical pollutants. Furthermore, the need for and appropriateness of such a hierarchy has been challenged. Wherever the research method ranks in the hierarchy, a well-designed study will produce results that are more plausible than those from a poorly designed study. It has also been suggested that rigid adherence to this hierarchy has seriously misrepresented, or under-reported, the evidence supporting the more widespread use of new imaging methods in oncology.[6]

In medical imaging, studies are commonly designed to measure the diagnostic accuracy of alternative imaging techniques and their combinations, or of the diagnostic performance of individuals or groups of observers/interpreters or even combinations of technology and observers. Diagnostic accuracy is usually based on the sensitivity of a test (the ability to detect disease when it is present) and the specificity of a test (the ability to exclude disease when it is absent). Although standards of good practice have been developed specifically for the design and reporting of such studies,[7] a diagnostic accuracy study can have the characteristics of either an RCT or an observational study and so can be evaluated broadly within the evaluation framework relevant to an RCT or observational study.

## Examples of different research designs in medical imaging and radiotherapy

Many different types of studies are published in the medical and health science literature and by no means are all of them are evaluations of patient outcomes or, in the case of medical imaging studies, diagnostic performance. The research literature is broad and may cover many aspects of professional practice, for example clinical audits, development of guidelines, developments in education and training, surveys of professional practice, surveys of user views and experiences, experimental studies relating to assessment of health technologies. Although many of the principles addressed in this chapter can be applied to the appraisal of such articles, the focus of this chapter is on research involving patient outcomes and diagnostic performance, because it is from such studies that changes can be made to clinical practice and improvements made in patient care.

Some examples from the medical imaging and radiotherapy/oncology literature that have used the primary research designs identified above are outlined in Table 4.2.[8–33] No attempt here is made to appraise these studies but they could serve as helpful examples to which you could apply an appropriate critical appraisal tool from the options presented in Appendix 4.1.

## Basic concepts in critical appraisal

There are some common concepts of critical appraisal that are relevant to most study designs. Some key pointers to evaluating a piece of published research are indicated below:

In appraising a research article you might ask:

- Are there clear aims and objectives?
- Is there a defined research question?
- Do the authors have a good grasp of previous research in this field?
- Is the study relevant to clinical practice and carried out in 'real world' circumstances?

- Is the method clear and well reported?
- Is the sample group sufficient and representative?
- Are there any obvious exclusions?
- Is the analysis of findings appropriate and do the results add up?
- Are there any possible sources of bias and are these identified by the authors?
- Are unexpected events or negative findings discussed?
- Are weaknesses in the study acknowledged by the authors?
- Are the authors balanced in their views and conclusions?
- Are there useful recommendations?

All research should be designed to produce *valid* results. Validity is concerned with the extent to which inferences can be drawn from a study, in particular generalizations extending beyond the study sample, having taken into account study methods and the representativeness of the study sample. Two types of study validity can be distinguished: a) *internal validity*, which means the ability of the research method to show a real relationship between cause and effect, such as whether observed differences in patient outcome can be attributed to the effect of the intervention under investigation; and b) *external validity*, which is concerned with how generalizable the findings from the study are to a wider population, based on the sample of patients included in the study.

Bias, confounding and chance can all reduce internal validity and may provide alternative explanations for an observed difference between study groups. Bias is often related to faults in the study design and can arise, for example, from an unrepresentative or skewed selection of patients for a study, or a partial or unbalanced collection of data. To prevent bias, good study designs will 'blind' (or mask) the patients, the clinicians and even the researchers so that they are kept ignorant of anything that could lead them to a change in behaviour that might affect study findings.

Confounding occurs when the apparent effect of the intervention on patient outcome is in fact due to the action of a variable other than the intervention. When confounding is known or suspected, it can be controlled for in the design (e.g. randomization, matching) or in the analysis (e.g. multivariable analysis). The effects of unknown confounders can be reduced by randomization. The effect of any intervention can also be explained by chance. Even a randomized trial which protects against systematic differences between groups does not prevent differences between samples arising

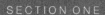

**Table 4.2 Examples of the different study designs used in medical imaging and radiotherapy research**

| Authors | Title | Purpose |
|---|---|---|
| **Systematic reviews** | | |
| Harris et al (1998)[8] | Systematic review of endoscopic ultrasound in gastro-oesophageal cancer. | To review the literature about the use of endoscopic ultrasound for the preoperative staging of gastro-oesophageal cancer, especially staging performance and impact |
| Bryant et al (2007)[9] | Cardioprotection against the toxic effects of anthracyclines given to children with cancer: a systematic review. | To conduct a systematic review of the clinical effectiveness and cost-effectiveness of cardioprotection against the toxic effects of anthracyclines given to children with cancer |
| Brealey et al (2005)[10] | Accuracy of radiographer plain radiograph reporting in clinical practice: a meta-analysis. | To quantify how accurately radiographers report plain radiographs in clinical practice compared with a reference standard |
| **Randomized controlled trials** | | |
| Bartholomew et al (2004)[11] | A randomised controlled trial comparing lateral skull computerised radiographs with or without a grid. | To investigate the effect on perceived image quality of the use or non-use of a secondary radiation grid for lateral skull radiography |
| Harrison et al (2001)[12] | Randomized controlled trial to assess the effectiveness of a videotape about radiotherapy. | To investigate whether the provision of a videotape, in addition to the standard information booklet, reduced pre-treatment worry about radiotherapy in cancer patients |
| Sala et al (2007)[13] | A randomized controlled trial of routine early abdominal computed tomography in patients presenting with non-specific acute abdominal pain. | To compare the effect of initial early computed tomography (CT) versus standard practice (SP) on the length of hospital stay, diagnostic accuracy and mortality of adult patients presenting with acute abdominal pain |
| Ravasco et al (2005)[14] | Dietary counseling improves patient outcomes: a prospective, randomized controlled trial in colorectal cancer patients undergoing radiotherapy. | To investigate the impact of dietary counselling or nutritional supplements on several outcome measures (nutritional intake, nutritional status and quality of life) in colorectal cancer patients |
| **Cohort studies** | | |
| Trakada et al (2006)[15] | Pulmonary radiographic findings and mortality in hospitalized patients with lower respiratory tract infections. | To identify whether specific radiographic findings in patients with lower respiratory tract infections predict mortality |
| Aktas et al (2007)[16] | Concomitant radiotherapy and hyperthermia for primary carcinoma of the vagina: a cohort study. | To evaluate the supplementary value of adding hyperthermia to radiotherapy in patients with primary vaginal cancer |
| Virtanen et al (2007)[17] | Angiosarcoma after radiotherapy: a cohort study of 332 163 Finnish cancer patients. | To evaluate the risk of angiosarcoma after radiotherapy among cancer patients in Finland |
| Jaremko et al (2007)[18] | Do radiographic indices of distal radius fracture reduction predict outcomes in older adults receiving conservative treatment? | To investigate whether radiographic deformities suggesting inadequate reduction would be associated with adverse clinical outcomes |

**Table 4.2 Examples of the different study designs used in medical imaging and radiotherapy research—cont'd**

| Authors | Title | Purpose |
|---|---|---|
| **Case-control studies** | | |
| Sernik et al (2008)[19] | Ultrasound features of carpal tunnel syndrome: a prospective case-control study. | To examine the most adequate cut-off point for median nerve cross-sectional area and additional ultrasound features supporting the diagnosis of carpal tunnel syndrome (CTS) |
| Cheng et al (2008)[20] | Yoga and lumbar disc degeneration disease: MR imaging based case control study. | To identify whether lumbar disc degenerative disease was reduced in practised yoga instructors compared to a control group |
| Spruit et al (2007)[21] | Regional radiotherapy versus an axillary lymph node dissection after lumpectomy: a safe alternative for an axillary lymph node dissection in a clinically uninvolved axilla in breast cancer. A case control study with 10 years follow up. | To compare disease-free survival and overall survival in patients with clinically uninvolved axilla undergoing radiotherapy or axillary lymph node dissection following lumpectomy for breast cancer |
| Finlay et al (2002)[22] | Advanced presentation of lung cancer in Asian immigrants: a case-control study. | To determine if Asian immigrants to the USA present with more advanced lung cancer compared to non-Asians |
| **Cross-sectional studies (surveys)** | | |
| Lutz et al (2004)[23] | Survey on use of palliative radiotherapy in hospice care. | Hospice professionals were surveyed to assess the need for palliative radiotherapy in the hospice setting |
| Davies et al (2005)[24] | Radiation protection practices and related continuing professional education in dental radiography: a survey of practitioners in the north-east of England. | To survey the opinion of practitioners on the availability of related postgraduate courses in the region |
| Jones & Manning (2008)[25] | A survey to assess audit mechanisms practised by skeletal reporting radiographers. | To survey the role of plain film reporting radiographers and the methods they employ to evaluate the quality of their performance |
| Power et al (2006)[26] | Videofluoroscopic assessment of dysphagia: a questionnaire survey of protocols, roles and responsibilities of radiology and speech and language therapy personnel. | To survey videofluoroscopic practice and identify the roles and responsibilities of radiology and speech and language therapy personnel |
| **Studies of diagnostic test accuracy** | | |
| Grisaru et al (2004)[27] | The diagnostic accuracy of [18]F-fluorodeoxyglucose PET/CT in patients with gynaecological malignancies. | To compare the diagnostic accuracy of PET/CT with standard imaging (CT/MRI/US) in patients with suspected recurrence of gynaecological malignancy |
| Burling et al (2008)[28] | Virtual colonoscopy: effect of computer-assisted detection (CAD) on radiographer performance. | To determine whether CAD as a 'second reader' improves polyp detection by trained radiographers reporting on virtual colonoscopy examinations |
| MERCURY Study Group (2006)[29] | Diagnostic accuracy of preoperative magnetic resonance imaging in predicting curative resection of rectal cancer: prospective observational study. | To assess the accuracy of preoperative staging of rectal cancer with magnetic resonance imaging to predict surgical circumferential resection margins |

*Continued*

**Table 4.2 Examples of the different study designs used in medical imaging and radiotherapy research—cont'd**

| Authors | Title | Purpose |
|---|---|---|
| Dai et al (2008)[30] | Does three-dimensional power Doppler ultrasound improve the diagnostic accuracy for the prediction of adnexal malignancy? | To investigate the diagnostic accuracy of 3-D power Doppler ultrasound in the differentiation between benign and malignant adnexal masses |
| **Qualitative studies** | | |
| Nagle et al (2008)[31] | Exploring general practitioners' experience of informing women about prenatal screening tests for foetal abnormalities: a qualitative focus group study. | To explore GPs' experience of informing women of prenatal genetic screening tests for fetal abnormality |
| Poulos & Llewellyn (2005)[32] | Mammography discomfort: a holistic perspective derived from women's experiences. | To use qualitative research methods to consider discomfort from a holistic perspective of the mammography experience derived from the women themselves |
| Colyer (2000)[33] | The role of the radiotherapy treatment review radiographer. | A qualitative study to gain an understanding of the role of the radiotherapy treatment review radiographer |

by chance although this does diminish as the sample size increases. The probability of an observed difference occurring by chance when no real difference exists is demonstrated by a p-value. A p-value of, for example, $P=0.01$, informs us that assuming there is no real difference between treatments, then the probability of uneven randomization explaining the difference is around 1 in 100. Therefore you would not expect the play of chance to explain your study findings. External validity is likely to be threatened when only a small sample of patients is obtained from a single geographical location or there is self-selection of patients into a study (e.g. volunteers). This is therefore addressed by conducting research at multiple sites, increasing the sample size and, when possible, selecting a random sample of patients into a study so that every eligible patient has an equal chance of being selected and thus the sample should be representative of the target population.

## The typical structure of a research paper

Most research articles are similarly structured, though the precise structure may vary according to the editorial policy of the journal and the design of the study. The general structure of a published research article is as follows:

*Title.* Making clear the purpose and design of the study.

*Authors.* Including names, qualifications and affiliations.

*Abstract.* Summarizing the background and purpose, structure, results and conclusions of the study.

*Introduction.* Presenting the background to the study and its rationale, including reference to previous relevant research.

*Methods.* Including a thorough description of the study design, an outline of the practicalities of how it was done, an explanation of how potential biases were addressed, and a description of the data analysis methods used.

*Results.* Presentation of the results, with the emphasis on the primary outcome measure identified for the study.

*Discussion.* Interpretation of findings, recognition of any limitations of the study, the discussion of the findings in the context of what was previously known and suggested implications for practice.

## Preliminary steps in a critical appraisal

When setting out to identify relevant research in an area of practice, the first task should be a systematic search of the literature using the methods discussed in Chapter 3.

From the outset, it is important to understand that there is no such thing as a perfect research study. Even the best conducted studies have potential flaws associated with them that are impossible to avoid. For example, almost all research involving patients or staff will need informed consent from the participants and if those who refuse to give that consent are over-represented in particular subgroups, such as gender, age or ethnicity, then the representativeness of the sample could be open to challenge. Also, all research is subject to logistical and economic constraints and so compromises have to be made when considering what is feasible. It is far easier to criticize the work of others than to design a study that is beyond criticism, so it is important when critically appraising a paper to consider the unavoidable constraints within which the researchers are working and to assess whether they have implemented all measures reasonably available to them to optimize the robustness of the study. A critical evaluation of a study is not just about finding fault – we should also praise when this seems appropriate.

Another issue to bear in mind is that there is a difference between the assessment of the method and findings of a research article and the assessment of the written presentation of that article, although both are important. Students often focus too much on the presentation of a research study when evaluating it, leading to a critique which is descriptive and uncritical. Published articles of high inherent quality may be poorly presented by the authors, meaning that some information may be lacking and a fair assessment of study quality is hard to undertake. Conversely, a weak study could be well presented, with strong structure and great detail, and yet could contain flaws so significant that no meaningful inferences can be drawn from it.

Once you have identified a research article that may be of relevance to you and that you may wish to critically evaluate there are a few preliminary steps and questions that should be considered before progressing further:

1. A reading of the abstract may clearly identify whether or not the paper is relevant to your purpose. If it is still unclear after reading the abstract, a quick reading of the full article may be necessary before you are able to make a decision. Is the nature of and emphasis within the study relevant to the purpose of your literature search and evaluation? Do not spend too much time on papers that are peripheral or irrelevant to your purpose.

2. Does the title accurately reflect the content of the study or is it uninformative or misleading?
   a. The title may give the impression that the study comprises fresh (primary) data but it may in fact be a review of previously published work. In this case the article may be of help to you in appraising some of the other pieces of published research to which it makes reference, but this is no substitute for your own independent assessment of the original studies.
   b. Is the study measuring the outcome(s) it says it is measuring, or are 'surrogate' outcome measures being used? (A surrogate outcome measure is one that is presumed – with or without good evidence – to be associated with the primary outcome of interest, but is usually easier to measure.)

3. Does the list of authors suggest that they have the relevant expertise in all important aspects of the research? You should never assume that eminence in a particular field guarantees the quality of the research, nor that an unknown author or an author from a different discipline should not be trusted or believed. All research should be appraised on its merits, but extra vigilance in the appraisal of the robustness of the research may be suggested where certain relevant expertise may appear to be lacking, for example the absence of a medical statistician from the list of authors of a paper that utilizes seemingly complex data analysis methods.

4. Is the study design what it says it is? Not all studies reported as RCTs are randomized or adequately controlled and some studies reported as cohort studies could more accurately be described as cross-sectional studies. The answer to this question is not always clear cut and the paper may require more thorough evaluation before it can be definitively answered.

5. Has the paper been commented upon already? Peer-reviewed journals normally include a letters section, in the printed edition and/or online, within which members of the health/scientific community pass informed comment on research previously published in the journal. In the online content pages of peer-reviewed journals, letters commenting on the research are often identified adjacent to the original article. It is always worthwhile to read the published views of other commentators on a research

article, though of course these comments themselves should also be subject to critical appraisal.

6. In the introduction to the paper, have the authors adequately identified and summarized the available evidence in the relevant subject area and justified the need for their own study? The Declaration of Helsinki, which governs the ethics of biomedical research, requires that research involving people should be underpinned by a thorough knowledge of the scientific literature in order that research volunteers are not subject to unnecessary harm or inconvenience.

# Critical evaluation strategies according to design method

We next consider the specific requirements for a critical evaluation of studies comprising the designs illustrated in Table 4.2. We have identified some key resources to assist students, and qualified practitioners alike, in performing the evaluation, including reference to key publications explaining the rationale for giving attention to specific aspects of the study design and an evaluation tool/checklist that provides a proforma for a systematic evaluation. A few of the key issues for each study design are briefly outlined but a more thorough explanation of the importance of each issue is provided in the essential resources indicated.

## Critical evaluation of systematic reviews

*Useful resources.* The QUOROM statement for improving the quality of reports of meta-analyses of randomized controlled trials.[34]

*Specific issues to consider.* The purpose of a systematic review is to help healthcare providers and other decision makers to make clinical decisions about best practice. Rather than reflecting the views of the authors or being based on a possibly biased selection of published literature, a systematic review involves locating all the available evidence in relation to a specific research question, appraising the quality of the evidence identified, to synthesize the available evidence, and if relevant, to statistically aggregate the evidence of all relevant studies. Systematic reviews should adhere to strict scientific design in order to

make them more comprehensive, to minimize the chance of bias (systematic errors) and random errors (mistakes occurring by chance), thus providing more reliable results from which to draw conclusions and make decisions. The following should therefore be considered when critically appraising the quality of a systematic review.

*Research question.* What question did the systematic review address? The main research question should be clearly stated and preferably describe the relationship between Population, Intervention (or test or exposure), Comparison intervention, and Outcome (PICO). Knowing the population is important for helping to decide whether the review applies to your specific patient group. The intervention is a planned course of action and the exposure is something that happens. These again need to be described in detail, as should the comparison intervention, to ensure clarity and to help you determine what contributed to the outcome. The most important outcomes, beneficial or harmful, should also be clearly defined. The title, abstract, or final paragraph of the introduction should clearly state the research question.

*Searching.* Is it unlikely that important, relevant studies were missed? The information sources searched should be clearly described (e.g. databases, registers, personal files, expert informants, hand searching) and any restrictions (e.g. years considered, publication status, language of publication). A comprehensive search for all relevant studies should include the major bibliographic databases (e.g. Medline, EMBASE, Cochrane, etc.), a search of reference lists from relevant studies, contact with experts to inquire about, in particular, unpublished studies, and the search should not include English language only. The search strategy should be clear, explicit, reproducible and be described in the methods section of the paper.

*Study selection.* Were the criteria used to select articles for inclusion appropriate? The inclusion and exclusion criteria (defining population, intervention, principal outcomes and study design) should be clearly defined before the search is undertaken to ensure the consistent and appropriate selection of eligible studies into the review. The methods section should describe in detail these criteria.

*Validity assessment.* Were the included studies sufficiently valid for the type of questions asked? There should be predetermined criteria used to assess the quality (e.g. randomization, blinding, completeness of follow up) of each included study depending on the type of clinical question being asked. The process of assessing validity should also be described, for example masking the reviewers to who were the authors of the study and whether two reviewers independently applied the quality criteria. The methods section should describe the quality criteria used and the process of applying the criteria, and the results section should provide information on the quality of studies and, if applicable, extent of agreement between reviewers when appraising studies.

*Study characteristics.* Were the study characteristics similar? The type of study design, participants' characteristics, details of intervention, and outcomes should be described. Heterogeneity, or inconsistency of results across different studies, could be explained by differences in study characteristics. The possibility of heterogeneity should be explored visually when interpreting forest plots of the results of studies or, more formally, with statistical tests such as chi-square (see Common statistical tests in Chapter 15.)

*Data synthesis.* Were the methods used to combine the findings of the relevant studies reported (if applicable)? The principal measures of effect (e.g. relative risk), method of combining results (statistical testing and confidence intervals), and a priori sensitivity and subgroup analyses should all be reported in the methods section and the findings in the results.

## Critical evaluation of randomized controlled trials

*Useful resources.* 'The revised CONSORT Statement for Reporting Randomized Trials: Explanation and Elaboration and the RCT-type specific Explanations and Elaborations',[35] where appropriate; an appropriate checklist from Appendix 4.1.

*Specific issues to consider.* A randomized controlled trial is usually regarded as the strongest type of primary research study in health care, although it may not be feasible in all situations. Subjects (usually patients) are allocated in a controlled but random way to two or more groups, receiving different interventions. One group may be a 'placebo' and receive no intervention. An RCT is generally the best available design to test: a) whether a healthcare intervention works at all (e.g. a drug, surgical technique, exercise regimen, radiotherapy treatment or diagnostic screening test), by comparing outcomes with the placebo control group; b) whether a new intervention is superior to existing treatment, by comparing outcomes with a group receiving

standard care; or c) whether a new, cheaper or less invasive intervention is equivalent in its effect to the current expensive or invasive procedure.

*Participants.* What are the eligibility criteria for participants? What are the settings (primary care, secondary care, community) and geographical locations from which recruitment is made? What are the specific inclusion and exclusion criteria and are they appropriate? Have participants been randomly *selected* (how subjects are randomly *allocated* is discussed later) or has a convenience sample been used (for example, all consecutive patients over a 1-month period)? Are the sample characteristics representative of the population of patients in whom you are interested, for example in terms of age, gender, ethnicity, socioeconomic characteristics, disease type and severity? If not, caution may be advised in generalizing the results to your patient population.

*Interventions.* Is the precise nature of the experimental and control interventions clear? How and when were the interventions administered? Is the control group receiving a placebo or standard care? Is this a comparison of a new intervention compared to standard care or is the new intervention in addition to standard care?

*Outcome measures.* Ideally there should be only one *primary* outcome measure, though occasionally more than one may be justified. Several *secondary* outcome measures may also be identified, but should be interpreted with more caution. Are the outcome measures adequately defined and accurately measured? Are they measured just the once or are repeated measures made over time? If the latter, then there will be important statistical issues to consider. Does the primary outcome measure evaluate the real concept of interest or are surrogate outcome measures being used?

*Sample size.* Has an appropriate prospective sample size estimation been undertaken? If so, has previous research been used to estimate a likely effect size (true difference in outcomes between the human groups included in the trial) or has a judgement been made regarding the minimum effect size that would represent a clinically important effect? If no sample size estimation has been undertaken, then there is a serious risk of the study being over-powered (an unnecessarily large sample) or under-powered (too small a sample to make any valid findings).

*Randomization.* Has the randomization method been adequately described and is it open to abuse? Were random number tables used, or a computer-generated random number sequence? Was simple randomization used or a restricted method, for example random number blocks, stratification or minimization (a method used to minimize differences in baseline characteristics between groups)? Was the group allocation of all participants adequately concealed?

*Blinding.* Ideally, the group allocation of all participants should remain unknown to participants and to those responsible for the administration of the intervention and data collection and for their general medical care, until after the data is analysed. Sometimes this is very difficult and sometimes it is not logistically feasible. Lack of blinding, or its inadequacy, can in some circumstances seriously compromise the validity of a study (due to complex psychological issues affecting both patients and those responsible for their care) but in other circumstances it may be of limited importance (for example, lack of blinding of the patient is unlikely to seriously compromise a study evaluating the diagnostic accuracy of alternative tests, since the outcome measure relates to observer interpretation of imaging signs rather than to the degree of improvement in the health status of the patient). Have all reasonable steps been taken to ensure adequate blinding? What more could have been done?

*Statistical methods.* Have appropriate statistical methods been chosen to analyse all outcome measures? For simple analyses the answer to this question should be within the scope of all readers. Although RCTs can be complex to undertake, the statistical methods chosen for their analysis (at least that of the primary outcome measure) is usually relatively simple because the groups should be fairly well balanced on all factors that may affect outcome, apart from the intervention group to which they have been assigned. More complex methods may be used for some secondary outcome measures. The primary analysis of a clinical trial should be based on 'intention-to-treat'. In other words, patients should be analysed within the group to which they were randomly allocated rather than according to the treatment they may actually have received.

*Results.* Is the flow of participants through each stage of the trial made clear? Have all important baseline characteristics of participants been summarized and are they very similar between trial groups? Have all participants been accounted for, with the number of dropouts evaluated and reasons given for all missing data? Have the results of statistical analyses been adequately reported (effect size, confidence intervals (where possible) and statistical significance)? Have secondary and further exploratory analyses been

identified as such? Has appropriate account been taken of multiple analyses in determining the threshold for statistical significance?

*Interpretation.* Are the researchers' claims justified by their results, in the context of what is already understood from previous research? Are the limitations of the study (in terms of inclusion criteria, uncontrolled potential biases, sample size and precision) adequately recognized by the authors? Is the evidence presented sufficiently strong to confirm, or warrant reconsideration of, current practice?

# Critical evaluation of observational studies

*Useful resources.* The STROBE Statement;[36] an appropriate checklist (see Appendix 4.1).

*Specific issues to consider:*

## Cohort studies

A cohort is a group of people with shared or common characteristics for the purpose of health research and is often followed *longitudinally*, over time. As in the case of an RCT, one cohort is often compared with another. A cohort study is usually the best available study design in situations where an RCT is either unethical or impractical. The main difference between an RCT and a cohort study is that, in the latter, subjects are not allocated at random to interventions or exposures. This lack of random allocation makes it harder to eliminate or control for biases due to systematic baseline differences between cohort subgroups to be compared. Otherwise, the characteristics of cohort studies are similar to RCTs. Cohort studies are not the most efficient design for studies investigating rare occurrences or diseases with long latency periods.

*Participants.* Settings, locations and periods of recruitment, follow up and data collection should all be stated. What were the eligibility criteria for inclusion and were they appropriate? If two or more sub-cohorts are to be compared, might there be any other systematic differences between them (e.g. different prior information, recruited at different times)?

*Exposure.* What is the nature of the 'exposure', how was it measured and how did it vary across the cohort? Was it measured reliably? In most cohort studies the exposure consists of some agent which the subject physically receives, for example a vaccine, drug, other medical intervention, or an environmental toxin such as a radiation exposure or inhalation of some toxic chemical agent. In many medical imaging studies, such as those by Trakada et al[15] and Jaremko et al[18] in Table 4.2, the role of the exposure is taken by imaging findings because we are wanting to assess the degree to which the imaging appearances can predict patient outcome.

***Outcome measures.*** Has a primary outcome measure been adequately defined and is it appropriately and adequately measured? What are the additional outcome measures? If the study is longitudinal (repeated measurements over time), has a specific time point been identified as the primary time point or is the trend over time of primary interest?

***Other variables.*** Unlike the case with RCTs, in a cohort study we cannot be assured of reasonable balance between groups in a cohort study, so baseline differences between groups may need to be accounted for in the analysis. There may be a number of potential confounders (other variables associated with both the exposure and the outcome measure) that need to be adjusted for in the analysis. All variables of importance in the study, their method of measurement/determination, and their role (measure of exposure, outcome measure or confounder) should be identified.

***Sample size.*** The same considerations are applicable as for RCTs, but the methods of estimation could potentially be more complex due to a necessarily more complex statistical analysis.

***Control of biases.*** Have the authors identified all serious potential sources of bias in the study and made all reasonable efforts to control them?

### Statistical methods

Although in some cohort studies the analysis methods used can be quite straightforward, often various types of regression model will be required to accommodate repeated measures on individuals and/or adjustment for confounders. The authors should explain clearly the nature of the analyses proposed.

***Results.*** All relevant details relating to the recruitment of participants should be reported, including the total number of people eligible for participation, the numbers declining consent, any missing data and the numbers lost to follow-up. Actual numbers, rather than just percentages, should be reported. The analysis process should be adequately described, including unadjusted and adjusted estimates, and the confounders adjusted for. Effect size and measures of uncertainty should be presented as well as statistical significance.

***Interpretation.*** As for RCTs, but the potential limitations due to uncontrolled biases require even more careful consideration.

## Case-control studies

Case-control studies involve comparing people with a disease or characteristic (the cases) with otherwise similar people who lack that disease or characteristic (the controls). They have proved very useful for establishing cause and effect, for example linking smoking with lung cancer. Case-control studies are most appropriately used in situations where the disease process being investigated is rare, though they are more prone to hidden biases than cohort studies. A cohort study in such cases would need to be inordinately large to ensure that sufficient cases of disease were included in order to effect comparisons between subgroups. In a case-control study the cases of disease are identified first; appropriate controls are then selected for comparison, and the focus is on a comparison of an exposure of interest between the two groups. Direct inference of causation cannot be made from case-control studies because our starting point is the identification of those who already have the disease of interest.

***Participants.*** Particular care is required in explaining how case ascertainment was determined because misclassification is a serious potential bias in studies of this type. Suitable controls are often also problematic to recruit. The control group should be similar in all its characteristics to the case group except with regard to their disease status and, potentially, their 'exposure'. Are there equal numbers of cases and controls or are two or more controls recruited for each case? Are controls matched or unmatched to cases? If matched, what are the matching criteria?

***Exposure, outcome, other variables, sample size and control of biases.*** As for cohort studies.

***Statistical methods.*** As for cohort studies. An additional issue for case-control studies arises when the cases and controls are matched. In this case the matching has to be specifically accounted for in the methods of analysis. For example, McNemar's test should be used, which analyses case-control pairs, rather than a simple chi-square test which compares groups at the aggregate level. Where a logistic regression model may be used for a cohort study, for a matched case-control study a *conditional* logistic regression model should be used which incorporates the matching variables.

***Interpretation.*** As for cohort studies.

## Cross-sectional studies

Studies of this type involve a 'snap-shot' investigation of some phenomenon of interest at a particular instant or over a short period of time. In epidemiology, they are often used to ascertain the prevalence of a particular disease at a moment in time in a well-defined geographical area or subject group. Surveys are usually examples of this design and are used widely in studies involving both patients and health professional groups.

*Participants.* Are the eligibility criteria for inclusion clearly stated? What are the settings and locations of recruitment? What are the methods of recruitment? Are the characteristics of the sample similar to those of your population of interest? What potential biases are present in the methods of sample selection?

*Variables.* In epidemiological studies this study design is often used to determine the prevalence of a disease in a population of interest. More broadly, surveys can be used to obtain information on a wide and complex range of issues using simple or complex, single or multiple questionnaires. Have all quantitative variables been adequately defined and are the measures valid? If a questionnaire is used, has it been previously validated and is it suitable for the purpose for which it is being used?

*Statistical methods.* Analyses could comprise simple evaluations of prevalence of disease (or other concept of interest), where confidence intervals should also be provided if a random sample of the population of interest is used. Commonly, surveys are based on non-random samples, in which case any statistical inferences should be treated with caution. Many surveys are essentially descriptive in nature, with assessment of responses to a large number of questions. The validity of any statistical comparisons in such circumstances are even more open to question unless efforts have been made to minimize the number of formal comparisons and account for multiple testing. It is not possible to ascertain causality from cross-sectional studies.

*Interpretation.* As for cohort studies.

# Critical evaluation of studies of diagnostic test accuracy

*Useful resources.* The STARD (standards for the reporting of diagnostic accuracy studies) statement is a checklist used to guide the reporting of studies of accuracy;[7] the QUADAS (quality assessment for diagnostic accuracy studies) is a generic tool used

to appraise the quality of primary studies in systematic reviews of diagnostic accuracy;[37] an appropriate appraisal tool from Appendix 4.1.

*Specific issues to consider.* Diagnostic accuracy studies are integral to the evaluation of new and existing imaging technologies and to the measurement of their ability to distinguish patients with and without the target disorder. Studies that assess the performance (or accuracy) of a medical imaging modality, such as magnetic resonance imaging of the knee, should apply the modality to a prospective and consecutive series of patients with and without the target disease, such as meniscal or ligamentous injury, and then the patients undergo a second gold standard or reference test, such as arthroscopy. The relationship between the results of the imaging modality (or index test) and disease status, as determined by the gold standard, is described using probabilistic measures such as sensitivity (correct abnormal diagnosis of patients with disease) and specificity (correct normal diagnosis of patients without disease). It is important that the results of the gold standard are close to the truth, or the performance of the imaging modality will be poorly estimated.

*Patient selection.* Was the setting for the evaluation described? Was the spectrum of patients representative of the patients who will receive the test in practice? Were selection criteria clearly described? Patient selection processes affect which patients enter the study and this can affect both its internal validity (in that a biased selection of patients could inflate the index test performance) and external validity (in that a narrow selection of patients could limit the generalizability of the findings). The setting, such as a specialized centre, could be referred rare or problem cases which could affect the prevalence and severity of disease in the patient sample and thus study generalizability. Similarly, an appropriate spectrum of patients should be selected in terms of demographics and clinical features as a limited spectrum can considerably bias the sensitivity and specificity of the test. Predetermined selection criteria should be described to ensure the explicit and reproducible selection of patients into the study.

*Observer selection.* Has the effect of the characteristics of observers on test performance been considered? Has observer variability been determined? The characteristics of the observers involved in the interpretation of images is important in diagnostic accuracy studies of imaging modalities, as they can affect estimates of test performance and generalizability. For example, a study that includes a single, highly specialist observer is likely to have low external validity. In contrast, such an observer could help to produce the best estimates of test accuracy and so increase internal validity. Characteristics of observers that have been considered important in the appraisal of a diagnostic accuracy study include: allocation of images to be read by observers; number, experience and training of observers; profession of observers; and assessment of observer variability and examination of its effect on test accuracy. The variability of an observer, or the reproducibility with which an observer interprets an image, can be assessed as different observers interpreting the same sample of images (interobserver) or the same observers interpreting the same images on separate occasions (intraobserver). The greater the observer variability, the less reliable are the results of the imaging modality. (See ROC, Chapter 8.)

***Choice and application of the reference standard.*** Is the reference standard likely to correctly classify the target condition? Is the time period between reference standard and index test short enough to be reasonably sure that the target condition did not change between two tests? Did the whole sample or a random selection of the sample receive verification using a reference standard diagnosis? Did patients receive the same reference standard regardless of the index test result? Was the reference standard independent of the index test? The reference standard is the method used to determine the presence or absence of the target condition and is assumed to be 100% sensitive and specific. Therefore the choice and application of the reference standard is very important for affecting estimates of the index test performance. A valid reference standard should be chosen that correctly classifies the target condition and is applied within a clinically acceptable timeframe after the index test to prevent a change in the target condition explaining a difference in the results between the index test and reference standard. The same reference standard should be applied regardless of the results of the index test and preferably to the whole or at least a random sample of patients. Not applying the same reference standard to determine the definitive diagnosis in the sample of patients could also explain differences in results between the index test and reference standard and thus estimates of test performance. Nor should the index test form part of the reference standard as this too will introduce bias.

***Independence of interpretation.*** Were the index test results interpreted without knowledge of the results of the reference standard? Were the reference standard results interpreted without knowledge of the results of the index test? Assessments that involve clinical judgement, such as the interpretation of medical images, are susceptible to bias owing to prior expectation. Therefore, the interpretation of the results of the test under evaluation should be done independently (or blind) to the results of the reference standard. Conversely, the results of the reference standard should be interpreted blind to the results of the index test. Not avoiding this bias may lead to inflated measures of diagnostic accuracy.

***Measurement of results.*** Were uninterpretable/intermediate test results reported? Were withdrawals from a study explained? Indeterminate index test results might arise due to factors such as technical faults or inferior image quality. Patients might also withdraw from a study before the results of either or both of the index test and reference standard are known. This could be for many uncontrollable reasons such as death, changing residency, or unwillingness to continue cooperation. A study should fully report these indeterminate test results and withdrawals and, as long as they are random and not related to the true disease status, they should not introduce bias but could affect generalizability.[38]

## Critical evaluation of qualitative studies

***Useful resources.*** The two articles by Giacomini and Cook[39,40] and the article by Barbour;[41] an appropriate appraisal tool from Appendix 4.1.

***Specific issues to consider.*** Qualitative research aims to provide an in-depth understanding of social phenomena such as people's experiences and perspectives in the context of their personal circumstances or settings. To explore the phenomena from the perspective of those being studied qualitative studies are characterized by: the use of unstructured methods which are sensitive to the social context of the study; the capture of data which are detailed, rich and complex; a mainly inductive rather than deductive analytic process; and answering 'what is', 'how' and 'why' questions. It employs a variety of methods including: interviews, focus groups, observations, conversation, discourse and narrative synthesis, and documentary and video analysis.

***Sampling.*** Are the criteria for selecting the sample clearly described? Was the sampling strategy comprehensive to ensure the generalizability of the analyses? Are the characteristics of the sample adequately described? As with quantitative studies, it is important for exclusion and inclusion criteria to be clearly specified. This will help you to judge whether the appropriate characteristics of patients according to age, gender, ethnicity and other relevant demographic features have been identified. Unlike quantitative research that requires the selection of a consecutive or random sample of patients that are representative of a population, qualitative research requires the selection of specific groups of people that possess characteristics relevant to the phenomena being studied. Convenience sampling might be used for pragmatic reasons and involves choosing the individuals that are easiest to reach, but this might introduce bias. Alternatively, there is purposive sampling when patients are deliberately selected because they possess a certain characteristic and this helps to ensure a range of viewpoints are represented. The characteristics of the sample must be described to help you judge whether an appropriate selection of patients has been included.

***Data collection.*** Were the data collection methods appropriate for the research objectives and setting? Common methods of data collection include observations, interviews or document analysis. Observation is used to record social phenomena *directly* by the investigators themselves or *indirectly* through audiotape or videotape recording. Direct observation requires the investigator to spend time in the social context under investigation and collects data through their nonparticipation or participation in a setting. In nonparticipant observation the researcher does not get involved in the social interactions being observed. It is therefore important to consider whether the observer is ignored or could inadvertently affect subjects' behaviour. In participant observation the researcher is part of the social setting, but again it must be considered whether their dual role as observer and participant influences social interactions. Collecting data using interviews might include semi-structured and in-depth interviews and focus groups. Individual interviews are more useful for evoking personal experience, in particular, on sensitive topics, whereas focus groups use group interaction to generate data, but their public forum might inhibit candid disclosure. You should consider the rationale for the choice of a particular method of data collection and its appropriateness for the topics being

studied. Finally, analysis of documents such as charts, journals and correspondence might provide qualitative data. This can be achieved by counting specific content elements (e.g. frequency of specific words being used) or interpreting text (e.g. seeking nuances of meaning). The former rarely provides adequate information for analysis. You should consider whether multiple methods of collecting data are included. This approach can improve the rigour of a study as it allows investigators to examine subjects' perspectives and behaviour from different angles and to capture information with one method that was not possible with another.

***Validity.*** Are the results of the study valid? This is concerned with whether the data collected truly reflect the phenomena under scrutiny. One method to achieve this is to use triangulation, which refers to the collection of data from different sources using different research methods to identify patterns of convergence. Another approach to validating data is to feed the findings back to the subjects to see if they consider the findings a reasonable account of their experience. There should also be appropriate consideration of 'negative' or 'deviant' cases by the researcher who should give a fair account of these occasions and explain why the data vary.

***Data analysis.*** Were the data appropriately analysed? Qualitative research begins with a general exploratory question and preliminary concepts. Relevant data is collected, patterns observed and a conceptual framework is developed. This process is iterative, with new data being incorporated that may corroborate or challenge the emerging framework. The process should continue until the framework stabilizes due to the incorporation of further data having minimal affect on its development. At this point 'theoretical saturation' or informational redundancy' is said to have been achieved. Qualitative data, and its interpretation, should be cross-referenced across multiple sources using triangulation in order to ensure the robustness of the analysis. Data synthesis should also, ideally, be undertaken by more than one person, and consensus agreement reached, to reduce the risk of researcher bias due to preconceived ideas about the phenomena investigated.

# References

[1] Greenhalgh T. How to Read a Paper: The Basics of Evidence Based Medicine. London: BMJ; 2001.

[2] Sackett DL, Haynes RB, Guyatt GH, et al. Clinical Epidemiology: A Basic Science for Clinical Medicine. 2nd ed. London: Little, Brown; 1991. p. 45.

[3] Sackett DL, Rosenberg WMC, Gray JAM, et al. Evidence based

medicine: what it is and what it isn't. Br Med J 1996;312:71–2.

[4] Sackett DL, Straus SE, Richardson WS, et al. Evidence-Based Medicine: How to Practice and Teach EBM. 2nd ed. Edinburgh: Churchill Livingstone; 2000.

[5] Daly J, Willis K, Small R, et al. A hierarchy of evidence for assessing qualitative health research. J Clin Epidemiol 2007;60:43–9.

[6] Hicks RJ. Health technology assessment and cancer imaging: who should be setting the agenda? Cancer Imaging 2004;4(2): 58–60.

[7] Bossuyt PM, Reitsma JB, Bruns DE, et al. The STARD statement for reporting studies of diagnostic accuracy: explanation and elaboration. Ann Intern Med 2003;138(1):W-1–W-12.

[8] Harris KM, Kelly S, Berry E, et al. Systematic review of endoscopic ultrasound in gastro-oesophageal cancer. Health Technol Assess 1998;2(18):1–134.

[9] Bryant J, Picot J, Levitt G, et al. Cardioprotection against the toxic effects of anthracyclines given to children with cancer: a systematic review. Health Technol Assess 2007;11(27):1–84.

[10] Brealey S, Scally A, Hahn S, et al. Accuracy of radiographer plain radiograph reporting in clinical practice: a meta-analysis. Clin Radiol 2005;60(2):232–41.

[11] Bartholomew AL, Denton ERE, Shaw M, et al. A randomised controlled trial comparing lateral skull computerised radiographs with or without a grid. Radiography 2004;10:201–4.

[12] Harrison R, Dey P, Slevin NJ, et al. Randomized controlled trial to assess the effectiveness of a videotape about radiotherapy. Br J Cancer 2001;84(1):8–10.

[13] Sala E, Watson CJE, Beardsmoore C, et al. A randomized controlled trial of routine early abdominal computed tomography in patients presenting with non-specific acute abdominal pain. Clin Radiol 2007;62:961–9.

[14] Ravasco P, Monteiro-Grillo I, Vidal PM, et al. Dietary counseling improves patient outcomes: a prospective, randomized controlled

trial in colorectal cancer patients undergoing radiotherapy. J Clin Oncol 2005;23:1431–8.

[15] Trakada G, Pouli A, Goumas P. Pulmonary radiographic findings and mortality in hospitalized patients with lower respiratory tract infections. Radiography 2006;12:20–5.

[16] Aktas M, de Jong D, Nuyttens JJ, et al. Concomitant radiotherapy and hyperthermia for primary carcinoma of the vagina: a cohort study. Eur J Obstet Gynaecol Reprod Biol 2007;133:100–4.

[17] Virtanen A, Pukkala E, Auvinen A. Angiosarcoma after radiotherapy: a cohort study of 332,163 Finnish cancer patients. Br J Cancer 2007;97:115–7.

[18] Jaremko JL, Lambert RGW, Rowe BH, et al. Do radiographic indices of distal radius fracture reduction predict outcomes in older adults receiving conservative treatment? Clin Radiol 2007;62:65–72.

[19] Sernik RA, Abicalaf CA, Pimental BF, et al. Ultrasound features of carpal tunnel syndrome: a prospective case-control study. Skeletal Radiol 2008;37:49–53.

[20] Cheng TC, Jeng C-M, Kung C-H, et al. Yoga and lumbar disc degeneration disease: MR imaging based case control study. Chinese Journal of Radiology 2008;33:73–8.

[21] Spruit PH, Siesling S, Elferink MAG, et al. Regional radiotherapy versus an axillary lymph node dissection after lumpectomy: a safe alternative for an axillary lymph node dissection in a clinically uninvolved axilla in breast cancer. A case control study with 10 years follow up. Radiat Oncol 2007;2:40.

[22] Finlay GA, Joseph B, Rodrigues CR, et al. Advanced presentation of lung cancer in Asian immigrants: a case-control study. Chest 2002;122 (6):1938–43.

[23] Lutz S, Spence C, Chow E, et al. Survey on use of palliative radiotherapy in hospice care. J Clin Oncol 2004;22:3581–6.

[24] Davies C, Grange S, Trevor MM. Radiation protection practices and related continuing professional education in dental radiography: a

survey of practitioners in the north-east of England. Radiography 2005;11:255–61.

[25] Jones HC, Manning D. A survey to assess audit mechanisms practised by skeletal reporting radiographers. Radiography 2008;14(3):201–5.

[26] Power M, Laasch H, Kasthuri RS, et al. Videofluoroscopic assessment of dysphagia: a questionnaire survey of protocols, roles and responsibilities of radiology and speech and language therapy personnel. Radiography 2006;12 (1):26–30.

[27] Grisaru D, Almog B, Levine C, et al. The diagnostic accuracy of 18F-fluorodeoxyglucose PET/CT in patients with gynaecological malignancies. Gynaecol Oncol 2004;94:680–4.

[28] Burling D, Moore A, Marshall M, et al. Virtual colonoscopy: effect of computer-assisted detection (CAD) on radiographer performance. Clin Radiol 2008;63:549–56.

[29] MERCURY Study Group. Diagnostic accuracy of preoperative magnetic resonance imaging in predicting curative resection of rectal cancer: prospective observational study. Br Med J 2006;333:779.

[30] Dai S, Hata K, Inubashiri E, et al. Does three-dimensional power Doppler ultrasound improve the diagnostic accuracy for the prediction of adnexal malignancy? J Obstet Gynaecol Res 2008;34 (3):364–70.

[31] Nagle C, Lewis S, Meiser B, et al. Exploring general practitioners' experience of informing women about prenatal screening tests for foetal abnormalities: a qualitative focus group study. BMC Health Serv Res 2008;28(8):114.

[32] Poulos A, Llewellyn G. Mammography discomfort: a holistic perspective derived from women's experiences. Radiography 2005;11(1):17–25.

[33] Colyer H. The role of the radiotherapy treatment review radiographer. Radiography 2000;6 (4):253–60.

[34] Moher D, Cook DJ, Eastwood S, et al. for the QUOROM group. Improving the quality of reporting of meta-analysis of randomised

controlled trials: the QUORUM
statement. Lancet
1999;354:1896–900.

[35] Altman DG, Schulz KF, Moher D,
et al. The revised CONSORT
statement for reporting randomized
trials: explanation and elaboration.
Ann Intern Med 2001;134
(8):663–94.

[36] Vandenbroucke JP, von Elm E,
Altman DG, et al. Strengthening
the reporting of observational
studies in epidemiology
(STROBE): explanation and
elaboration. Epidemiology 2007;18
(6):805–35.

[37] Whiting P, Westwood M, Rutjes
AWS, et al. Evaluation of
QUADAS, a tool for the quality
assessment of diagnostic accuracy
studies. BMC Med Res Methodol
2006;6:9.

[38] Kelly S, Berry E, Roderick P, et al.
The identification of bias in studies
of the diagnostic performance of
imaging modalities. Br J Radiol
1997;70:1028–35.

[39] Giacomini MK, Cook DJ. Users'
Guides to the Medical Literature:
XXIII. Qualitative Research in
Health Care A. Are the results of

the study valid. JAMA 2000;284
(3):357–62.

[40] Giacomini MK, Cook DJ. Users'
Guides to the Medical Literature:
XXIII. Qualitative Research in
Health Care B. What are the results
and how do they help me care for
my patients. JAMA 2000;284
(4):478–82.

[41] Barbour RS. Checklists for
improving rigour in qualitative
research: a case of the tail wagging
the dog? Br Med J
2001;322:1115–7.

## Further reading

Boutron I, Moher D, Altman DG, et al.
Extending the CONSORT statement
to randomized trials of
nonpharmacologic treatment:
explanation and elaboration. Ann
Intern Med 2008;148(4):295–309.

Crombie IC. The Pocket Guide to
Critical Appraisal. London: BMJ;
1996.

Egger M, Davey Smith G, Altman DG.
Systematic Reviews in Health Care:
Meta-analysis in Context. London: Br
Med J; 2001.

Evans D. Hierarchy of evidence: a
framework for ranking evidence
evaluating healthcare interventions. J
Clin Nurs 2003;12:77–84.

Feinstein AR. Meta-analysis: statistical
alchemy for the 21st century. J Clin
Epidemiol 1995;48(1):71–9.

Hicks RJ. Health technology assessment
and cancer imaging: who should be
setting the agenda? Cancer Imaging
2004;4(2):58–60.

Kelly S, Berry E, Roderick P, et al. The
identification of bias in studies of the
diagnostic performance of imaging
modalities. Br J Radiol
1997;70:1028–35.

Mays N, Pope C. Qualitative research:
rigour and qualitative research. Br
Med J 1995;11:109–12.

Spencer L, Ritchie J, Lewis J, et al.
Quality in Qualitative Evaluation: A
Framework for Assessing Research
Evidence. Crown Copyright 2003.

Stolberg HO, Norman G, Trp I.
Fundamentals of clinical research for
radiologists: randomized controlled
trials. Am J Roentgenol
2004;183:1539–44.

Whiting P, Westwood M, Rutjes AWS,
et al. Evaluation of QUADAS, a tool
for the quality assessment of
diagnostic accuracy studies. BMC
Med Res Methodol 2006;6:9.

## Appendix 4.1  Resources for critical appraisal

The following resources have been developed to assist medical and health practitioners in the critical appraisal of research appropriate to their practice:

- BestBETs (Best Evidence Topics) – critical appraisal worksheets for a wide range of study types: http://www.bestbets.org/links/BET-CA-worksheets.php (accessed 23 September 2009)
- Boynton PM, Greenhalgh T. Hands-on guide to questionnaire research: selecting, designing, and developing your questionnaire. BMJ 2004; 328: 1312–1315 – checklists for questionnaire design and the critical evaluation of a questionnaire based studies. Table E, Critical appraisal checklist for a questionnaire study, available at: http://www.bmj.com/cgi/content/full/328/7451/1312/DC1 (accessed 23 September 2009)
- Centre for Evidence-based Medicine – critical appraisal tools for systematic reviews, RCTs and diagnostic accuracy studies. Available at: http://www.cebm.net/index.aspx?o=1157 (accessed 23 September 2009)
- NHS Public Health Resource Unit – appraisal tools developed by the Critical Appraisal Skills Programme (CASP) for the appraisal of systematic reviews, randomized controlled trials (RCTs), qualitative research, economic evaluation studies, cohort studies, case control studies and diagnostic test studies. Available at: http://www.phru.nhs.uk/Pages/PHD/resources.htm (accessed 23 September 2009)
- Centre for Health Evidence – a collection of user guides on the critical appraisal and contextual interpretation of all forms of evidence encountered in healthcare practice. Available at: http://www.cche.net/usersguides/main.asp (accessed 23 September 2009)

# Reflective practice

5

Pauline Reeves

## CHAPTER POINTS

This chapter reviews a range of skills which link clinical practice with research methods. These are:
- reflection
- critical incident technique
- research appraisal
- reflexivity
- evidence-based practice.

We have attempted to show how this range of skills can help you to develop as a practitioner and life-long learner in radiography.

This chapter will examine the meaning of the term *reflective practice* and will then outline a research method which can be used to encourage you to reflect clinically, even at a very early stage in training. We will show how this research method can be used in the classroom as a way of demonstrating the relevance of research to clinical practice and illustrating the fact that doing research can be a simple process, accessible to all.

The chapter will then look at *reflexivity*, contrasting it with clinical reflection and discussing how and why it should be used in the teaching of research methods to radiography students. We will also look at the need to be critical about written research. This will lead into a definition of the term *evidence-based practice* and what this means in radiography. These are presented as a developmental series of skills with the overall aim of this chapter being to demonstrate how knowledge of research methods and the associated skills can be the key to your development as a full autonomous professional practitioner.

Those responsible for teaching research methods to trainee practitioners often comment that students (even at postgraduate level) can find the topic difficult and boring and question its relevance to medical imaging and radiotherapy. This has been reported by those teaching other social science subjects to health care students.[1] Another area of difficulty has been identified around the teaching of reflective practice to health care students.[2]

A study of undergraduate research in UK radiography education centres concluded that the broad aims for the teaching of research methods were the development of the following:

- an understanding of the skills and knowledge required to undertake research
- a questioning attitude toward clinical practice (*reflection-in-action*)
- the ability to develop appropriate research questions for the current and future needs of the radiography profession.[3]

## Research methods and their contribution to course outcomes and professional development

As stated above, this chapter offers a hierarchy of skills which link clinical radiographic practice to the study of research methods. For most people, the acquisition of these skills is likely to come as part of the pursuit of particular qualifications as you train as a practitioner then climb up the career ladder.

The different levels in degree courses and how they relate to research methods are summarized below.[4] These level descriptors are also integrated with the College of Radiographers' levels of practice and their descriptors for the skill of reflection;.[5]

## Level 4 (Year 1 undergraduate/Cert HE-Assistant Practitioner)

Primarily about knowledge of the concepts and principles underlying radiography together with the ability to evaluate both quantitative and qualitative data; to reflect on and learn from experience within own scope of practice.

## Level 5 (Year 2 undergraduate/DipHE/ Foundation degree-Assistant Practitioner)

Display knowledge, critical understanding and the ability to apply concepts and principles in a radiographic context. Students should be able to demonstrate knowledge of the main methods of enquiry used within medical imaging and radiotherapy.

## Level 6 (BSc (Hons)-Radiography Practitioner)

The ability to synthesize knowledge, often from the forefront of the field, and to deploy techniques of research while also being able to comment upon published findings; to reflect on and learn from research evidence and experience and apply to own and others' working practices.

## Level 7 (MSc-Advanced Practitioner)

Display a systematic understanding of knowledge and critical awareness, with the ability to develop this to a high level. The ability critically to evaluate current research and advanced scholarship with a comprehensive understanding of applicable research techniques. Reflect on and learn from relevant research evidence, policies and legislation and apply across professional and organizational boundaries.

## Level 8 (PhD/Consultant Radiographer)

Be responsible for the creation and interpretation of new knowledge, through original research or other advanced scholarship, of a quality to satisfy peer review, extend the forefront of the discipline, and merit publication. Acquire a systematic acquisition and understanding of a substantial body of knowledge

which is at the forefront of an academic discipline or area of professional practice. Within the area of individual practice/expertise, be able to reflect on and learn from other practices, political, economic and social contexts and use to effect changes to service delivery.[4,5]

The descriptors outlined above help to demonstrate the importance of the study of research methods to the achievement of a degree qualification, whether a foundation degree (assistant practitioner), honours degree (radiography practitioner), Master's degree (advanced practitioner) or Doctorate (consultant practitioner).

# Reflective practice as a skill

Reflective practice has been identified as one of four generic skills which are relevant at all levels of practice within the profession, from assistant practitioner to consultant practitioner. These levels and skills were outlined in the previous section. The levels of knowledge and understanding of reflective practice should be such as to allow the 'Practitioner to reflect on, and learn from, research evidence and experience and apply to own and others' working practices'.[5]

The process of reflection gives you the tools to resolve apparent inconsistencies between theoretical teaching and clinical practice, something which troubles students, especially in the early stages of training.[6] This is mirrored in the definition of reflection presented by Johns:[7]

> Reflection is being mindful of self, either within or after experience … in order to … move toward resolving contradiction between one's vision and actual practice.[7]

The stimulus for written reflection may come from any number of events, for example changes in rotation to include a new work area, a promotion, a specific interaction with a patient or member of staff or from a news item or journal article.[2] In two recent studies of communication styles in radiography, the first presents observational data outlining how practitioners communicate and relates this to the theory of transactional analysis; in the second paper the author outlines how transactional analysis can be used as a tool to help you reflect on your own communication styles and thus relate better to patients.[8,9]

Reflection on practice allows you to create your own body of theoretical experiential knowledge to underpin your clinical skill base and the intuitive aspects of clinical work.[10] Reflection can be via a portfolio or a reflective diary,[2] but one way to start out is to recall significant (critical) events and to focus on those as a learning tool. Once you have described the incident itself, then try and write down your reactions and feelings about what happened. Why were things different than you expected? This may lead you to conclude that there is knowledge missing; this may be behavioural (as with the example of communication skills given above) or you may conclude that you have a gap in your theoretical knowledge, which may lead you to research that gap in your knowledge. In both medical imaging and radiotherapy there is a need to reflect on the working environment – diagnostic practitioners may reflect on their experiences of working in the accident and emergency environment (and especially on call), for example. Radiotherapy practitioners are urged to examine their beliefs and attitudes to working in the cancer setting.[2]

# Critical incident technique as a tool for reflection

Critical incident technique (CIT) has been defined as:[11]

> A set of procedures for systematically identifying
> behaviours that contribute to success or failure
> of individuals or organisations in specific situations.[11]

Data may be collected via interviews or by observer reports.[12] In nursing research the technique has typically been used to highlight aspects of best and worst practice by asking respondents to write about critical incidents themselves.[13] One of the advantages of focusing on specific incidents is that atypical incidents facilitate recall and they allow participants to clarify both their perceptions and feelings about the incidents identified.[14,15] CIT can be a very effective tool in this respect but has not been commonly used in radiography studies so far.[16] It also has the advantage of encouraging you to focus on good practice, rather than the tendency to recall only negative events.

# Methods

While the student can be made to recognize the importance of research methods, it is the duty of the lecturer to make the subject matter relevant to the study of radiography as a discipline. One example of this is

set out here. This section sets out to outline teaching methods previously used in an undergraduate module in research methods. The sessions were organized with two overall aims: to introduce the students to the use of critical incident technique (CIT) and to introduce them to the principles of qualitative data analysis.[17]

The lessons set out to fulfil a number of objectives for the students:

1. to demonstrate the relevance of research to radiography practice
2. to give them actual practical experience of the use of research methods
3. to demonstrate that research could be easy and straightforward
4. to encourage active reflection on practice.

*Critical incidents* have been described as 'any incident which made an emotional impact,'[6] either positively or negatively (maybe because it was very emotional or stressful). Critical incidents are alluded to in a recent paper which defines reflective practice as 'a process that is undertaken in response to a positive or negative event that may be initiated consciously or subconsciously, that requires analysis to provide an answer or insight'.[2]

CIT was first described by John Flanagan in 1954.[12] Flanagan stated that there were five steps in the use of the technique, as described below:

## 1. Determining the general aim of the study

Critical incident technique was outlined to the student groups as a methodology and it was explained that they were going to use critical incident technique to look at the concept of patient care.

## 2. Planning and specifying how data will be collected

The students were then asked to take a sheet of A4 paper and divide it lengthways and annotate it to form a response sheet, as shown in Table 5.1. One of the advantages of the technique is that this response sheet is easy to design, unlike structured questionnaires.

## 3. Collecting the data

The students were then asked to consider the factors that make for good or bad patient care. The sessions were all with first year radiography students in their second semester. They had all undertaken clinical placements.

**Table 5.1 The design of a response sheet**

| |
| --- |
| Good |
| Good |
| Bad |
| Bad |

The students were asked to think about incidents that they had witnessed during their clinical placements and to describe them in the boxes on their response sheet, adding the reasons why they classified them as either 'good' or 'bad' critical incidents of care. The group members were given time to formulate their responses and were asked to give four incidents if at all possible, but not to worry if they could not think of four. They were asked not to mention any names or hospitals and the forms were anonymous. It was explained that the data generated would be used for an exercise in the next lecture session.

When the students had finished writing, the forms were collected in. They were then passed to a clerical assistant who cut the forms up into individual responses; classified them into *good* and *bad* piles and then stuck the responses onto A3 sheets of paper, according to their classification. A full set of the students' responses (both good and bad) was then photocopied for each individual. Actual examples of critical incidents generated are given below:

*Examples of critical incidents*

**Good:** 'Patient was v.v.v.v. scared due to ?spinal # – the practitioner stayed with the patient reassuring all the time while another took X-rays.'

**Good:** Breast boards with adjustable features such as tilt angles, and arm and wrist indexed positions allow the practitioner to set up a patient for a breast treatment more accurately each day and also ensure that each individual patient is more comfortable during the procedure. This increases set-up accuracy and reduces the risk of overdosing the underlying lung of the affected side or compromising the healthy breast on the other side.

**Good:** 'I was present during the examination of a still-born baby being X-rayed. All staff members present treated the baby as a live baby which I thought showed great respect to the baby and its family.'

**Bad:** 'There was an incident with a member of staff where the staff member referred to a female patient as a "beached whale" within earshot of the patient. This was a disgraceful thing for the staff member to say and did not show any positive patient care skills.'

**Bad:** There are still many traditional practices being used regarding the skin care of patients undergoing radiotherapy. Many of these practices have little or no objectively based foundation and are inherently flawed but are still stressed as important to the patient, i.e. not to use soap in the affected area. Even though much research has been undertaken practice has not always followed the evidence.

**Bad:** 'An elderly gentleman was having a barium enema. The catheter fell out three times and the table was covered in barium. The practitioners tried to keep him decent while cleaning him up but the radiologist ripped the gown off and left him naked on the fluoroscopy table, covered in barium sulphate solution.'

## 4. Analysing the data

For the next session the students were asked to bring highlighter pens or crayons with them. One of the collated response sets was given to each student. A short lecture session on qualitative data analysis then followed (see Chapter 16). The students were asked to go through the response sets with highlighter pens looking for the reasons why each critical incident represented either good or bad patient care. They were advised to look for keywords and highlight them and that the aim of the session was for the group (via the lecturer) to generate theories on the board at the end as to what factors made for good or bad patient care. The students were advised to write down their keywords on separate sheets of paper.

## 5. Interpreting and reporting the outcomes

Towards the end of the 2 hour session, the lecturer then asked the students as a group to list on the whiteboard the factors or themes that they had identified with respect to patient care. Poor (bad) patient care was looked at first as this was thought to be easier. Students were each asked to come up with one factor from their analysis which was then written on the board. Once this exercise had been completed (and any keywords which they felt had been left out were added) the group were asked to identify factors which meant the same thing (in other words to collapse the data down). The keywords were thus gradually whittled down so that what remained was a list of discrete concepts or factors which contributed to bad patient care in their opinion. This exercise was repeated to generate keywords relating to the provision of good patient care.

## Discussion

The overall aims of the exercise were as follows:

1. to demonstrate the relevance of research to radiography practice
2. to give actual practical experience of the use of research methods
3. to demonstrate that research can be easy and straightforward
4. to encourage active reflection on practice.

This discussion will examine each of the aims in turn.

### To demonstrate the relevance of research to radiography practice

Exercises such as this can help participants see the relevance of learning about research and how research can relate to radiography. In this exercise the students were specifically asked to reflect on their experiences of radiographic clinical practice. Research suggests that reflection on specific events is easier than attempting to reflect on practice overall.[2]

### To give actual practical experience of the use of research methods

The participants used critical incident technique to generate the data and then undertook manual analysis of qualitative data (see Chapter 16) in the second session. Over the two sessions (3–4 hours in length) they had thus participated in a discrete piece of research. With a class of 30 students this exercise will generate 100 or more separate critical incidents reflecting both good and bad examples of clinical practice.

### To demonstrate that research can be easy and straightforward

Research is sometimes seen as being difficult and wrapped in mystique. The exercise allows students to see that research can be relatively easy to carry out and need not be very time-consuming. The exercise can be used at all levels, from foundation degree to professional doctorate.

### To encourage active reflection on practice

Reflection on practice is a key aim of any undergraduate programme and marks out the independent practitioner. The exercise requires participants both to reflect on practice and to link that clinical reflection to the practice of research.[18,19] The exercise used is in line with the use of the critical incident technique in published studies[6,14] and with the College of Radiographers' definition cited above.[5] As a research method, critical incident technique can also be used with patients as participants.[14] This is in line with the definition of evidence-based radiography presented later in this chapter; that is, our clinical practice should include consideration of patient preferences.

Once the class exercise had been completed, copies of the data sets were sent out to clinical tutors so that they could use them for discussion group work within the clinical setting. The class exercise could also be followed up with a written assignment using the data to encourage individuals to reflect in more depth on the critical radiographic incidents generated or as an assignment in research methods. In one educational study using critical incidents, small group work was used after data generation to examine role expectations, belief systems, coping strategies and a range of issues such as power, autonomy, caring, ethics and patients' rights.[6]

## Critical analysis of research

Throughout both your course and your career you will be expected to search for and appraise research papers. Unfortunately it is the case that the quality of research 'evidence' varies dramatically. Reasons for this have been cited as being selective reporting (including the tendency to report positive results but not negative ones) and issues of bias, including the viewpoint of a particular medical speciality.[20] Radiology research has been argued to be of poor quality and very variable. This is said to be partly because of the pace of technological change and the need for rapid assessment of potential new technologies. This means that randomized controlled trials are very infrequent in radiology.[20] Chapter 4 will help to advise you on how to appraise research carefully and what to look out for; suffice to say, it is important to be critical and not merely accept the veracity of the papers that you utilize in your studies.

## Reflexivity

At the culmination of any radiography degree course (whether BSc or MSc) you will normally be required to undertake some form of research project. This may include active research but, increasingly, at undergraduate level, it is likely to be an extended study or literature review (referred to as a dissertation). A study in 1999 showed that all radiography education centres at that time required their undergraduates to undertake primary research but this has become much more difficult as the ethical climate has changed.[3]

There is often a lot of stress generated in deciding what topic to undertake. Unlike a doctoral project, the research (whether for BSc or MSc) does *not* have to be original. The project can be a reworking of another study in a new setting or a review of existing literature. Indeed it can be argued that the actual topic chosen for the research study is, to some extent, immaterial since the aim of such a study is to allow you to demonstrate the ability to carry out research (be it primary/active or secondary/documentary) and to critically analyse the findings. It must be remembered that those who gain a degree classification of 2.1 or higher are eligible to go straight on to a doctoral programme, should they wish to do so.[21] Research methods training is a preparation for postgraduate research. It should also be remembered that the College of Radiographers includes the ability to learn from research evidence as part of their definition of reflection.[5]

In the context of this chapter, the term *reflexivity* is taken to refer to reflection upon the research process itself. The term may be defined as follows:[22]

> Reflexivity is the project of examining how the researcher and intersubjective elements impact on and transform research.[22]

The concept of reflexivity in research arose from qualitative methods, principally ethnography. Ethnographic methods utilize the concept of *researcher as instrument*; the researcher immerses him- or herself in the setting and collects data via a variety of methods but including participant observation.[23] Many qualitative healthcare research projects may be classified as participant observation since they take place in the workplace. Reflexive critique forms part of the research report in order for the researcher to determine, and make explicit, the effect that *they themselves* have had upon the research, since they have been a participant within the setting. Has their participation introduced bias (contamination) into the research (especially where the setting is also the researcher's own workplace)?[24]

In the context of the student research project the inclusion of a reflexive chapter at the end of the project report has the function of requiring you to explicitly audit your own research. Guideline questions here would include: 'What did you learn from the research process?', 'What would you do differently if you were to approach the research again?', 'Can you identify any flaws in your research?' This section readily leads in to recommendations for further research and to the final conclusions.

The inclusion of a reflexive section allows you to demonstrate critical analysis and to show whether you have understood the research process. It can also help those marking the project to differentiate between gradings.

## Evidence-based practice

The definition of reflective practice stated earlier encompasses the need for evidence-based practice.[5] It is argued that the generation of an evidence base in radiography lags behind that of other allied health professions such as physiotherapy and nursing.[25,26] Several reasons have been given for this, including low self-esteem of practitioners, reliance on tradition and subjectivity and a focus on clinical competence to the exclusion of all other professional attributes.

Many recently qualified practitioners now have experience of problem-based learning whereby the focus of student learning is shifted away from passively sitting in lectures to active, focused investigation and analysis. It is argued that the ability to undertake this form of learning will equip you to become a life-long learner.[25] This is now very important given the changes in health care in the 21st century. In the UK all National Health Service (NHS) employees are now required to demonstrate their competence annually as part of an individual review using the knowledge and skills framework (NHS KSF).[27] The Health Professions Council (HPC) and the College of Radiographers also have their own mandatory requirements for continuous professional development (CPD),[28,29] as do other professional bodies worldwide such as the Australian Institute of Radiography (AIR).[2] Registrants with the HPC are required to keep a portfolio documenting their learning activities and showing that those activities are relevant to current or future practice (e.g. for someone studying to become a sonographer). These learning activities do not just consist of attending courses. They can include research and activities such as critical analysis of original journal articles:[25]

> Evidence-based radiography is informed and based on the combination of clinical expertise and the best available research-based evidence, patient preferences and available resources.[25]

This step forms the final link in the chain. Reflection on practice begins the process; this should lead to identification of gaps in knowledge or clinically related questions that need answering; this in turn leads the practitioner into the research literature, being careful to be critical of what is found in that literature. The final step is to integrate those findings into everyday practice.

This process was triggered for me shortly after starting my most recent clinical post; I received a request for acromioclavicular joints for a patient from the orthopaedic outpatients' clinic. The request did not stipulate the views to be undertaken and I did anteroposterior weight-bearing comparison views and sent the patient back to clinic. A few minutes later I was summoned to see the consultant, who criticized me in no uncertain terms and instructed me to do a Zanca view, which I had never heard of, even though I had taught radiographic technique for many years as a radiography lecturer. I did some research on the subject and eventually published a paper on the topic. The research revealed that weight-bearing views were regarded by orthopaedic surgeons as being of little use.[30]

Current literature seems to be divided as to whether radiography practice is indeed evidence based,[25] although a recent study into research utilization in ultrasound found that 72.9% of the sonographers surveyed claimed that they had integrated research findings into their clinical practice.[31] The researchers note, however, that this group largely comprised higher grade sonographers rather than younger staff and/or recently qualified sonographers. This raises concern for the future research base of the profession.

## Conclusions

Any radiography student who graduates in the 21st century will have been equipped with the skills described above. You will have been encouraged to reflect on your practice as you developed your clinical skills. You will have been introduced to a variety of research methods and the ability to critically appraise them, as this book sets out to do. You will have been given the understanding and skills of evidence-based practice. The extent to which you use those skills once you have qualified, by choosing to make your clinical practice evidence based and by pursuing higher qualifications, is likely to determine how far in your profession you progress. Mandatory continuous professional development (CPD) requires all practitioners to demonstrate life-long learning, but certainly anyone wishing to become an advanced and/or consultant practitioner needs to make a positive choice regarding the use of research methods, appraisal skills, and the drive to implement the resultant knowledge into changing clinical practice. Those who adopt evidence-based practice are said to be professional role models, whether they be clinicians or academics.[25] Research methods are the key to the higher levels of the profession and to safe and effective radiographic practice. They are also the answer to those who still doubt that radiography is truly a profession.[25,26,32]

## Acknowledgement

The cooperation of Rachel Harris in the preparation of this chapter is gratefully acknowledged.

## References

[1] Culmer P, Bundy C, Iphofen R. The teaching of behavioural science to undergraduate radiography students. Res Radiogr 1995;4 (1):13–6.

[2] Chapman N, Dempsey SE, Warren-Forward HM. Workplace diaries promoting reflective practice in radiation therapy. Radiography 2008;15(2):166–70. Available online: doi:10.1016/j.radi.2008.4.008 (accessed 21 August 2008).

[3] Nixon S. Undergraduate research: theory or practice? Radiography

1999;5(4):237–49. Available online: doi:10.1016/S1078-8174(99)90056-1 (accessed 24 September 2009).

[4] Quality Assurance Agency. The framework for higher education qualifications in England, Wales and Northern Ireland – August 2008, London: QAA; 2001. Available at: http://www.qaa.ac.uk/academic infrastructure/fheq/EWNI08/FHEq08.pdf (accessed 24 September 2009).

[5] College of Radiographers. Learning and development framework for clinical imaging and oncology, London: CoR; 2008. Available at: http://doc-lib.sor.org/learning-and-development-framework-clinical-imaging-and-oncology (accessed 24 September 2009).

[6] Smith A, Russell J. Using critical learning incidents in nurse education. Nurse Educ Today 1991;11:284–91.

[7] Johns C. Becoming a Reflective Practitioner. 2nd ed. Oxford: Blackwell; 2004.

[8] Booth L, Manning DJ. Observations of radiographer communication: an exploratory study using transactional analysis. Radiography 2006;12(4):276–82. Available online: doi:10.1016/j.radi.2005.09.005 (accessed 24 September 2009).

[9] Booth L. Observations and reflections of communication in health care – could transactional analysis be used as an effective approach? Radiography 2007;13(2):135–41. Available online: doi:10.1016/j.radi.2006.01.010 (accessed 24 September 2009).

[10] Rolfe G, Freshwater D, Jasper M. Critical Reflection for Nursing and the Helping Professions: A User's Guide. Basingstoke: Palgrave; 2001.

[11] EMMUS (European MultiMedia Usability Services). Critical incidents technique. 1999. Available at: http://www.ucc.ie/hfrg/emmus/methods/cit.html (accessed 12 May 2008).

[12] Byrne M. Critical incident technique as a qualitative research method. AORN J 2001; Available at: http://findarticles.com/p/

articles/mi_m0FSL/is_4_74/ai_80159552/pg_1 (accessed 12 May 2009).

[13] Aveyard H, Woolliams M. In whose best interests? Nurses' experiences of the administration of sedation in general medical wards in England: an application of the critical incident technique. Int J Nurs Stud 2006;43(8):929–39.

[14] Redfern S, Norman I. Quality of nursing care perceived by patients and their nurses: an application of the critical incident technique. Part 1. J Clin Nurs 1999;8(4):407–13.

[15] Schluter J, Seaton P, Chaboyer W. Critical incident technique: a user's guide for nurse researchers. J Adv Nurs 2007;61(1):107–14.

[16] Iedema R, Flabouris A, Grant S, et al. Narrativizing errors of care: critical incident reporting in clinical practice. Soc Sci Med 2006;62(1):134–44.

[17] Boyes C. Discourse analysis and personal/professional development, Radiography 2004;10(2):109–17. Available at: http://dx.doi.org/10.1016/j.radi.2004.02.003 (accessed 24 September 2009).

[18] Reeves P, Murphy F. Oral history as a technique for the professionalisation of student radiographers. J Diagn Radiogr Imag 1998;1(2):97–104.

[19] Decker S, Iphofen R. Developing the profession of radiography: making use of oral history. Radiography 2005;11(4):262–71.

[20] Halligan S, Altman DG. Evidence-based practice in radiology: steps 3 and 4 – appraise and apply systematic reviews and meta-analyses. Radiology 2007;243:13–27.

[21] Reeves P, Hardy M, Stewart-Lord A. Doing your PhD – how to get started. Synergy 2007; November: 26–8.

[22] Finlay L, Gough B. Reflexivity: A Practical Guide for Researchers in Health and Social Science. Oxford: Blackwell; 2003.

[23] Streubert HJ, Carpenter DR. Qualitative Research in Nursing: Advancing the Humanistic

Imperative. Philadelphia: Lippincott; 1995.

[24] Malterud K. Qualitative research: standards, challenges and guidelines. Lancet 2001;358(9280):483–8.

[25] Hafslund B, Clare J, Graverholt B, et al. Evidence-based radiography. Radiography 2008;14(4):343–8. Available online: doi:10.1016/j.radi.2008.01.03 (accessed 23 August 2008).

[26] Sim J, Radloff A. Profession and professionalisation in medical radiation science as an emergent profession. Radiography 2009;15(3):203–8. Available online (2008): doi:10.1016/j.radi.2008.05.01 (accessed 23 August 2008).

[27] Department of Health. The NHS knowledge and skills framework (NHS KSF) and the development review process, London: DOH; 2004. Available at: http://www.dh.gov.uk/en/Publicationsand statistics/Publications/Publications PolicyAndGuidance/DH_4090843 (accessed 23 August 2008).

[28] Health Professions Council. Your guide to our standards for continuing professional development. London: HPC; 2006. Available at: http://www.hpc-uk.org/publications/index.asp?id=101 (accessed 23 August 2008).

[29] Society of Radiographers. CPD Now. London: SoR; 2008. Available at: http://www.sor.org/members/effective-practice/cpd.htm (accessed 23 August 2008).

[30] Reeves P. Radiography of the acromioclavicular joints: a review. Radiography 2003;9(2):169–72. Available online: doi:10.1016/S1078-8174(03)00041-5 (accessed 24 September 2009).

[31] Elliott V, Wilson SE, Svensson J, et al. Research utilisation in sonographic practice: attitudes and barriers. Radiography 2008;15(3):187–95. Available online: doi:10.1016/j.radi.2008.06.03 (accessed 24 September 2009).

[32] Nixon S. Professionalism in radiography. Radiography 2001;7(1):31–5. Available online: doi:10.1053/radi.2000.0292.

# Research governance and ethics

6

Lisa Booth   Paul Brown

## CHAPTER POINTS

- The concept of ethics and patient care or rights is not new.
- Minimum levels of research rights for participants are laid out in the Declaration of Helsinki and the ICH Harmonised Tripartite Guideline for Good Clinical Practice.
- Ethical review in the UK is only compulsory for healthcare research undertaken in the NHS. For clinical trials that that are undertaken outside the NHS different ethical processes apply.
- Ethics applications often fail because of poor quality information and explanation given within the application and on the participant/patient information sheet.
- Researchers should not raise participants' expectations or anxiety.
- While the basic premise of ethical review is to protect the participant/patient from any potential harm, at the same time respecting their dignity, rights and well-being, it may also seek to safeguard the researcher and/or institution undertaking the study.

Research governance and ethics have become an important part of healthcare practice in determining quality of service (audit) and the creation of new knowledge (research). This chapter considers how research, particularly clinical research, is governed by looking at the historical development of the underlying ethical principles and the practical aspects to be taken into account when undergoing ethical review. In addition, a glossary of relevant terms is provided (p. 59).

Research governance should not be confused with clinical governance, although the two can be linked, in that clinical governance may be supported, investigated and measured utilizing research/audit. Clinical governance looks at the activities involved in delivering high-quality care to patients whereas research governance encompasses a 'broad range of regulations, principles and standards of good practice that exist to achieve, and continuously improve, research quality across all aspects of healthcare in the UK and worldwide'.[1]

## A brief history

The rights of patients have long been a part of medical and healthcare practice:

> I will use those … regimens which will benefit my patients according to my greatest ability and judgment, and I will do no harm or injustice to them.
>
> Hippocratic oath (4th century BC)[2]

However, it was not until 1947 and the development of the Nuremburg Code, that the rights of participants were recognized as an important consideration in how medical research was conducted.[3] The Nuremberg Code was a consequence of the Nuremberg trials, where 23 Nazi doctors who had carried out inhumane experiments in the name of medical research were tried for crimes against humanity.[3] It summarizes the rights of research participants, which should be considered by all researchers prior to conducting research, i.e.: 'voluntary and informed consent; autonomy in decision making; risk/benefit; the avoidance of harm'[4] and, in particular, that participants should have the right to withdraw from research at any time with no repercussions.[3] Many thought that the Nuremburg Code would see the end of unethical research practices carried out in the name of medical science, but in fact it took many years and many examples of unethical research for the legacy of the Nuremburg trials to become a part of the ethical review system that we have in the UK today.[4]

The Declaration of Helsinki, originally developed in 1964 by the World Medical Association, built on the principles of the Nuremberg Code and issued 11 statements relating to ethical practice in research. Since this time it has undergone six revisions, mainly in response to examples of unethical research practices. The current declaration, adopted in October 2008, now contains 25 statements relating to how medical research should be undertaken and it makes explicit that 'research . . . must be submitted for consideration, comment, guidance and approval to a research ethics committee before the study begins'.[5] Although the 1964 declaration of Helsinki was an effort to remove unethical practices from research involving human subjects, evidence of unethical practices continued well after this date. For example, in 1966, Henry Beecher detailed 22 examples of research where the lives of the participants taking part had been put at risk,[6] one of these examples was the Tuskegee Syphilis study.[6,7] The Tuskegee Syphilis study, sponsored by the US Public Health Service, took place between 1932 and 1972. The aim of the study was to monitor the natural progression of Syphilis if left untreated. The participants were 399 African-American males, who were never told they had the disease, and despite a cure (Penicillin) becoming available in the 1940s, this treatment was withheld from the study participants.[7,8] Although it is known that more that 100 participants died of the disease, the true cost of this study – i.e. how many wives/children became infected – may never be known.[8]

In 1975, eleven years after the Declaration of Helsinki, and due to pressure from the Royal College of Physicians in 1967 and 1973, the then Department of Health and Social Security incorporated the recommendations of Helsinki into the UK research framework. It was recommended that all UK hospitals should have an ethics committee to review research applications, although the optional nature of these recommendations meant that these committees tended to be self-governing and so there was much variation in their quality.[3,9]

This arrangement persisted until 1990 when the International Conference on Harmonisation of Technical Requirements for the Registration of Pharmaceuticals for Human Use (ICH) guidelines were formulated.[3] Although the main aim of these guidelines were to streamline the processes involved with registering new medicinal products, they importantly included guidance on how clinical trials should be conducted, namely that all clinical trials should be reviewed by an independent Research Ethics Committee (REC).[3] It was at this point, in 1991, that a centralized system for reviewing and advising on the ethical suitability of a research project was first introduced to the UK. The Department of Health (DOH) issued a new set of guidelines stipulating that each health authority should appoint an REC; who should be appointed to these RECs; and the function and remit RECs.[3] However, even with this centralised system, 'ethics were acknowledged but occasionally disregarded' in the research practices that followed.[9]

It should be noted here that in the late 1990s devolution took place within the UK, and responsibility for health care within the four member countries (England, Scotland, Wales and Northern Ireland) was formally devolved. Although all follow similar ethical guidelines, there are some differences with regard to the age of consent and the ultimate reporting structure and researchers will need to consider these variations when applying for ethical approval in the UK.

In 2001 the European Clinical Trials Directive (2001/20/EC) made it a requirement across the countries of the European Community that all clinical trials had to be approved by an appropriately constituted ethics committee. The UK Research Governance Framework/s, which were created around the same time, took this one step further, stipulating that all 'research [conducted in the National Health Service (NHS)], whether a clinical trial or not, receive advice from an NHS REC.'[10] This may have been a response to the optional nature of research ethics review that had been the case until this point which led to the much publicized scandals that followed the research undertaken at Alder Hey Children's Hospital, Liverpool, and the Bristol Royal Infirmary in the early 1990s, where organs and tissues of dead children were removed and retained for research purposes without parental consent.[11]

What was interesting about Alder Hey and Bristol is that they both highlighted how UK law and medical ethics are often at odds with each other. For example, in English common law, the removal and retention of organs without the consent of relatives is not unlawful: 'there is no property in a corpse . . . relatives and executives of the estate have no right to retain the body or dispose of it as they wish' (Williams *v*. Williams (1882), cited in Plomer 2005).[11]

Therefore researchers at Alder Hey and Bristol did not do anything unlawful; in fact the ambiguous Anatomy Act of 1984 and the Human Tissue Act of 1961 were unclear on such practices.[11] Many would argue that the medical advances we enjoy today are a consequence of research carried out on organs and tissues that were collected in this way. What Alder Hey and Bristol really exposed was how the removal of organs and tissue for research purposes, a practice which was acceptable to the medical profession, was actually distressing to the parents and relatives involved, 'exposing a cultural and moral schism between the medical establishment and the rest of society'.[11] The legacy of Alder Hey and Bristol has been to ensure that ethics are institutionalized into all research conducted in the NHS today, in an effort to ensure that the moral implications, not just the lawful ones, are fully considered.

Many outdated and ambiguous acts were reformed around this time, all of which made more explicit the rules and regulations that govern research activities; the Department of Health's 12 Points of Consent: The Law in England (2001)[12] and the Human Tissue Act (2004) replaced the Human Tissue Act (1961), the Anatomy Act (1984), and the Human Organs Transplant Act (1989).[13] Amendments have also been made to the Children Act (1989),[14] the Mental Health Act (1983),[15] and the IR(ME)R regulations (2000).[16] It is important for any researcher who is applying for ethical approval to ensure that they are compliant with these Acts (where applicable) if they are to be successful in their applications. Researchers also need to be aware that although their research project may fall outside the remit of NHS Research Ethics Review (explained later), if they wish to use; participants who lack capacity; human tissue; or radiation, by law they will need to apply to an appropriately constituted Research Ethics Committee. Currently in The UK only NHS RECs or the newly formed Social Care Research Ethics Committees (mental capacity only) can review such applications. In 2004, the Medicines for Human Use (Clinical Trials) Regulations came into force and the necessity to apply to a NHS Research Ethics Committee to conduct research within the NHS became UK law.[17]

## Ethical standpoints

NHS Research Ethics Committees (RECs) are coordinated by the National Research Ethics Service (NRES), the remit of which is to ensure that the standards and operating procedures of RECs are consistent throughout the UK.[10] Each REC must have a particular constitution of medical and lay members who are trained to review research applications (NRES provides training annually for all REC members to ensure that knowledge is up to date). Although the function of the NRES is to ensure a standard approach to ethical review in the NHS, there have been many complaints about the process, owing to what is considered to be an inconsistent approach to reviewing research applications;[17] the evidence from a small number of applications appears to support this view.[18,19] Given the nature of ethics this inconsistency is perhaps not surprising, as ethical views vary depending on the moral standpoint of an individual; the nature of the dilemma; and they also change over time.[19] Sayers[19] argues that to remove this inconsistency would require there to be only one decision maker, or for committee members to have their moral outlook screened before appointment, or for committee members to be told which ethical standpoint should be applied to all research applications, all of which presume that one particular ethical standpoint is superior to another, which is of course not the case.

For example, the utilitarian or consequentialist philosophical approach sees an action as good if it produces, on balance, the greatest good for the greatest number of people.[20] If we apply this approach to the research of Edward Jenner (1749–1823), who investigated the smallpox vaccine, we might feel that the benefits of ridding the world of smallpox outweighed any risks associated with his methods. Jenner's research investigated the belief that milkmaids did not catch smallpox, a disease which, at the time, killed 400 000 people every year in Europe.[21] He believed that this was because milkmaids caught a mild, non-threatening form of smallpox known as cowpox. To test this theory Jenner inoculated the 8-year old son of his Gardener, James Phipps, with the pus from a cow pox blister (Phipps had never contracted cow pox or small pox). Some weeks later Jenner inoculated the boy again, this time with live smallpox material; no disease occurred. Phipps was immune to the smallpox disease.[22] Further vaccinations proved Jenner's theory further and by 1800 vaccination against smallpox had spread to Europe. Jenner's work eventually resulted in the worldwide eradication of the disease.[21] The question is, were Jenner's methods ethical? If we agree that the risk to one research participant, James Phipps, was outweighed by the research outcome, namely the eradication of smallpox, it can be said that we have a utilitarian moral outlook. However, it could also be argued that the research conducted upon concentration camp prisoners by Nazi doctors in the Second World War led to the development of the yellow fever vaccine,[6] which is still responsible for 30 000 deaths each year in unvaccinated populations;[23] can the same utilitarian outlook that was applied to Jenner's research be applied here?

Those who think of themselves as having a Kantian or deontological moral outlook do not perceive actions to be about consequences, but consider that certain actions are inherently right or wrong,[20] e.g. lying, breaking a promise, stealing. A Kantian might feel that no individual should be put at risk for the sake of research, whatever the research outcome might be, as to put an individual at risk is in itself morally unjustifiable.

We can test this by presuming that the following principle is true (adapted from Sayers[19]). 'Breaching a participants confidentiality would be wrong' with the reasoning that:

1. breaching confidentiality, when it has been promised, is wrong
2. this is a situation where a participant's confidentiality has been breached
3. therefore this situation is wrong.

But would breaching a participant's confidentiality, even when promised, still be wrong if during the course of your research you uncovered practice that was harmful to the participant themselves, or others? Radiography practitioners in the UK, as members of the allied health professions, have a duty of care under the Health Professions Council to report colleagues who act inappropriately, in both clinical and research capacities. For example, if a practitioner was investigating the use of lead protection in pelvic examinations in a diagnostic imaging department and found that one of the radiographers was persistently misplacing the lead, this would have to be reported to a senior member of staff, even if anonymity had been promised.

These two standpoints alone demonstrate that ethical decisions cannot easily be standardized, just as any decision cannot be standardized,[19] and as such it is likely that there will always be some inconsistency in the ethical review process, although there are certain procedures that applicants can follow to increase their chances of a favourable opinion (see Aspects to be considered when undertaking research and ethical review, later in this chapter).

# Research governance and ethical review: the formal process

The first consideration that any researcher has to determine is whether their proposed study is likely to require ethical review. All formal enquiry has some ethical component, even if it is only that researchers conduct themselves honestly in undertaking their study and do not deliberately influence (bias), copy (plagiarize) or even make up the work. However, not all clinical studies require ethical review. Within the UK, formal NHS ethical review is not required if the proposed study is deemed to be an audit and/or service evaluation rather than research.[24] This is dependent upon the intention of the researcher – i.e. are they aiming to obtain new knowledge through rigorous and systematic approaches (research), or measuring existing practice/undertaking quality assurance (service evaluation/audit)? Table 6.1 outlines some of the determinants that can be used in deciding which category a proposed study may fall into and whether it requires formal NHS ethical review.

While the basic premise of ethical review is to protect the participant/patient from any potential harm, and at the same time respecting their dignity, rights and well-being,[25,26] it may also seek to safeguard the researcher and/or institution undertaking the study. However, the process of implementation differs around the world, and not all countries have a formalized committee structure.[27] For example, within the European Union (EU) all member states should adhere to the Clinical Trials Directive;[28] in the USA the regulation of clinical research comes under the auspices of the Food and Drug Administration (FDA); in Turkey there is no ethical review based on the rights of the patient.[27] The Good Clinical Practice (GCP) [29] guidelines were developed to standardize the quality of clinical trials across the European Union,[30] Japan and the USA and have subsequently become an indicator of researcher capability, with ICH-GCP often being taken as the minimum level of training that shows awareness of good research/ethical practice.

The research governance framework within England,[26] and to a major extent across the rest of the UK, lays out a two-phase process: internal review within the NHS Trust/social services and independent external review by a REC.[31] Where the researcher is a student or member of staff in a

**Table 6.1 Determining need for ethical approval**

| | | Researcher's intent | Questions | Data collection | Allocation/randomization | Decision |
|---|---|---|---|---|---|---|
| Service evaluation | | To evaluate service delivery and/or current care | What is the standard met by the service? | Measures service only; can only be tested on treatments/investigations/techniques in practice | None | May require NHS Trust R&D review but not usually ethical review |
| Clinical audit | | To evaluate service delivery and/or current care against best practice | Does the service meet predetermined standard/s? | Measures service against standard; can only be tested on treatments/investigations/techniques in practice | None | May require NHS Trust R&D review but not usually ethical review |
| Research | Quantitative approaches | To derive new knowledge, test hypotheses and interrogate research questions | Based on hypothesis | Evaluation or comparison of new treatments/investigations/techniques using existing or new data | May use both (probability sampling) | Formal NHS Trust R&D and ethical review required |
| | Qualitative approaches | | Research questions to identify and explore themes | Understanding the implications of new treatments/investigations/techniques and/or relationships using existing or new data | May use both (non-probability sampling) | |

Adapted from National Patient Safety Agency – National Research Ethics Service.[24]

university, internal review may also occur within the institution. For academic or non-clinical research this may be the only review that takes place, but in the case of the student/staff member wishing to undertake clinical research in the health and social care sector, an application to a NHS REC *must* be made.[32] Currently this covers any proposed research involving:

**a.** patients and users of the NHS. This includes all potential research participants recruited by virtue of the patient or user's past or present treatment by, or use of, the NHS. It includes NHS patients treated under contracts with private sector institutions

**b.** individuals identified as potential research participants because of their status as relatives or carers of patients and users of the NHS, as defined above

**c.** access to data, organs or other bodily material of past and present NHS patients

**d.** fetal material and IVF involving NHS patients

**e.** the recently dead in NHS premises

**f.** the use of, or potential access to, NHS premises or facilities

**g.** NHS staff recruited as research participants by virtue of their professional role.

However, the governance regulations covering ethical review are often reviewed; for example, there is current debate about whether NHS staff and the use of premises will require formal review in the future. While there may be no requirement for formal ethical review (if the study is considered to be an audit or service evaluation[27,31]), the basic tenets of research ethics apply in any study.

NHS Trust hospital research and development (R&D) committees generally review applications, whether research, audit or service evaluation, for scientific validity and the potential impact of the proposed study on service provision in the hospital/Trust. This covers the use of premises, clinical tests, staff resources, revenue implications, etc. The role of the R&D committee is not to carry out ethical review; this should only be undertaken by the REC. Conversely, ethical review by the REC does not usually include a review of the scientific basis for a study, although this may be taken into account if the proposed method is thought to be inappropriate.[18] It would be unethical to subject patients/ participants to a poorly designed study, particularly if it was deemed that no real benefit would accrue, or more importantly, that harm could occur.[27] An example of this would be a survey of patients' reactions to barium enema examination where it was proposed to interview the patients 15 minutes after the end of the investigation. Patients are unlikely to be in a position to answer questions at this time as they will be recovering from the examination. The study might be better served utilizing a questionnaire for the patient to complete in their own time at a later period, or interviewing patients after they have fully recovered, an hour or so after the procedure.

## Aspects to be considered when undertaking research and ethical review

Application for ethical review of clinical research within the UK through NRES has become clearer, and arguably easier, with the introduction of electronic forms. In 2008, the Integrated Research Application System (IRAS)[32] was introduced, combining forms from several agencies into one online application. It is designed in the main for NHS R&D and Research Ethics committees, but also covers research applications involving administration of radioactive substances (ARSAC), criminal offenders, gene therapy and medicinal products among others. Further information and support can be obtained from the NRES website,[33] which has large amounts of useful advice and guidance for applicants as well as links to other sources. The IRAS form has been designed to reduce the amount of repetition in completing required information via automated filling in of boxes throughout the form. However, novice and even experienced researchers sometimes struggle with the various and numerous questions they are confronted with when making an application. Once the form has been completed it is electronically locked by the researcher for onward submission. However, you normally only have 4 days in which

to then get the required signatures and submit a paper copy through to NRES, though this may be extended by prior arrangement. If an application is being made to an NHS Trust R&D Committee the form will automatically be forwarded. Once the application has been accepted for review by a REC, they must give a response on its ethical acceptability within 60 days, although on one occasion only, the committee is able to 'stop the clock' if it requires further expert advice to help it come to a decision or if the researcher is asked to submit further information. It is advisable, if offered the opportunity, to attend the meeting of the Research Ethics and/or R&D Committee as being on hand enables the researcher to give direct answers to queries that the committee may have and to correct any misunderstandings that may arise from the application. The decision of the REC may or may not be given at the time of the meeting, but you should receive it within 10 working days of the meeting. Decisions range from favourable (where no amendments are required), favourable/provisional (minor amendments required and if fulfilled then a favourable decision is given) to unfavourable, where the application is rejected. Where an unfavourable opinion is given then the researcher has the option to have it reviewed by another committee or will need to submit a new application. When a favourable opinion is given it only relates to the specific investigation or research study covered in the application; it does not give the researcher carte blanche to set up related studies. This would generally require a new application for each study. The whole process of research governance and ethical review can take several months and if not factored into the research timetable this can cause slippage within the project, a complaint often cited by researchers.[34]

In the experience of the authors of this chapter, as members of Research Ethics committees within UK universities and the NHS, the most successful applicants are those who think carefully about the ethical implications of their proposed work and address these in the application itself, especially the supporting documentation. It is perhaps worth noting that the most common reason for not giving a project a favourable opinion is the poor quality of the information given in the participant/patient information sheet (PIS) and the consent forms; researchers often give information which is too complicated for the average lay person to understand.[17] A classic use of this is the overuse of technical and professional jargon. The concept of measuring radiation dose in millisieverts will not be understood by the lay participant, and thus it may be useful to use a comparator, the most commonly used being units/level of background radiation, or the equivalence to a number of chest X-rays, or the level of radiation you would receive in a plane crossing the Atlantic.

The remainder of this chapter highlights areas and topics which occasionally cause issues in relation to applications and review for ethics/R&D approval, which are presented using a glossary style to enable readers to utilize this section as a quick answer to a query. It is not envisaged to be a panacea for ethical review, only an overview of some areas where problems may arise. For ease of writing the term 'participant' is used to cover all individuals or groups who act as subjects, respondents, interviewees, informants, etc. within any type of research design, whether it be quantitative or qualitative in nature.

## Areas where problems may arise in relation to applications for ethics and R&D approval

**Anonymity** Researchers sometimes offer the participant 'anonymity and confidentiality' in order to gain their cooperation to take part in their research. The participant's identity and views are then hidden in any subsequent report or publication. Occasionally this term is incorrectly used. For example, in face to face interviews the participant cannot be anonymous; however, their identity remains confidential in that they are unknown to others. Anonymity may be achieved in a variety of ways, for example the use of pseudonyms to protect the identity of participants/locations and the use of codes to identify participants, with the information that relates to this code (participant) being kept on a separate central list (key).

**Assent** The acceptance to be involved in the research study given by a participant under the age of consent for research purposes (16 years of age in Scotland and 18 years in the rest of the UK). In order to obtain assent the participant information sheet should be age-appropriate with respect to the language and explanations utilized. It has no legal standing but where the participant is old enough to understand what taking part in the research entails, it is good practice to interact with the young person as an individual as well as with the adult (parent/guardian/legal representative) who gives the formal (legal) consent. It should be noted that research on children should be avoided if the data can be obtained by using only adult participants.

**Coercion** Payments, either in monetary terms or in goods such as vouchers, are sometimes offered by researchers to thank participants for taking part in research.

Payment may also be made to investigators, usually by pharmaceutical companies, for their time in taking part in a clinical trial. These are governed by the Association of British Pharmaceutical Industry (ABPI) and British Medical Association (BMA) guidelines on levels of payment. However, if the level offered is considered to be too high this may be viewed as coercive, in that it may induce investigators to sign up numbers of participants purely for monetary return. A similar situation may happen with participants. Coercion may also be considered to be taking place when researchers, in whatever way, pressurize participants into taking part in research. This can inadvertently occur when researchers attempt to recruit participants into a study without allowing them time to consider the implications of their involvement in the research before they consent to take part. Usually a minimum period of 24 hours after initially discussing the research should be given to potential participants in order that they can consider whether or not they want to take part. It is recognized that there are circumstances where consent may have to be obtained immediately, for example in an accident and emergency X-ray department a randomized controlled trial could be taking place to compare a new technique for imaging scaphoid fractures (e.g. tomography) against the standard two-view radiographic technique. Patients would have to have the study explained, and consent given, prior to being randomized to either technique. However, if this type of research were to proceed it would require the approach to be fully justified in the application and shown that the same results could not be obtained on any other population (i.e. one that has time to consider participation). Coercion may also occur in respect to the nature of the relationship between researchers and participants, especially where the research is being undertaken by clinical staff or by academics with their own students. It may be difficult for a patient to refuse to participate when the surgeon who is going to perform his operation asks if he would like to take part in a clinical trial, or a first year student is invited by his professor to be interviewed as part of her research. In circumstances where participants have a particularly dependent relationship with the researcher, consideration should be given to asking another member of the clinical/research team to take consent.

**Confidentiality** Similar to anonymity, confidentiality is the promise that it will not be possible to attribute/connect the findings of the research to the participants themselves, unless participants have given permission for this prior to consenting to take part. If the researcher wishes to utilize anonymous direct quotations from participants it is good practice to gain express permission from the participants to do this prior to them taking part in the research.

**Conflicts of interest** A conflict of interest may arise where there is some form of relationship between various individuals or groups within a study that could possibly affect the outcome of the research through bias, coercion, etc. The relationship should be declared and clearly identified in an application and also, if appropriate, in the patient/participant information sheet (PIS). An example of this could be the source (and amount) of funding provided to a researcher – participants may not want to take part if they are unhappy about the research funding body, for example patients with lung cancer being asked to participate in a research study funded by a tobacco manufacturer. It is also good practice for researchers, particularly undergraduate practitioners, to declare on the PIS if they will receive an academic qualification as a consequence of undertaking the research. In some ways this may have a beneficial impact, with altruistic patients wanting to help the student to fulfil their research, although this could also be construed as possibly being coercive.

**Consent** The formal acceptance given by a participant to be involved in a research study. Any consent should as far as possible be fully *informed* and *written*, in that the potential participant should be made aware of what the research is about, and of methods and implications in taking part. This is normally given in the form of a written leaflet (see Patient/participant information sheet later in this chapter) which sets out the details of the proposed research; researchers usually base their PIS on the NRES guidelines, although this is not compulsory. Informed consent becomes difficult when the participant is unable to give consent because of their age (young and old), mental capability, or physical state (e.g. unconscious). In these situations consent should be obtained as far as possible from the individual concerned but if it cannot be obtained then another person such as a parent/guardian, carer or legal representative may be asked to give the consent on behalf of the prospective participant. However, if the participant is only temporarily incapacitated it is important that consent be obtained from the participant once they regain their full faculties.

Written, informed consent is taken to be the standard but there are others forms of consent that may occur in research practice. *Implied consent* is taken to occur when a participant does not expressly give their consent but this is inferred through their actions. In a research sense this generally occurs with survey methods utilizing questionnaires, when consent is not specifically asked for by the researcher but is taken to be given (implied) if the questionnaire is returned. *Presumed consent* has little basis within research, whereby the participant is assumed to give consent unless they opt out of the study. An example of this could be a cytological research study utilizing tumours surgically removed from patients, the assumption being the tumour is waste material that the patient would not want after the operation. While this premise may be generally true, after the Alder Hey and Bristol inquiries, the ethics committee will generally prefer the opposite, in that participants should opt in to research rather than being pressured into or presumed to consent to taking part.

Once given, consent does not become permanent; participants may withdraw from the study without being required to give any reason and may also be able to ask that their data not be used. This is should be indicated on the consent form. However, if data have been anonymised and aggregated it would be difficult for an individual participant's information to be to be separated out. This may also occur with data obtained from focus groups because it is the group interaction that generates the data; withdrawing one participant's data would therefore make the remaining data difficult to interpret. In cases such as these it needs to be made clear on the PIS that data collected up to the point of withdrawal will need to be retained. In addition, ethical approval is only given for any one named project at a time; it does not cover future studies where the subjects being identified have not been clearly stated. Research which evolves from current work will require separate ethical approval and consent from participants at some time in the future; the current authorization will not apply. As well as the various types of consent, researchers also need to consider who is to take/obtain consent from the participant as there may be issues of *coercion* and a possibility of power bias, as outlined above. Conversely, the person taking the consent must be aware of the implications of the study in order to be able to answer any queries, thus enabling the participant to make a decision as to whether to take part, by being fully informed.

**Data Monitoring Committee (DMC)** In clinical trials, the role of the DMC is to review the study while it is in progress to assess the impact of the intervention (e.g. drug/new technique) upon the participants. If it is shown that serious side-effects are beginning to occur in large numbers then the trial should be stopped to avoid exposing future participants to harm. On the other hand when a study shows overwhelming positive results then it might be suggested that enough data have been collected to show benefit, thus it would be unethical to inconvenience or recruit further participants and therefore the study should be stopped.

**Data** In respect to any research data collected in the UK, researchers must operate in accordance with several legislative acts governing data protection and access to medical records. Researchers should indicate how and where data are to be stored (usually in a locked cabinet or password protected computer), who has access to it (usually the researchers), how long it is to be stored (a minimum of 3 years if data are to be published), and what will happen to it post-study (i.e. destruction, etc.). Any data that are to be sent outside of the UK and/or Europe should be anonymised. As outlined in the section on anonymity, the use of codes/keys can be used to separate identifiable data.

**Interviews/focus groups** The use of focus groups to generate and discuss data as a research tool is very helpful; however, participants may get carried away with the situation and say too much but later regret what they have said. It is good practice to allow participants editing rights over what is recorded (although this is not possible in focus groups) as well as the right to withdraw from the study. This could and should be agreed when interviewing individual participants but would not be feasible in focus groups, so researchers must make this clear in the PIS and on the consent form.

**Long-term studies and follow-up** Longitudinal research studies taking place over a period of time rather than the one-off snapshot, and studies conducted in a research population which has a high possibility of mortality, for example those using participants with cancer, may face difficulties in making repeat contact with participants. Physical mortality as opposed to research mortality (where a participant withdraws from a study) requires the researcher to be sensitive to the distress that future contact may cause to relatives, friends and carers of the participant who may have died during the period of the study. The researcher may need to consider alternatives to direct contact prior to starting the study, possibly by getting in touch with the participant's GP (assuming consent has been given for this) to check that the participant is or is not alive.

**Participant/patient information sheet (PIS)** The PIS is arguably the most important document within a research study in that the information contained within it explains and invites participants into the study. It will receive particular scrutiny at the REC meeting. A clearly written, well defined and appropriate PIS should give participants enough information on the nature of the proposed study for them to be able to make an informed choice about whether to take part or not. Guidelines and a template are given on the NRES website and while RECs prefer the PIS to be in this format, it is not compulsory. However, if not using the template, then researchers should make sure that the appropriate sections relevant to their study are included in whatever alternative format they utilizes, such as a letter. The PIS must be written in lay terms and in a language style that is understandable to the possible participants. The average reading age within the UK is thought to be that of someone between the ages of 9 and 12 years old; hence the PIS should use language appropriate to this age range. If assent is being sought from someone under the age of 16/18 years, then again it is necessary to amend the level of reading ability. For younger children, around 8 years of age, it can be beneficial to use drawings or diagrams to explain the information. Language again may be an issue with respect to multinational studies; the PIS may have been written outside of the UK so the language may be inappropriate, with different terminology and meaning than in UK English and should therefore be anglicized. Similarly, if a PIS is required for non-English speakers it must be translated. Unlike clinical practice, it is not enough to get relatives to translate or act as interpreters for participants, the participants must have the relevant information available directly to them in order to be able to make an informed choice, and so professional services should be utilized. With respect to research documentation, applications, etc., and in particularly the PIS, the researcher should make sure that all paperwork is devoid of errors in spelling and grammar, and that all sections have been completed correctly with the information required, otherwise the decision of the REC may be delayed.

**Radiation** Research studies involving the use of radiation will generate specific sections of the IRAS form to be completed detailing the type of radiation and particularly the dose to be received. This will need to be substantiated by the local radiation protection adviser who will be required to sign the form confirming the proposed level of radiation exposure. Researchers will also need to give information about any possible radiation effects to participants on the PIS. This should be related in terms that the participants may be able to understand, e.g. units of radiation equated to levels of radiation received as numbers of chest X-rays or by pilots of airplanes crossing the Atlantic.

**Recruitment** The mechanism for study recruitment is another area to which RECs give particular attention in an application. All access should initially come through clinical staff if the study is based in an NHS Trust hospital – it is not appropriate for researchers to contact prospective participants directly in clinics, etc. The clinician has a greater understanding and awareness of the patient's condition and their capacity to take part than the researcher. Likewise if the proposed route of contact is via the participant's address, under the Data Protection Act and Access to Medical Records Act, the researcher would be unable to obtain these from the hospital/clinic without the patient's consent. One approach may be to send a flyer or letter via the clinician or data protection guardian, either separately or with the hospital appointment, but this would be sent out by the clinician; the researcher should not have access to addresses at this stage. The flyer/letter would outline the study and ask the prospective participant whether they would like further information, along with the contact details of the researcher. The prospective participant can then opt in to asking for further information via telephone or a reply slip on the letter before making a decision to take part. Similarly the use of a poster displayed in the clinic/hospital or GP surgery may be used to initiate contact, with participants replying for further details. If this approach is to be utilized the poster will need to be reviewed by the REC.

**Respondent distress/expectation** As explained earlier, one of the basic tenets of research ethics is the protection of the participant, and there may be times when participants become distressed or require further information about topics that are highlighted as a result of their participation within a study. The researcher will need to detail, both in the application and on the PIS, how these situations will be dealt with, usually by giving advice on access to further information and support services or, if appropriately qualified, undertake this directly themselves. In determining the suitability of the PIS an ethics committee may be concerned that a study is not artificially raising the participants' expectations of a particular treatment or examination, or causing unnecessary anxiety and stress through the information given. For example, a researcher may want to ask patients with prostate cancer their views on which treatment they would prefer to have (radiotherapy or surgery). However, while both options are available in one hospital, only surgery is available in another. For the patients in the second hospital equity is not apparent and it may thus be deemed unethical as the research could be raising expectations that the patient should have a choice of treatment.

**Researcher issues and responsibilities** While the primary purpose of any research ethics system is to protect the participant, researchers also need to be aware that there may be times when their own actions/circumstances need to be considered within a study. This could include visiting a participant in their home or collecting data alone in a city centre, etc. The REC will look for some indication that the researcher is aware of these issues (risk assessment undertaken) and that they have put into place a mechanism to protect themselves (e.g. lone-worker policy). This is particularly important for research involving radiation, and prospective researchers must show that they are aware of the implications of their actions with regard to any use of radiation, complying with the principles of ALARA (as low as reasonably achievable) and ALARP (as low as reasonably practicable). In addition, researchers have a responsibility to participants and to society as a whole by the very nature of what they are undertaking, in that they should not copy (plagiarize) or falsify data, and should act fairly (unbiased) in their approaches to all participants, measurements, etc. in order for good quality findings to be obtained, otherwise it becomes unethical to subject participants to poor research practice.

**Sponsor** Inexperienced applicants are sometimes confused regarding questions as to whether their research has a sponsor and often answer no because they take this to relate to someone who has provided them with money to undertake the study. In governance terms this is taken to be a person or company, usually the employer, who accepts responsibility for the actions of the researcher in respect of any claims for negligence or harm as a result of the research. In most cases the answer therefore would be yes, particularly for researchers working within the NHS. In respect of student researchers, the university should take responsibility as sponsor but this would be through the research supervisor as it is they who are directly employed rather than the student.

# References

[1] What is research governance? London: Imperial College London; 2010. Available at: http://www3.imperial.ac.uk/clinicalresearchgovernanceoffice/researchgovernance/whatisresearchgovernance (accessed 19 March 2010).

[2] North M. 'I swear by Apollo the Physician ...'. Greek medicine from the Gods to Galen. National Library of Medicine, National Institutes of Health; 2002. Available at: http://www.nlm.nih.gov/hmd/greek/greek_oath.html (accessed 19 March 2010).

[3] Hilditch WG, Pace N. Ethics of research. Foundation Years 2006; 2(3):110–3.

[4] Erler CJ, Thompson CB. Ethics, human rights, and clinical research. Air Med J 2008;27(3):110–3.

[5] World Medical Association. Declaration of Helsinki: Ethical Principles for Medical Research Involving Human Subjects. WMA; 2008. Available at: http://www.wma.net/en/30publications/

10policies/b3/index.html (accessed 19 March 2010).

[6] Neuberger J. Nazi medicine and the ethics of human research. Lancet 2005;366:799–800.

[7] Reverby SM. Tuskegee: could it happen again? Postgrad Med J 2001;77:553–4.

[8] Baker SM, Brawley OW, Marks LS. Effects of untreated syphilis in the negro male 1932–1972: a closure comes to the Tuskegee study 2004. Urology 2005;65:1259–62.

[9] Neville L. A response to Martin Johnson's editorial 'Research ethics and education: a consequentialist view'. Nurse Educ Today 2003;23:549–53.

[10] Dixon-Woods M, Angell E, Ashcroft RE, et al. Written work: the social functions of research ethics committee letters. Soc Sci Med 2007;65:792–802.

[11] Plomer A. The Law and Ethics of Medical Research: International Bioethics and Human Rights, vol. 93. London: Routledge Cavendish; 2005. p. 99.

[12] Department of Health. 12 Key Points on Consent: The Law in England. London: HMSO; 2001.

[13] Department of Health. Human Tissue Act 2004. London: HMSO; 2004.

[14] Children Act 2004. London: HMSO; 2004.

[15] Mental Health Act 2007. London: HMSO; 2007.

[16] Ionising Radiation (Medical Exposure) Regulations 2000 (together with notes on good practice). London: HMSO; 2007.

[17] Dixon-Woods M, Angell E, Tarrant C, et al. What do research ethics committees say about applications to do cancer trials? Lancet Oncol 2008;9:700–1.

[18] Angell E, Sutton AJ, Windridge K, et al. Consistency in decision making by research ethics committees: a controlled comparison. J Med Ethics 2006;32:662–4.

[19] Sayers G. Should research ethics committees be told how to think? J Med Ethics 2006;33:39–42.

[20] Moldoveanu MC, Stevenson H. Ethical universals in practice: an analysis of five principles. J Socio Econ 1998;27(6):153–62.

[21] Riedel S. Edward Jenner and the history of smallpox and vaccination. Proc (Bayl Univ Med Cent) 2005;18(1):21.

[22] McNally J. A brief life of Doctor Edward Jenner. Semin Pediatr Infect Dis 2001;12(1):81–4.

[23] World Health Organization. Yellow Fever. Geneva: WHA; 2001. Available at: http://www.who.int/mediacentre/factsheets/fs100/en (19 March 2010).

[24] National Patient Safety Agency – National Research Ethics Service. Defining Research. Issue 3. London: NRES; 2008. Available at: http://www.nres.npsa.nhs.uk/EasysiteWeb/getresource.axd?AssetID=355&type=full&servicetype=attachment (accessed 19 March 2010).

[25] Governance arrangements for NHS Research Ethics Committees, Department of Health; 2001. Available at: http://www.dh.gov.uk/en/Publicationsandstatistics/Publications/

PublicationsPolicyAndGuidance/DH_4005727 (accessed 19 March 2010).

[26] Research Governance Framework for Health and Social Care. 2nd ed. Department of Health; 2005. Available at: http://www.dh.gov.uk/en/Publicationsandstatistics/Publications/PublicationsPolicyAndGuidance/DH_4108962 (accessed 19 March 2010).

[27] Tschudin V. European experiences of ethics committees. Nurs Ethics 2001;8(2):142–51.

[28] Official Journal of the European Communities. Directive 2001/20/EC of the European parliament and of the council of 4 April 2001. European Union. L 121/34–44 Available at: http://www.eortc.be/Services/Doc/clinical-EU-directive-04-April-01.pdf (accessed 19 March 2010).

[29] ICH Harmonised Tripartite Guideline for Good Clinical Practice. London: European Medicines Agency; 2006.

[30] Official Journal of the European Communities. Commission Directive 2005/28/EC of

8 April 2005. European Union; 2001. L 91/13–19 Available at: http://ec.europa.eu/enterprise/pharmaceuticals/eudralex/vol-1/dir_2005_28/dir_2005_28_en.pdf (accessed 26 September 2009).

[31] NHS Research and Development Forum. Notes on developing procedures within NHS organisations for appropriate authorisation and management of research and related projects. 2006. Available at: http://www.rdforum.nhs.uk/docs/categorising_projects_guidance.doc (accessed 19 March 2010).

[32] Integrated Research Application System, IRAS; 2008. Available at: http://www.myresearchproject.org.uk (accessed 19 March 2010).

[33] National Research Ethics Service Homepage. National Patient Safety Agency; 2008. Available at: http://www.nres.npsa.nhs.uk (accessed 19 March 2010).

[34] Duley L, Antman K, Arena J, et al. Specific barriers to the conduct of randomized trials. Clin Trials 2008;5:40–8.

# Section **2**

## **Research planning**

# Planning your research study

7

## Barbara Wilford   Susan Cutler   Peter Williams

## CHAPTER POINTS

- The research question posed will determine the orientation of the research.
- Make sure that you factor in time for unexpected events.
- If you are working in a group, discuss and establish the ground rules at the beginning.
- Make sure you see your supervisor regularly throughout the project.
- Write your proposal and refer back to it at regular intervals.
- Ensure that you have sought and gained appropriate ethical approval for your study.
- Make sure that you are aware of the advantages and disadvantages of the method used to collect your data.
- Ensure the instruments used are appropriate for the task, and if need be, have been calibrated.
- Check the validity and reliability of your chosen method.
- Ensure your sample size is appropriate for the project.
- Check that there are no omissions in your data collection.
- Keep an account of each piece of data generated.
- Use appropriate statistical tests to analyse quantitative data.
- Use appropriate reduction techniques to analyse the data generated in qualitative designs.
- Ensure that you follow the guidelines for writing up and presenting your research.
- Refer back to the guidelines at each stage of writing up your project.

This chapter provides insight into good practice measures when planning your study of work. Qualitative and quantitative research designs are mentioned briefly with tabulation of the advantages and disadvantages of each design. The various stages of the research process are described briefly to give you a good overview of the anticipated amount of time and effort that is required to undertake a research project. Those stages are then discussed in detail throughout other chapters within the text.

## Introduction

One of the challenges of research, particularly for new researchers, is thinking about an area for research that is valid, worthwhile and researchable; this is the first step in the research design. Exploration of the predominantly peer-reviewed published and to a lesser extent unpublished literature is a good place to start. It will help you evaluate what research has already been carried out and give you an indication of any gaps in your current research area. Even if a study has been carried out before, it may still be valid to repeat the study if the new research will add additional knowledge. Guidance on searching, evaluating and critiquing can be found in Chapters 3 and 4.

Once you have considered an appropriate area you would then need to frame a specific question or questions. The process of developing and refining your research question is discussed in Chapter 2. The research question is fundamental to the research approach adopted, and throughout this book a number of research approaches are explored. It is, however,

© 2010, Elsevier Ltd.

important to learn the difference between the method and methodology. The method relates to the tools of data collection or analysis, such as questionnaires or interviews. Methodology refers to the approach or paradigm that underpins the research. For example, an interview conducted within a qualitative approach that seeks to explore, say, feelings or experiences will have a very different underlying purpose and produce different data from an interview conducted within a quantitative design.

For example, you may want to explore patients' experiences of a visit to the medical imaging or radiotherapy department and you could explore this in two quite distinct ways, qualitatively and quantitatively. First we will look at a qualitative approach, and then at a quantitative one.

'Tell me about your recent visit to the medical imaging/radiotherapy department.' This open question gives the patient the opportunity to tell you about the issues, concerns and experiences that are important to them. The narrative produced will be rich in data that may highlight issues, experiences or concerns that you had not considered. The data will be in the patient's own words. The first stage will be identifying some themes, and following the first read through of the data, you will have a list of words or phrases beside each issue or concept.

*Patient A*: 'They all seemed very busy, I was worried that I might have to wait a long time for my appointment, but I was only 5 minutes late. I was then taken to another waiting area, where I had to get changed and then I had to wait again. I wasn't expecting that.'

When you look at this transcript there are possibly a few words that you could highlight, for example 'busy', 'worried' 'waiting' 'unexpected'. When you have explored other interviews you may find there are similar issues arising that will enable you to develop categories and themes.

Using a quantitative approach, on the other hand, you might ask 20 randomly selected patients to complete a questionnaire using a rating scale. An example of a question from the questionnaire might be phrased, 'How would you rate the efficiency of your recent visit to the medical imaging/radiotherapy department?' You may want to distribute this to two different patient groups, for example those who utilize an open access service and those patients with appointments (Table 7.1). You will give these patients one of five options from which they are required to select their response:

**Table 7.1  Data gathered using a quantitative approach**

| Efficiency rating | Open access patients | Patients with appointments |
|---|---|---|
| 5 | 2 | 5 |
| 4 | 4 | 8 |
| 3 | 6 | 5 |
| 2 | 7 | 1 |
| 1 | 1 | 1 |
| | $n=20$ | $n=20$ |

**5.** Excellent
**4.** Very good
**3.** Average
**2.** Poor
**1.** Very poor.

The data produced will appear in a very different form. The raw data would be as follows:

Patients with appointments: 54333454454344342551.

Open access patients: 33343224422522334521.

As you can see, these two different approaches will result in very different data; the first will highlight issues that are pertinent to the patient, while the second will give you numerical data which illustrate how many patients rated the department as efficient.

In order for your project to be successful you will need to have a clear plan of action. Making changes as you go along could be a recipe for disaster. You therefore need to think about the research process and the actions that you need to undertake this. Often the ideal is superseded by what is practicable and this needs to be taken into consideration at the beginning of the project. Ironing out potential issues at the beginning of the process will reap benefits later on in the project. It is during the planning process and selection of the appropriate tools that the researcher must acknowledge and recognize potential pitfalls that could arise. As you will be committing a great deal of time and effort to this endeavour, we think an important consideration of undertaking research is choosing a research topic that has personal interest or is of professional significance, to help motivate you. It is suggested that you consider your own skills set and which ones you will be using to conduct your research. For example, if you like talking to people you might want to consider using interviews, or observing people to maximize your skills.

Whether you realize it or not, you, as the researcher, will have a powerful influence on the research project. What you have read in the past will influence your thinking. How you phrase or ask questions will influence the data collected,[1] as discussed earlier. You do need to take a reflective approach to your project and should try and maintain a sceptical approach to the evidence provided by respondents and other data sources.[2]

In order to plan your work, it is good practice to have a structure or a framework to work from, as given below.

1. orientation of the research
2. research design and methodology
3. data analysis
4. reporting and writing up the research

## Orientation of the research

The generation of the research idea and the specific research question, aim or hypothesis is discussed in detail in Chapter 2. However, there are some practical issues that are worth considering during this initial phase.

Time is one of the key resources available to the researcher. However, as with all the best laid plans, things can – and do – go wrong. Therefore it is imperative that time is assigned in the overall plan to account for any potential problems. This is particularly important if the research is undertaken as part of undergraduate or postgraduate studies as the time line is often very tight and is frequently the main factor in determining the research design. A longitudinal study will not be feasible if the project needs to be completed in a set number of weeks. For example, it would be unrealistic to try and undertake a research project exploring practitioners' attitudes to continued professional development activities and their career projection, which cannot be undertaken in only 20 weeks.

The timescale will affect the research question and the way the data are collected. You may only be able to use one instrument, but would have ideally liked to validate your data further with the use of another data collection instrument. The number of researchers undertaking the project will also influence the focus of the project and the research question. You may be undertaking the project on your own or be working as part of a research group. If

undertaking the research as a group, careful planning and ground rules must be identified at the planning stage to ensure all group members are aware of the timescale, targets and deadlines. You will need to consider the amount of time needed to undertake the data collection, for example conducting interviews can be very time consuming and this may constrain the number that an individual can undertake.

The cost of the project also needs to be considered at this early stage. If your research is being undertaken as part of your degree, one of your priorities will probably be to keep costs to a minimum. Therefore travel to interview participants from diverse geographical areas as part of a qualitative project is likely to preclude this type of question. This will impact on your time also. Similarly, if you are considering testing a hypothesis that requires the use of equipment not available at your university, this too may exclude a particular research focus.

Whether you are a first time researcher or someone with experience, the importance of regular meetings with your supervisor cannot be overemphasized. Your supervisor is also a key resource as he or she will have experience of the research process from guiding other students.[3] These meetings will give you an opportunity to discuss or clarify each stage of your project. This is especially useful once you have collected the data and can discuss the implications of your findings. If you are a pre-registration student studying at either undergraduate or postgraduate level, these meetings will also help you keep on schedule by ensuring you submit your work on time.

## Research design and methodology

This is the stage where your idea or theory moves towards a concrete project, where aims are translated into specific questions that can be answered, and when you decide how the questions are going to be answered, i.e. what instruments are going to be used to gather the data. A detailed planning of the project should be written up in a document called the 'research proposal', which may be submitted as part of the ethics approval process and should be presented to your supervisors (Box 7.1). It is prudent to keep referring back to this document as the project progresses.

It is acknowledged that your area of research would not be fully developed at this stage and this proposal serves as your guide to completion.

**Box 7.1**

## What should you include in your proposal?

The main headings in the proposal should include:

- Aims and objectives – what are you going to do, broken down into measurable objectives?
- Background – why is this topic interesting or important? What is the clinical relevance of the study?
- Methods – you will need to justify your chosen methodology and approach. How will you carry the research out? This should include a detailed description of the data you will collect, including sample size, access and if applicable, statistical tests that will be applied. How are you going to ensure the validity and reliability of the study? Have you thought about credibility, transferability and trustworthiness of the research?
- Literature review – this should be a brief outline of the current literature that relates to your study. This is essential to enable the researcher to assess research already undertaken in a specific area. This should include your key references.
- Ethical issues – those related specifically to your study should be identified in this protocol. Submission of this protocol is usually an integral aspect of your ethical approval process.

- Resources – costing of staff, travel, materials. This may have to be very explicit, especially if your project is funded and you are accountable for all the monies spent. Often new researchers underestimate the costs of staff time particularly. It is easy to underestimate how long tasks will actually take. Normally in an undergraduate project there are no significant cost implications and the materials and equipment required are usually supplied by the university.
- Pilot study – if applicable, a pilot study should always be undertaken and you will need to describe in this protocol how this will be conducted and what your sample size will be.
- Timescale – this should include the important milestones such as the start and completion of the data collection process; data analysis; chapter drafts and time allocated for amendments. It is always worthwhile to include some contingency time, as well as a completion date.
- Dissemination – how are you going to inform others, including participants, of the findings?[4]

Research design is an essential consideration in any research project. There are two main paradigms that are employed in research studies today and they are quantitative and qualitative research designs. Depending on the nature of your aims and objectives, your study would usually fall within one of these two categories of research design. These are revisited in Chapter 16 as well as elsewhere in the text (see Chapters 8 and 15).

*Quantitative research* is usually structured to test a hypothesis. A hypothesis consists either of a suggested explanation for a phenomenon or a reasoned proposal suggesting a possible correlation between multiple phenomena. It is a methodology that aims to determine the relationship between one thing (independent variable) and another (dependent variable) in a specific population. Quantitative research is often described as being reductionist[5] and collects a range of numerical data in an effort to answer a research question. Though this may not always be the case, you may be seeking to describe a specific set of circumstances or characteristics of a study sample or target population.[6] The designs used in this paradigm are experimental and non-experimental designs

such as surveys, epidemiology and quasi-experimental designs.

## Experimental designs

In experimental design the investigator deliberately controls and manipulates the conditions which determine the events in which they are interested.[7] An experiment involves making a change in the value of one variable. These are often undertaken in a laboratory, but in health care the experiments often need to be undertaken in the hospital or clinical setting and this is when a randomized controlled trial may be undertaken. This is an experimental design aimed at assessing clinical effectiveness. It is quite often used when ascertaining the effectiveness of new drugs. The population is defined by the researchers, for example men over the age of 60 with prostatic disease, and the study sample is then selected from that population. Using a randomized assignment procedure participants are allocated to a group and followed by the intervention. The outcomes are measured; you need to be aware of this type of design, though it is not often used in medical imaging and radiotherapy.

## Non-experimental designs

In non-experimental designs surveys are often used. In medical imaging and radiotherapy practice they can be employed to ascertain the attitudes, opinions and beliefs of people using the services we provide. The participants could be patients, but also doctors, dentists or other healthcare practitioners who refer patients, or they could be radiographers. Questionnaires are often used to collect the data and these surveys can used, for example to give us an overview of the use of imaging services or radiotherapy in a given community.

Epidemiology is an approach used particularly in public health and is concerned with the population as a whole or a particular group within the population. They can use comparison studies, comparing responses of different cultural groups to an intervention, for example. They also undertake correlation studies, which are used to identify interrelationships. Epidemiological methods are discussed in Chapter 9.

Quasi-experimental designs resemble experiments, but the participants are not randomly assigned. Also, such research may include time-series designs. These are when the sample may have an intervention allocated and are then observed over a period of time. For example, some patients may be recruited to this type of experiment and have radiotherapy while another group may have radiotherapy in addition to a new drug.

*Qualitative research* does not usually test hypotheses. It is concerned with understanding personal meaning through specific questions which aim to guide the investigation. This method seeks to make sense of, or interpret, phenomena in terms of the meanings people bring to them. Qualitative research is used to help us understand how people feel and why is it that they feel as they do. Samples tend to be much smaller as compared with quantitative projects which tend to include larger samples. A good qualitative study addresses a clinical problem through a clearly formulated question and often uses more than one research method, known as triangulation. Analysis of qualitative data can and should be done using explicit, systematic methods and should be reproducible.[8] Interviewing, focus groups and observations are common techniques used in qualitative research and these are discussed in Chapter 16. Qualitative methodology is a useful method to assess individual feelings, experiences and knowledge. For example:

- How do student practitioners perceive the role of the personal tutor?
- How do students feel about distance learning while on clinical placement?

The interview is defined as a two-person conversation initiated by the interviewer with the specific purpose of gathering information relevant to the research objective. Some interviews may be quite formal, where a series of questions are asked and the responses recorded and the researcher is quite directive. Or they could be less formal, where the researcher raises a number of issues in a conversational way and the researcher is less directive.

Focus groups or group interviews can also be used to generate data. One of the advantages is that they can generate a wider range of responses than individual interviews. They are often quicker but they do not really allow personal matters to emerge or to be explored in any great depth. So individual interviews would be appropriate to find out how diagnostic and therapeutic practitioners cope with death and dying, but a focus group would be useful to ascertain what support diagnostic and therapeutic practitioners need for continued professional development.

Observations allow gathering of live data from live situations and enable the researcher to look at what is happening in situ rather than at second hand. A structured observation will know in advance what it is looking at, for example the hand washing technique undertaken by practitioners. An unstructured observation, on the other hand, will be less clear about what it is looking for and will have to go to a situation and observe what is taking place and from that determining what is significant. For example you may have made available some patient information in your waiting room, and you could observe whether and how patients engage with it over a period of time.

The advantages and disadvantages of both these approaches are listed in Table 7.2.

Let us look in more detail at each approach:

## Advantages of a quantitative approach

- Eliminates or reduces subjectivity of judgement or interpretation. Subjectivity affects all research to some extent. Even before a study begins it is already influenced by factors and constraints such as the researcher's desires, interests and preoccupations. Quantitative research eliminates

**Table 7.2 Advantages and disadvantages of quantitative and qualitative approaches**

| Advantages | |
| --- | --- |
| **Quantitative approach** | **Qualitative approach** |
| Objectivity – the elimination or reduction of subjectivity of judgement or interpretation | Interviews yield much richer data than a questionnaire might |
| Independent and dependent variables clearly and precisely specified | Can handle complex topics |
| Data reliability high – due to controlled observations, laboratory experiments, mass surveys, or other form of research techniques | Interviews help where the topic is new or unfamiliar |
| Representative – often more representative of a wider population and can compare similar studies more easily | |
| Results are usually statistically reliable | |
| **Disadvantages** | |
| Not appropriate for learning why people act or think as they do | Inconsistency: It is very possible to be inconsistent in the way you ask questions, what questions you ask, and how you interpret answers |
| Questions must be direct and easily quantified | Generalizability – difficult to generalize from interviews |
| Participants may answer differently in a structured survey than they would in a real life situation | Low validity/reliability – the data-gathering measure may not measure what you want it to, or may not give the same results if repeated |
| Very difficult to prevent or detect researcher induced bias in quantitative research | Experience – conducting interview or managing focus groups effectively does require a high level of experience from the researcher to obtain the required information from the respondent |
| | It is time-consuming to immerse yourself in the wealth and volume of data generated |

some of these factors due to the fact that it clearly states the research problem in specific and well defined terms resulting in numerical data which can be statistically analysed.[9]

- Clearly and precisely specifies both the independent and the dependent variables under investigation. The independent variable is the variable that is changed or manipulated by the researcher. The dependent variable is the response that is measured. An independent variable is the presumed cause, whereas the dependent variable is the presumed effect.
- Achieves high levels of data reliability owing to controlled observations, laboratory experiments, mass surveys, or other forms of research technique.
- Is often more representative of a wider population and can compare similar studies

more easily. This is due to the fact that sample sizes are larger.
- Results are usually statistically reliable.

Consider the example mentioned earlier in the chapter, in which a questionnaire was distributed to patients who were asked to rate the efficiency of the department. They had to choose from one of five categories. The numerical data collected from this question could then be analysed statistically. The example used in this illustration is a small sample, but a questionnaire could be distributed to a much larger sample which might be several hundred patients. You might collect demographic information, and providing the participants had completed this information correctly, the number of men and women who completed our questionnaire, alluded to earlier, could be clearly defined. If you were using interview data from a few participants, statistical tests could not be applied.

## Disadvantages of quantitative approach

- Not appropriate for learning why people act or think as they do.
- Questions must be direct and easily quantified. It is vital that the questions are unambiguous or the responses with detract from the focus of the research and will reduce the validity of the study.
- Participants may answer differently in a structured survey than they would in a real life situation. There is no opportunity to probe respondent's answers.
- It is very difficult to detect researcher-induced bias in quantitative research.

## Advantages of qualitative approach

- Rich data: as discussed in more depth in Chapter 16, interviews yield much richer data than a questionnaire might. It allows in-depth analysis of phenomena and is not limited to the rigid parameters of definable variables. If you refer back to the example mentioned earlier in the chapter, where patients talked about their experiences, think about how a patient's meaning of the issues they alluded to can be explored further.
- Complex subjects: sometimes it is difficult to construct a questionnaire as the issues are too complex to encapsulate in a series of relatively closed questions. Interviews allow a comprehensive exploration of such issues.
- Unknown territory: where you as a researcher/ interviewer may not have a good grasp of a particular phenomenon, interviews are excellent as a way in. For example, the interview proved perfect for one of the writers many years ago when undertaking a study of the (then) new phenomenon of the world wide web, and its impact on journalistic practices.

## Disadvantages of a qualitative approach

- Inconsistency: it is very possible to be inconsistent in the way you ask questions, what questions you ask, and how you interpret answers. Of course, if your brief is wide, and you are exploring people's wider views and experiences, the interviewee leads to an extent, so you may not always ask the same questions, but you must try and adopt the same (disinterested) approach.
- Generalizability: it is difficult to generalize from interviews, but that is not a problem if your aims do not suggest you want to. The paper by Davies and Bath, 'Interpersonal sources of health and maternity information for Somali women living in the UK: information seeking and evaluation', for example,[10] used only thirteen participants, eight in a focus group and five individuals, and made no attempt to generalize beyond postnatal Somali mothers receiving maternity care in a particular city in the UK, or beyond the specific (maternity information) topic examined.
- Low validity/reliability: validity is, according to Hammersley,[11] 'truth: interpreted as the extent to which an account accurately represents the social phenomena to which it refers'. In other words, does the data-gathering measure what you want it to measure? As for reliability, this is, also according to Hammersley,[12] 'the degree of consistency with which instances are assigned to the same category by different observers or by the same observer on different occasions'. For example, does the data-gathering produce the same results if repeated? These are consistency issues it is wise to be aware of when planning and delivering your interviews (see Chapter 10 and interviews in Chapter 16).
- Time-consuming: in order to immerse yourself in the wealth and volume of data that are generated when undertaking qualitative research you need a great deal of time. Trawling through the data can be labour-intensive.
- Experience: conducting interviews or managing focus groups effectively does require some experience from the researcher to obtain the required information from the respondent.

Let us go back to the interview with the patient about their recent visit to the medical imaging department; the patient says they are worried. It is not clear from this initial response why they were worried. An open interview would allow you to explore this further with the patient. The patient also says there were aspects of their experience they were not expecting. You might want to find out more about this. If you were using the questionnaire, the fact that the patient was worried might not be captured or explored any further.

## Instrumentation

Refers to how the data will be collected. This may be questionnaires, interviews, accounts, observation and tests. Some research is based on an observation made with instruments (such as recording electrodes, microscopes, and standardized clinical tests, weighing scales); but other research may not require the use of instruments to collect the data. You will need to think about the practicalities of using instruments (which may include the cost to use them), time and also the reliability of the instruments. You should use standardized tools, or if you are using a new tool you will need to establish the reliability and validity of the tool. If you are weighing patients before a radiographic test or therapeutic intervention, for example, you will need to ensure that the scales are calibrated and checked regularly. A feature of scientific observation is the accuracy and reliability of the equipment employed. Instrumentation relates to the situation when the instrument changes over the period of the study thus invalidating comparison of measured results,[6] and this may compromise the internal validity of the study.

## Selecting your sample

As part of the process you will be required to select your sample from the subject population. Generally for qualitative studies the sample tends to be smaller and for quantitative data collection the sample tends to be larger. As discussed earlier, if you are interviewing patients about their experiences you may only have the resources and opportunity to interview five or six participants, but they need to be representative of the population. If the focus of your study is the experience of adolescents you will need to define adolescent and ensure you interview participants who meet the criteria. But if your design is quantitative and your instrument is a questionnaire, and you are looking at the over 60s population, there is the potential to distribute this to much larger numbers.

You will want to ensure your sample size is sufficient for the purpose of the analysis you intend to perform. You also need to ensure your sample is representative of the population you are studying.

Before gathering your sample, it is important to find out as much as possible about your population. Population refers to the larger group from which the sample is taken and you will need to know some of the overall demographics of the population, such as age, sex, etc., before commencing the sampling. To some extent, when undertaking a project as part of a degree, your sample size will be determined by your available population and the time frame of the study. You also need to consider how much it might cost to interview a large sample or send out a large number of questionnaires. The context of the sample should be considered. If the sample is selected from a population of practitioners working within a rural setting, how applicable is it to generalize the findings to those practitioners who work in large urban environments? A sample is a subset of the population, so you could consider all practitioners registered with the Health Professions Council in the UK and select 50 therapeutic radiographers as your sample. But the sample should be representative of the population; a biased sample does not adequately represent the key groups.

## Validity and reliability

Cohen et al[7] describe validity as an important aspect of effective research and it is a requirement of any research paradigm (see Chapter 10). Reliability refers to the ability of the research to be replicated over time and over different samples. A reliable instrument will produce similar data when similar respondents are used. Validity and reliability of a study can be maintained by careful sampling, using the correct instruments and the application of correct statistical tests (see Chapter 15). Conversely, using qualitative data, the validity might be addressed through honesty, depth, the participants and the extent of triangulation. So it is important that the researcher have confidence in the elements of research planning, data collection, processing and analysis, interpretation and judgement.

## Mixed method designs

This is the combination of at least one qualitative and one quantitative method in a single research project. This approach should be used if you think it will give you greater objectivity and could help you reduce bias in your data collection.[13] It is often used when conducting social research, for example; you may wish to use questionnaires as the initial tool, but to get more detail these could be followed up by an interview.[14] The advantages and disadvantages of the quantitative and qualitative approaches should be considered; however, you need to think about some of the practical consequences of using a mixed method approach in that it will require additional resources to collect and analyse the subsequent data. Triangulation techniques are often used to explain more fully the richness and complexity of human behaviour by studying it from more than one viewpoint, hence the use of both quantitative and qualitative methods. It is also useful in confirming the concurrent validity, i.e. where the data or results of the test concur with the data or results from other tests. For example, if you were to investigate practitioners' perceptions of their role as mentors to undergraduates, a predominantly qualitative mixed method approach could be used as this is an exploratory study rather than testing a hypothesis. A series of interviews could be conducted in the first instance in order to generate data from which a rating questionnaire could be developed. In order to triangulate the data collected a focus group could be conducted to confirm the concurrent validity.

## Data analysis

It does not matter which research paradigm you use for data collection, you will find out very quickly just how much data you generate. This information needs to be organized and you will need to account for each piece of data generated. Information such as a person's age and gender are important data points. An interview that has lasted an hour could generate 50 pages of transcript. So whether the data are written or numerical, you need to manage them.[15] On a practical note, you will need to find a secure place to keep your data and also have a second copy as a back-up. Security is particularly important if you are using audio or video to collect your data when the participants could be readily identified. In addition you will need to keep the consent sheets somewhere away from your raw data so that there is no risk of the participants being identified.

If your approach has been experimental you will need to input your data into a computer programme. DePoy and Gitlin[15] suggest a staged approach, the first being to check the data collection form for omissions, and then try addressing the missing data. You will need to label each variable and then decide which order you would need to enter the variables into the computer programme. Guidance on quantitative data analysis is provided in Chapter 15. Once you input your data, it is good practice to carry out a systematic check to ensure you have submitted the data correctly. It is very easy to hit the wrong key on your keyboard, especially if you are spending long hours working at your computer. The check also ensures that you have input all your data and that no information has been omitted.

For qualitative data, you tend to undertake the analysis while sorting out your data, unlike the quantitative approach, but the information will still require sorting and analysing. This approach generates enormous amounts of data and this will essentially be narrative, but could be videos. Information from interviews is transcribed, for example, or as data from videos is analysed frame by frame. These data are verbal or nonverbal rather than numerical. Most analysis is designed to transform the data collected into meaningful categories, taxonomies or themes that explain the meanings or underlying patterns of the phenomenon of interest.[16] But whether the data are numerical or written they still need to be managed. Usually the first stage for interview data is transcription of the interview. You can do this yourself or get professional transcribers to undertake this task; the interviews should be transcribed verbatim.

One advantage of transcribing data yourself is that you do get to listen to them over and over again and therefore start to get a feeling for what is being said, which helps you start the analysis of the data. However, it can be very time-consuming and tedious, though there is voice to text software available now. It may take you approximately 6–10 hours to type up just 1 hour of interview. Once the transcription has been undertaken, you will need to check that you typed the data accurately and verbatim, and to ensure that there are no misspellings or missing data. Once this is complete you then need to immerse yourself in the data, which requires you to read it or listen to it several times. As you start to generate categories of information, you need to establish a way of accessing the key passages that reflect these categories. How you organize this is to a great extent up to the individual; you might like to use cards, or word processing programmes. These can help you to catalogue and store and manipulate the information, but cannot help you analyse it. This is something you need to allocate time to do. It is useful while you are undertaking this task to keep a note book so that you can make your comments regarding the data. Once again you will need to refer back to your original questions and aims to ensure that your analysis tries to address the focus of the research. You can often generate further questions during this process.

# Reporting and writing up the research

This stage is the culmination of all your hard work. Your project may have quite a strict word count assigned to it and therefore you might have to consider carefully what you want to write about. Clearly you will have to address the questions you posed, but you can also include some discussion of the limitations and constraints of your project. Your research may have highlighted some unexpected findings and this should be considered as a possible area for further research. Evidence-based practice does serve to decrease the uncertainty that patients and healthcare professionals experience in a complex healthcare system. Your research, if in the public domain, will be scrutinized. It is worth considering what practitioners will be looking for when critiquing your work as this should be considered when developing your protocol. Beaven and Craig[17] suggest you should consider the following:

- Are the results of the study valid – is the quality of the study good enough to produce the results that can inform clinical decisions?
- What are the results and what do they mean?
- If your research relates to practice, you might also consider whether the results of the research can be applied in the clinical setting.

Structure and presentation of your project is considered fully in Chapter 17 and writing for publication in order to disseminate your findings is considered in Chapter 18.

# References

[1] Blaxter L, Hughes C, Tight M. How to Research. 3rd ed. Maidenhead: Open University Press; 2006.

[2] Carter S, Henderson L. Approaches to qualitative data collection in social science. In: Bowling A, Ebrahim S, editors. Handbook of Health Research: Investigation, Measurement and Analysis. Maidenhead: Open University Press; 2005.

[3] Marshall G, Brennan P. The process of undertaking a quantitative dissertation for a taught MSc: personal insights gained from supporting and examining students in the UK and Ireland. Radiography 2008;14:63–8.

[4] Green J, Thorogood N. Qualitative Methods for Health Research. London: Sage Publications; 2004.

[5] Parahoo K. Nursing Research: Principles, Process and Issues. 2nd ed. Basingstoke: Palgrave Macmillan; 2006.

[6] Polgar S, Thomas SA. Introduction to Research in the Health Sciences. 5th ed. Edinburgh: Churchill Livingstone; 2008.

[7] Cohen L, Manion L, Morrison K. Research Methods in Education. 6th ed. London: Routledge Falmer; 2007.

[8] Greenlaugh T, Taylor R. How to read a paper: papers that go beyond numbers (qualitative research). BMJ 1997;315:740–3.

[9] Gerrish K, Lacey A. The Research Process in Nursing. 5th ed. Oxford: Blackwell Publishing; 2006.

[10] Davies MM, Bath PA. Interpersonal sources of health and maternity information for Somali women living in the UK: information seeking and evaluation. J Doc 2002;58(3):302–18.

[11] Hammersley M. What's Wrong with Ethnography: Methodological Explorations. London: Routledge; 1992.

[12] Hammersley M. Reading Ethnographic Research: A Critical Guide. London: Longmans; 1990.

[13] Bergman MM. Advances in Mixed Methods Research. Los Angeles: Sage; 2008.

[14] Blaxter L, Hughes C, Tight M. How to Research. 3rd ed. Maidenhead: Open University Press; 2006.

[15] Depoy E, Gitlin LN. Introduction to Research: Understanding and Applying Multiple Strategies. 3rd ed. Baltimore: Mosby; 2005.

[16] Grbich C. Qualitative Research in Health: An Introduction. London: Sage; 1999.

[17] Beaven O, Craig JV. Searching the literature. In: Craig JV, Smyth RL, editors. The Evidence-based Practice Manual for Nurses. 2nd ed. Edinburgh: Elsevier; 2007.

# Types of information

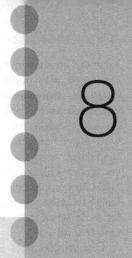

Alan Castle

## CHAPTER POINTS

- When attempting to find answers to questions, different approaches need to be adopted.
- While quantitative data are concerned with measurements that can be statistically treated, qualitative data are concerned with trying to understand the thoughts, feelings and experiences of individuals.
- Not all research exclusively uses either quantitative or qualitative approaches; some use a mixture of both (triangulation) in an attempt to improve quality of results and validity of findings.
- Quantitative data lend themselves to statistical analysis as a means of understanding numerical data that enable the researcher to reduce, summarize, organize, evaluate and interpret data and involve the use of both descriptive and inferential statistics.
- Descriptive statistics help visualize any patterns in the data such as averages, frequency distribution, measures of spread and correlation.
- Inferential statistics are concerned with hypothesis testing, making relationship between variables, and significance testing.
- Qualitative data generally take the form of loosely structured narrative material, such as dialogue between an interviewer and interviewee or field notes of an observational study and, while not amenable to statistical analysis, still have to be organized, interpreted and presented in a meaningful way.
- Using a range of tables, graphs and charts allows both quantitative and qualitative findings of research to be presented in the most effective way and can enhance the quality and accessibility of your work.
- The performance of diagnostic tests can be measured and compared using ROC curves.

Attempting to find answers involves looking for, analysing and evaluating quantitative (factual) and qualitative (perceptual) information and this chapter will discuss both types of data, using appropriate examples, and how this may be collected and displayed. These areas are revisited in Chapters 15 and 16.

## Introduction

Research in diagnostic imaging or radiotherapy is concerned with a systematic and rigorous search for knowledge and information to provide a sound basis for the development of practice. Ultimately, such research aims to enhance the health of the population by improving individual health outcomes and the delivery of health services.[1] The process of research means different things to different people, as does the type of information or data collected. To some it implies a large-scale undertaking lasting many years and collecting vast amounts of numerical data. For others, it is simply about exploring a little more deeply into why, for example, radiographers hold certain views on particular topics. For all of us though, research is about trying to *find answers to questions*.

## Quantitative and qualitative information

There are essentially two broad approaches to collecting information or data, namely quantitative and qualitative, as mentioned in Chapter 7. Data are generally considered to be quantitative if they are concerned with numbers (giving opportunities for statistical analysis) and qualitative if they are concerned with words (providing description and insight).[2,3] Since statistical analysis is more effective with larger numbers, quantitative approaches tend to favour more substantial studies, where the researcher is likely to be more detached. Conversely, qualitative approaches, partly because words take longer to analyse than numbers, tend to be on a smaller scale where the researcher may be more intimately involved.[3]

*Quantitative* data arise from a natural science approach which is based on the premise that things are measurable and the aim is to predict what will happen by stating a *hypothesis* or assumption, measuring outcomes and making appropriate changes based on the outcomes. For example, in radiotherapy you might state a hypothesis that 'topical products containing steroids are more effective than homeopathic products at preventing radio-dermatitis'. You could design a randomized controlled trial to test this hypothesis, whereby the study population was randomly assigned to an experimental or a control group. Those in the experimental group would use a product containing steroids and those in the control group a homeopathic product. You could then measure the outcomes by comparing the effect each topical product had on controlling the level of radio-dermatitis. In this case the variable you manipulated (topical product) is called the *independent variable* and the effect each product had on controlling the level of radio-dermatitis is called the *dependent variable*. Subsequently, the variables can be enumerated, tabulated and subjected to statistical procedures.[4] Depending on whether the hypothesis was accepted or rejected, you might either maintain or change the product you prescribe to patients following their radiotherapy treatment.

*Qualitative* data is essentially sociological in nature and is concerned with trying to understand human activity. Therefore doing qualitative research is rather like going exploring,[5] because it is a process of discovery rather than one of measuring variables. It involves obtaining material, mainly in the form of the written or spoken word. For example, in diagnostic imaging you may want to find out why some people are reluctant to attend their breast screening appointment. This might involve you conducting interviews with women focusing on practicalities such as appointment times and access, as well as anxieties such as the anticipated experience of pain during the procedure and the fear of detecting breast cancer, issues which may be invisible to a quantitative researcher using standardized indicators of health and health care.[6]

While making a distinction between quantitative and qualitative data is useful, placing too much emphasis on this division can be confusing, as in reality there is a considerable amount of crossover between the two approaches, despite the fact that quantitative researchers may argue that their data are more scientific and credible and qualitative researchers that their data are more sensitive and contextual. In the end the choice between different approaches should depend upon what you are trying to find out.[7]

Most quantitative data are based upon qualitative judgments, including decisions over which methodological approaches to choose and the levels of acceptable statistical significance to be applied to the results. For example, measuring changes in the weight of a patient during a course of radiotherapy treatment to the head and neck involves making decisions about how often to measure and what significance to place on the data obtained. Therefore what may look like a simple, straightforward quantitative measure is actually based on qualitative judgments.

Similarly, although qualitative data cannot be measured directly, it may be possible to assign numbers to certain attributes such as attitudes, values and adjectives used by respondents for describing feelings and convert this data by rating or categorizing the information obtained so that it can be organized and analysed more efficiently.[4] For example, you could ask patients to rank their level of anxiety prior to a magnetic resonance imaging (MRI) scan on a scale ranging from 1 (no anxiety) to 5 (extremely anxious) and use these data to produce quantitative results.

Quantitative and qualitative data are therefore intimately related to each other, and there are occasions when qualitative researchers draw on quantitative approaches and vice versa.[1] Sometimes it is advisable to employ more than one approach to collect data (*triangulation*), as mentioned in Chapter 16, as frequently a limitation of both approaches is their reliance on a single tool. Triangulation involves locating the true position by referring to two or more coordinates.[3] For example, if you wanted to know the 'truth' about what practitioners think about the human resources made available to run their department, you could use different methods of data collection to provide different angles on the topic. You could firstly ask practitioners in a questionnaire to rate their response to the following statement:

> The budget provided for this department in terms of human resources is not sufficient for us to provide a high quality service.

| 1 | 2 | 3 | 4 | 5 |
|---|---|---|---|---|
| Strongly agree | Agree | Don't know | Disagree | Strongly disagree |

Suppose you subsequently found that 75% of respondents rated the statement a '2', it would be difficult to place much validity on this result without understanding the assumptions that underlie it. For example, what does 'agree' mean? How do we interpret the value '2'? Thus, it is difficult to really understand this quantitative value unless we explore some of the judgements and assumptions that underlie it, such as:

- Did the respondent understand the term 'human resources'?
- Did the respondent understand that a '2' means that they are agreeing with the statement?
- Did the respondent read carefully enough to determine that the statement was limited only to human resources (for instance, equipment and buildings were not included)?
- Does the respondent care or were they just circling anything arbitrarily?
- How was this question presented in the context of the survey (e.g., did previous statements or questions immediately before this one bias the response in any way)?
- Was the survey anonymous and confidential?

As a follow-up you could, for example, use interviews in the triangulation process to explore some of these assumptions which would mean that different kinds of data on the same topic could be collected which is likely to improve the quality of the results and ultimately the validity of the findings.[3]

Thus, although the terms quantitative and qualitative may be well understood, there is no clear dividing line between the two approaches. The choice of approach you use depends on the nature of your study, whether you feel more comfortable working with numbers or words, large or small samples, or depth or breadth of investigation.[3]

# Data collection

The data that you might collect using quantitative and qualitative approaches include physical measurements (interval data), the use of rating scales (ordinal data), categorization of characteristics (nominal data) and the written or spoken word (non-numerical data).

*Interval data* obtained from physical measurements such as radiation dose, blood pressure or body mass index (BMI) are common in much medical research aimed at investigating relationships or testing hypotheses. Interval data are usually obtained from experiments where the numerical data are derived from accepted scales in which regular, measurable intervals can be recognized, thus giving an absolute measurement and producing continuous data.[4] Such research is generally concerned with testing a hypothesis whereby the researcher changes the independent variable and measures the effect on the dependent variable. For example, a hypothesis could be stated that the introduction of a new digital radiography system will reduce the mean radiation dose to a patient population by 10%. The independent variable is the one that is deliberately manipulated (new digital radiography system) and the dependent variable the one that is looked at for signs of change (radiation dose). The radiation dose received by a sample of 1000 patients is measured for a given radiographic procedure over a period of time and the mean dose compared to a similar sample of patients who were examined using the existing computed radiography system. Descriptive statistics may show a mean reduction in radiation dose of only 5% and therefore the hypothesis is rejected. However, inferential statistics can be used to assess whether there is any significant difference, variance or correlation between the two sets of data obtained using *parametric tests* (which can be used when it is assumed that there will be a normal distribution or variance of scores). Interval data therefore greatly expand the possibilities of undertaking subsequent statistical analysis.

*Ordinal data* are collected in such a way that they can be ordered, positioned or ranked. The intervals between the categories are not known and cannot be assumed to be equal, but they can be placed in a meaningful sequence.[4] For example, you could use a questionnaire to ask radiographers to rank-order a series of six medical images (A–F) in terms of their perceived level of resolution from highest to lowest. Here, the measurement does not tell us anything about how much better the definition of one medical image is than another, but does provide a relative measurement, which can be subsequently analysed using *non-parametric tests* (which can be used when it cannot be assumed that a normal distribution or variance of scores will be obtained). However, while ordinal data cannot be converted into interval data they can be converted into nominal data. Closed-ended questionnaires are probably the most familiar research method used to obtain ordinal data, as they can offer respondents a number of alternatives from which to choose the most appropriate answer. Table 8.1 illustrates some examples of closed-ended questions.

*Nominal data* are obtained by assigning numbers to classify characteristics into, for example, gender categories (male/female) and weight categories (small/medium/large), to compare the radiation dose received by different groups of patients for the same diagnostic imaging examination. Any numerical codes assigned to nominal measurements do not convey any quantitative information, but rules can be established such as assigning males = 1, females = 2, small = 3, medium = 4 and large = 5, etc. However, the numbers themselves have no meaning as clearly, for example, 2 does not mean more than 1 and 4 is not twice 3. Also the numbers can equally be reversed, thus they are merely symbols used to represent attributes and the numbers are useful for subsequent analysis. Thus, while there is no limit to the number of categories that can be included on a nominal scale, the numbers generated cannot be meaningfully added, subtracted, multiplied, etc.[4] A statistical test of significance (Pearson's chi-square) could be carried out on nominal data of this type to ascertain whether there

**Table 8.1 Examples of closed-ended questions**

| Question type | Example | Answer |
|---|---|---|
| Continuous scale | How important is it that you are seen within 10 minutes of your appointment time? | 1. Of utmost importance<br>2. Very important<br>3. Not sure<br>4. Of minor importance<br>5. Not at all important |
| Cafeteria | People have different opinions about the breast screening programme. Which of the following statements best represents your view? | 1. Is expensive and should be discontinued<br>2. May have some undesirable effects that suggest the need for caution<br>3. No opinion<br>4. Has many beneficial effects that merit its continued use<br>5. Has saved many lives and should be extended to the whole population |
| Categorical scale | Which of the following most closely resembles how you felt after your radiotherapy treatment? | 1. Tired<br>2. Light-headed<br>3. Sore<br>4. Sick<br>5. Other (please specify) |
| Visual analogue scale (VAS) | How would you describe the pain you now experience? | ←————————————→<br>5 Pain as severe as it could be    1 No pain at all |
| Rating | On a scale of 0 to 5 (where 0 = extremely dissatisfied and 5 means extremely satisfied), please circle the number that reflects your satisfaction with the information provided to you by the radiology department before your recent examination | 0  1  2  3  4  5 |

is a significant difference between the radiation dose received by males and females of different weight ranges for a particular diagnostic imaging examination.

*Non-numerical data* can be collected either as part of an information gathering exercise or used to generate their own theories (*grounded theory*). Grounded theory is concerned with attempting to develop theory from the data, rather than looking to existing theory into which the data has to be fitted.[8] There are many ways of collecting non-numerical data, but most commonly used in health care are open-ended questionnaires, interviews, observation and written documents.

*Open-ended questionnaires* allow subjects to respond in their own words, for example, 'What was the biggest problem you faced during your radiotherapy treatment?' Open-ended questions are easier to ask than closed-ended questions, but are more difficult for the respondent to answer and for the researcher to analyse. Questionnaires in general are relatively cheap to administer (especially electronically) and they offer the possibility of complete anonymity. Additionally, the absence of an interviewer assures that there will be no bias in the responses, such as when the respondent may say what they think the interviewer wants to hear (see also Chapter 16).

*Interviews* can involve either individual interviews (e.g. one-on-one) or group interviews (including focus groups) and the data obtained recorded in a wide variety of ways including audio/video recording or written notes. The purpose of the interview is to probe the ideas of the interviewees about the topic of interest and this could take the form of a structured or unstructured approach. A *structured interview* involves you developing an interview schedule in the form of a questionnaire, where questions are asked in a consistent and sequential way to ensure each respondent is asked the same questions in the same order. Table 8.2 is an example of an interview schedule that you could use when interviewing practitioners to seek their opinion about a course they had undertaken on image interpretation. This is the simplest approach to adopt and produces data that are easy to analyse (see also Chapter 16).

An *unstructured interview* is more complex and best used by more expert hands. Although you may have some initial guiding questions or core concepts to ask about, there is no formal structured instrument or protocol and you are free to move the conversation in any direction of interest that

**Table 8.2 Example of an interview schedule for a structured interview**

| Question number | Question |
| --- | --- |
| 1 | What have you gained by undertaking the course? |
| 2 | Can you give me examples of topics that were of particular interest? |
| 3 | Can you identify aspects of the course that you had problem with? |
| 4 | In what ways will you be able to practise your new skills? |
| 5 | Can you suggest ways in which the course could be improved? |

may come up. Consequently, unstructured interviewing is particularly useful for exploring a topic broadly and may produce a wealth of valuable data. However, because each interview tends to be unique with no predetermined structure, the data obtained are usually more difficult to analyse. For example, you could undertake interviews with practitioners (individually or as a group) to ascertain their views on a new government pay deal which might involve probing such issues as acceptability of the offer, staging of awards, effect on staff morale, employment opportunities, promotion prospects, etc.

*Observation* differs from interviewing in that the observer does not actively query the respondent, but watches rather than taking part and witnesses events first hand.[3] *Direct* or *systematic observation* usually produces more quantitative data, while participant observation usually produces qualitative information. For example, with direct observation you could draw up an observation schedule aimed to provide objective data about how long patients had to wait for their examination/treatment from the time of their actual appointment to the commencement of the procedure. This would involve recording the time they check in to the reception desk, the scheduled appointment time and the actual time of the commencement of the procedure. Such a schedule is illustrated in Table 8.3. Here it can be seen that such data could provide information about mean waiting times, consequences of arriving early or late, etc., and might be used to attempt to improve service delivery.

**Table 8.3 Example of results obtained from direct observation schedule**

| Patient number | Check-in time | Scheduled appointment time | Time of commencement of procedure |
|---|---|---|---|
| 1 | 11.47 | 12.00 | 12.10 |
| 2 | 11.59 | 11.45 | 12.15 |
| 3 | 12.00 | 12.00 | 12.30 |
| 4 | 12.15 | 12.30 | 12.20 |
| 5 | 12.30 | 12.45 | 12.45 |
| 6 | 12.45 | 12.50 | 12.55 |

*Participant observation* requires that the observer become a participant in the culture or context being observed and this often involves months or years of intensive work because you need to become accepted as a natural part of the culture in order to ensure that the observations are of the natural phenomenon. For example, in order to explore the culture of a specific diagnostic imaging or radiotherapy department, it would be necessary to make observations about what it is like to work in the department, observe other members of staff doing their work, talk to staff and patients, etc. In this way it would be possible to observe record, analyse and interpret the data you gather. However, this approach is beyond the scope of the type of small-scale study in which you are likely to be involved, but the literature on participant observation discusses how to enter the context, the role of the researcher as a participant, the collection and storage of field notes, and the analysis of field data.[2,3]

*Written documents* (as opposed to transcripts of interviews) can include journals, textbooks, newspapers, websites, annual reports, etc. Usually these written documents are analysed using content analysis, whereby the text is broken down into smaller components (such as words or sentences) and categories are developed (such as key words or phrases) associated with the theme. For example, you could conduct a content analysis of different NHS Trust mission statements to make some inferences about what they hold as their primary reasons for existence and their aims for the future (Table 8.4).

Here, content analysis would reveal such wide-ranging statements as: 'best care', 'patient-centred',

'best employment practice', and 'clean and pleasant environment'.

Ultimately, all qualitative data you obtain needs to be organized before it can be analysed, and the question of how to analyse subsequent transcripts often poses a problem.[9] The solution involves *coding* the data by extracting concepts from the raw data so that units such as specific words, ideas or events can be classified and ultimately collapsed down into more manageable, broader *categories* or *themes* so that interconnections that recur can be identified.[3] The categories themselves may come from theory, intuition or the data themselves.[10] Thus, for example, using a semi-structured interview to explore students' experience of a teaching programme might reveal categories such as: 'has increased my knowledge', 'there was a lack of practical examples', 'would be better in the morning' and 'venue too hot'. From these categories, themes might emerge such as content, delivery, timing and venue (see also Chapter 16).

## Data display

Having collected the data, the next stage is to look at the data to provide, for example, a description of what has been found and any relationship between variables or emerging patterns, before possibly going on to undertake more sophisticated statistical analysis. Illustrations such as tables, graphs and charts can be used to present certain types of information more clearly and in less space than written text.[11] Tables can be used to organize much of the numerical data obtained during the research process and allow the reader to rapidly identify the information collected, while graphs and charts can be used to illustrate complicated relationships more clearly. Most importantly, any illustration should not simply be a repetition of text or vice versa and thus appropriate methods of data display should be carefully considered so that they enhance rather than confuse the reader.[11]

## Tables

Tables can be used for most types of numerical data and their level of complexity depends on the audience for whom they are intended. In general they should be as simple as possible, but where they do contain a lot of information divisions marked by horizontal and vertical lines will help the reader interpret the data.

**Table 8.4 Examples of NHS Trust mission statements**

| Hospital | Mission statement |
|---|---|
| A | 'Our vision is of — as a confident, high performing organization, in the top 10 per cent of NHS Trusts, working in partnership to provide the highest possible quality of services to patients and their families' |
| B | '— NHS Trust aims to provide a high quality, integrated health care service for the people of —' |
| C | '— NHS Trust will provide first class services in state of the art hospital facilities, which deliver choice, exceed patients' expectations and meet the changing needs of the growing communities in —' |
| D | 'The — NHS Trust's mission statement is to provide the very best care, for each patient, on every occasion' |
| E | 'The — Healthcare NHS Trust aims to provide high quality integrated health care services locally by promoting and investing in best clinical and employment practice' |
| F | 'The — Trust is a patient-centred organization delivering high quality health care to the community. In the pursuit of excellence we are committed to providing an environment which is responsive to the needs of patients, staff and visitors' |
| G | 'Putting patients first, treating them with dignity and respect – offering safe, skilled, sensitive care delivered by conscientious, committed staff in a clean and pleasant environment' |
| H | 'We want to be your hospital of choice' |
| I | 'We will ensure the – Hospital NHS Trust is a locally, nationally and internationally renowned centre of excellence for patient care, education and research. We will deliver this vision by ensuring we employ the best possible staff and invest in their development' |
| J | 'To provide to all users and staff a quality service which strives to meet the best standards of professional care, that is sensitive and responsive to their individual needs. Our aim is to be innovative in the treatment provided and in the environment created' |
| K | 'To provide a high level of service and quality previously unknown in this country' |
| L | 'To be the best district general hospital' |

The data set in Table 8.5 was obtained during a clinical audit on a sample of 30 patients to measure the dose they received during an antero-posterior (AP) projection of the pelvis. The dose-area product (DAP) is obtained by multiplying the dose and area of exposure (measured in $Gy.m^2$) and is used in a clinical setting to approximate the absorbed dose received by the patient.

While the data may be said to be clearly presented in Table 8.5, it would be possible to analyse, for example, the gender, mean age, % frequency and mean DAP reading data and present this as a smaller table (Table 8.6).[11] This clearly shows that two-thirds of patients were female, had a lower mean age and a higher mean DAP reading.

Tables can also be used to clearly and effectively summarize data that have been subjected to statistical analysis. Table 8.7 summarizes pre- and post-test data scores for two groups of practitioners. The cohort of 80 radiographers was randomly ascribed to either study group A or control group B. Group A ($n = 40$) completed a sequence of a pre-test of their image interpretation skills, structured teaching of a revised image interpretation course and a post-test of their image interpretation skills. Group B ($n = 40$) completed a sequence of a pre-test of their image interpretation skills, structured teaching of the old image interpretation course and a post-test of image interpretation skills.

As can be seen from Table 8.7, the mean pre-test scores for both groups were similar, but the mean post test scores for group A were significantly higher ($P = 0.001$) than those for group B ($P = 0.5$),

**Table 8.5 Data set obtained from clinical audit**

| Gender | Size (estimated by radiographer) | Age (years) | mAs | kVp | DAP (cGy.cm$^2$) |
|---|---|---|---|---|---|
| Female | S | 79 | 13.4 | 70 | 153 |
| Male | M | 74 | 11.9 | 75 | 153 |
| Male | S | 71 | 14.2 | 70 | 164 |
| Male | M | 66 | 15.6 | 70 | 177 |
| Female | S | 59 | 17.5 | 70 | 203 |
| Female | M | 41 | 18.8 | 70 | 212 |
| Male | M | 53 | 17.4 | 75 | 222 |
| Female | M | 32 | 17.7 | 75 | 224 |
| Female | S | 75 | 20.9 | 70 | 242 |
| Female | M | 68 | 22.3 | 70 | 255 |
| Female | M | 55 | 20.3 | 75 | 258 |
| Female | M | 31 | 21.0 | 75 | 269 |
| Male | M | 50 | 22.5 | 75 | 286 |
| Female | M | 51 | 26.1 | 70 | 296 |
| Female | M | 68 | 25.4 | 75 | 325 |
| Male | L | 50 | 26.2 | 75 | 335 |
| Female | M | 58 | 32.7 | 70 | 374 |
| Male | M | 63 | 30.3 | 75 | 383 |
| Female | M | 70 | 35.5 | 70 | 408 |
| Female | M | 55 | 33.0 | 75 | 419 |
| Female | M | 70 | 36.4 | 70 | 421 |
| Male | L | 66 | 37.9 | 70 | 431 |
| Female | M | 38 | 39.2 | 70 | 452 |
| Female | M | 58 | 39.6 | 70 | 457 |
| Female | L | 49 | 36.3 | 75 | 459 |
| Male | L | 44 | 40.2 | 75 | 506 |
| Female | L | 48 | 54.1 | 70 | 627 |
| Female | M | 73 | 54.5 | 70 | 633 |
| Male | L | 51 | 57.6 | 70 | 670 |
| Female | L | 25 | 66.4 | 75 | 828 |

Small (S) = <60 kg; medium (M) = 60–80 kg; large (L) = >80 kg.

**Table 8.6 Analysis of patient gender, mean age, % frequency and mean DAP readings obtained from the clinical audit**

| Gender | Mean age (years) | % Frequency | Mean DAP (cGy.cm$^2$) |
|---|---|---|---|
| Male | 59 | 33.3 | 333 |
| Female | 55 | 66.7 | 376 |

indicating that the post-test performance of the study group was greater than think of the control group.

Tables can also be used to illustrate how non-numerical data can be coded and categorized, such as data obtained from in-depth interviews undertaken with a group of students to ascertain their opinions on the success of a teaching programme aimed at improving their communication skills. Among other questions, students were asked:

- How has this programme helped you?
- How could the programme be improved?

Following reading of the transcripts of the interviews, Table 8.8 illustrates how six of the student responses to these questions could be coded.

From this is can be seen that four categories or themes emerge, namely:

- Improved my confidence ($n = 4$).
- Needs a better venue ($n = 4$).
- Needs to happen earlier in the day ($n = 2$).
- No benefit ($n = 2$).

All data from the interview transcripts of all 12 students could then be examined to ascertain how many of them referred to each category, as shown in Table 8.9. The X means that the particular

student mentioned this category in their interview transcripts.

Thus we can see that tables are a very flexible method of presenting both numerical and non-numerical data.

# Graphs

## Line graphs

Line graphs are used to present a change in one variable as a function of another variable. This is particularly useful in demonstrating a trend or interaction and the most common use of a line graph is where a time sequence can be displayed on the x-axis (horizontal) as the independent variable and the variable change measured is displayed on the y-axis (vertical) as the dependent variable.[11,12] For example, Figure 8.1 illustrates how there has been a general increase in the number of patients attending a medical imaging department over a 10-year period.

More complicated line graphs can be used to compare a series of data over the same time period. Figure 8.2 shows how three imaging departments compare in terms of the number of patients attending over a 10-year period. This illustrates that imaging department A has had a relatively consistent number of patients attending since 2002, B has had a steady increase up until 2004 but this has since started to reduce, and C has had a steady increase over the last 10 years, which has increased more markedly since 2004.

Line graphs are a common way of displaying certain types of data, particularly when showing changes over time, so that any emerging patterns can clearly be identified. They generally work better with large data sets and big variations.[3]

**Table 8.7 Scores (%) obtained in the test before and after teaching to a group of student practitioners**

| Group | Number of students ($n$) | Pre-test | | Post-test | | P |
|---|---|---|---|---|---|---|
| | | Mean ($\bar{x}$) | Standard deviation (SD) | Mean ($\bar{x}$) | Standard deviation (SD) | |
| Study group A | 40 | 68 | 8 | 74 | 6 | 0.001 |
| Control group B | 40 | 66 | 13 | 68 | 6 | 0.5 |
| P | | 0.5 | | 0.001 | | |

### Table 8.8 Coding of interview transcripts

| Student | Notes from transcript | Coding |
|---|---|---|
| 1 | • Made me more confident in my dealings with people, at the moment I tend to be a bit defensive and aggressive if I am criticized<br>• The room was set out as a lecture theatre and it would have been better if the room was set out more appropriately for small group work | • Improved my confidence<br><br>• Needs better venue |
| 2 | • I feel more confident and I feel I can deal with difficult patients more effectively now<br>• I think having this session earlier in the morning would be better as by 4 p.m. most of us had already had enough for the day | • Improved my confidence<br><br>• Needs to happen earlier in the day |
| 3 | • Nothing as I was quite good at dealing with patients anyway and the time could be used learning more radiographic techniques<br>• The room was very cold | • No benefit<br><br>• Needs better venue |
| 4 | • I am not so shy as before. I tended to be rather withdrawn and passive in my dealings with patients and I think this has helped me improve my self-esteem<br>• Having a session like this at the end of the day is a bad idea as we're all tired by then and just want to get away | • Improved my confidence<br><br><br>• Needs to happen earlier in the day |
| 5 | • I suppose most people need to improve their communication skills as it is important when dealing with patients and I think effective communication is a key clinical skill. I found the bit about being able to say 'no' effectively was particularly useful and I will try to use this more in the future<br>• I didn't like the room we used, it was too cold and bleak. Also this type of session is better earlier on when we are fresh. By the end of the day all we want to do is go home | • Improved my confidence<br><br><br><br><br>• Needs better venue |
| 6 | • I think I'm good at communicating with people already so I didn't learn much and found it all a waste of time<br>• I didn't like the room we used as a lecture theatre is not appropriate for this type of course | • No benefit<br><br>• Needs better venue |

### Table 8.9 Categorization of codes emerging from interview transcripts

| Category | Student number | | | | | | | | | | | |
|---|---|---|---|---|---|---|---|---|---|---|---|---|
| | 1 | 2 | 3 | 4 | 5 | 6 | 7 | 8 | 9 | 10 | 11 | 12 |
| Improved my confidence | X | X | X | X | X | | X | X | | X | | X |
| Needs a better venue | X | | X | | X | X | | X | X | | X | X |
| Needs to happen earlier in the day | | X | | X | X | | X | X | X | X | X | X |
| No benefit | | | X | | | X | | | X | | | |

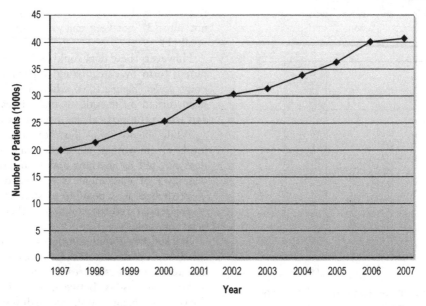

**Figure 8.1** • Line graph to illustrate how the number of patients have increased over the last 10 years.

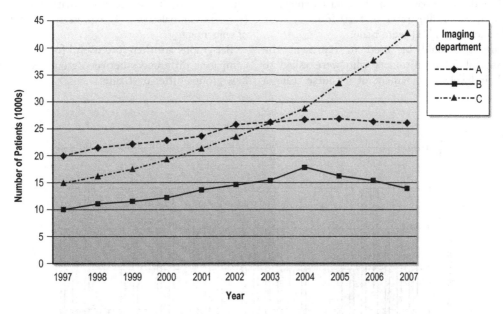

**Figure 8.2** • Line graph to show comparative patient numbers attending three imaging departments over the last 10 years.

## Bar graphs

Bar graphs are an effective way of presenting discrete data, such as frequency, with bars being of equal width and the height representing the frequency. Conventionally there are gaps between each bar and therefore a minimum of two bars is required for comparison. Ten bars should be used as a maximum otherwise the illustration can look too crowded.[3] For example, a simple bar graph (Figure 8.3) could be used to illustrate the numbers

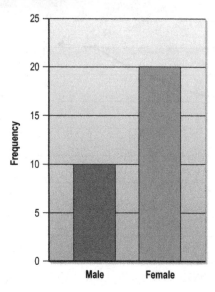

**Figure 8.3** • Bar chart comparing number of male/female patients in clinical audit.

of male and female patients in the data set shown in Table 8.5, which illustrates that 20 (66.7%) were female and 10 (33.3%) were male.

Figure 8.4 could be used to represent the responses of 30 practitioners who were asked to rate their level of enjoyment of a course using a five-point scale: very enjoyable (5), enjoyable (4), not sure (3), not very enjoyable (2), not enjoyable at all (1).

However, these data could be presented in a simplified form by categorizing responses into a five-point scale (Figure 8.5), where the bar chart has been turned on its side to make it easier to label and where the vertical axis becomes the *x*-axis.

While Figure 8.5 illustrates overall reported levels of enjoyment, since the data are ordinal it does not tell us anything about how much greater one level of enjoyment is compared to another. Nevertheless, it is possible to state that 17 (57%) respondents rated the course as either enjoyable or very enjoyable.

Stacked bar graphs can be used to illustrate the relative proportions of the factors that make up the total, giving the reader the opportunity to make comparisons between overall frequencies. For example, Figure 8.6 shows the difference between male radiographers ($n = 15$) and female radiographers ($n = 15$) in terms of their levels of enjoyment of a course, where it can be seen that more females ($n = 9$) than males ($n = 4$) expressed a positive level of enjoyment.

Bar graphs are therefore useful for presenting or comparing differences between groups, or showing how groups differ over time.

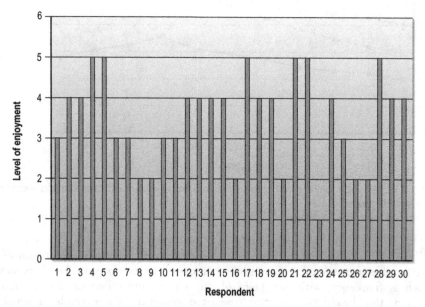

**Figure 8.4** • Analysis of expression of level of enjoyment.

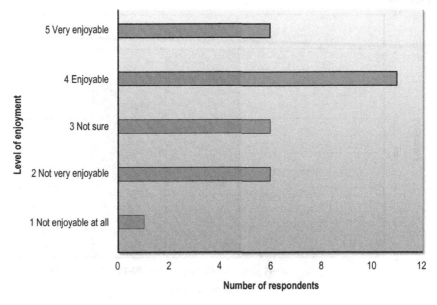

**Figure 8.5** • Summary of expression of level of enjoyment.

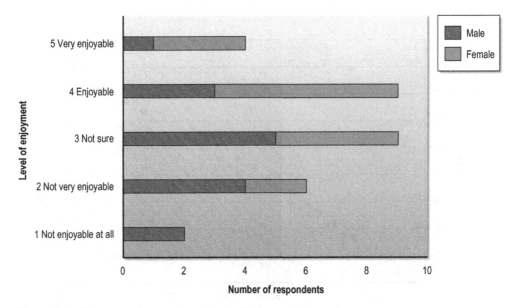

**Figure 8.6** • Summary of expression of level of enjoyment by gender.

## Histograms

Histograms are similar to bar graphs except that they are better at displaying continuous, rather than discrete, data. For example, the age distribution of the sample group in the data set shown in Table 8.5 (Figure 8.7) shows that 22 patients (73%) were aged between 45 and 74 years.

## Scatter plots

A scatter plot can be used to explore the relationship between two variables. It consists of one axis for each variable, and each data value is represented by a symbol positioned at the appropriate distance along each axis. For example, Figure 8.8 demonstrates the relationship between the mAs and DAP data from Table 8.5.

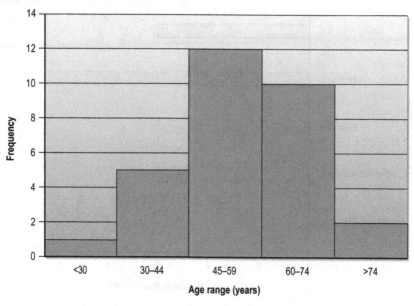

**Figure 8.7** • Histogram demonstrating age distribution of sample in clinical audit.

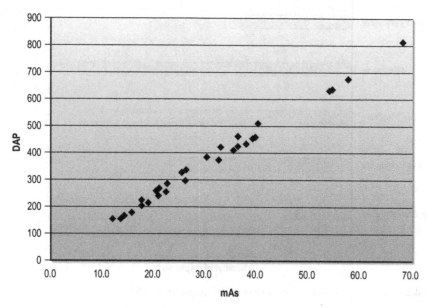

**Figure 8.8** • Scatter plot to demonstrate the relationship between mAs and DAP readings.

This shows a positive correlation between the mAs selected and the DAP obtained where the more closely the individual plots come together, the closer the relationship between the variables and vice versa. This type of illustration is particularly good at showing patterns and deviations, but it does require a reasonable amount of data to be plotted.[3]

# Charts

## Pie charts

Pie charts are useful for illustrating percentages and proportions in relation to each other and to the whole.[11] They consist of a circle representing the total data (100%), with each segment of the pie being proportional to the percentage of a particular category. For example, Figure 8.9 illustrates the size distribution of the sample of 30 patients in the clinical audit data shown in Table 8.5, where 64% ($n = 19$) of patients were estimated as being medium, and only 13% ($n = 4$) estimated as being small.

To enhance their impact, either individual segments or all the segments can be pulled away from the core as an exploded pie chart (Figure 8.10).

Alternatively, three dimensional (3-D) pie charts allow the volume of each segment to be represented, as illustrated in Figure 8.11.

Pie charts are visually very powerful, but can only be used with one data set. As a general rule there

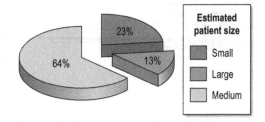

**Figure 8.11** • (3-D pie chart) Percentage of patients in each patient size group (as estimated by the practitioner).

should be no more than five segments in a single pie chart (to avoid visual overload), no single segment should account for less than 2% of the total, each segment should be easily distinguishable from another, and a legend should be provided to identify each segment.[12]

## Flow charts

All diagrams are visual devices that depict relationships between analytic concepts.[13] Charts can be used to present models or flowcharts and consist of enclosed boxes or circles connected by lines or arrows. They can be used to illustrate conceptual models as, for example, a chart to illustrate the key components important in assessing the critical thinking skills of students (Figure 8.12). Here, the concept of critical thinking is placed centrally with the seven key components represented as subdivisions. In addition, each of the key components has two related dimensions which state the evidence required to assess the extent to which each component has been achieved.

A flow chart could also be used to demonstrate the course of patients through a clinical trial. Figure 8.13 shows an example of such a flow chart. This type of chart makes it easy to see how many patients entered the study, how many completed, and how many were excluded.

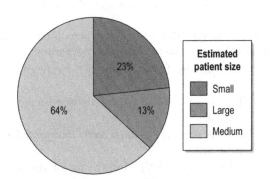

**Figure 8.9** • (Simple pie chart) Percentage of patients in each patient size group (as estimated by the practitioner).

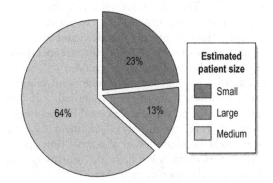

**Figure 8.10** • (Exploded pie chart) Percentage of patients in each patient size group (as estimated by the practitioner).

# Receiver operating characteristic (ROC) curves

In addition to collecting data, you may wish to test the performance of diagnostic applications, procedures[14] or individuals[15] and this might be done using receiver operating characteristic (ROC) testing, plotted on graphs known as ROC curves. These are often used in medicine to assess the performance and

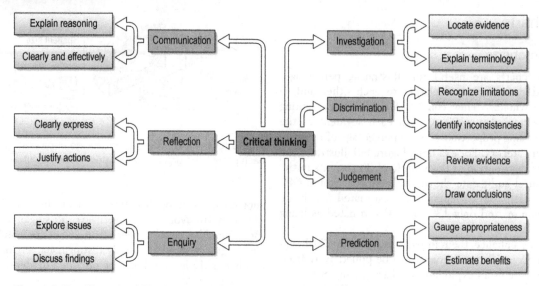

**Figure 8.12** • (Flow chart) The key components of critical thinking.

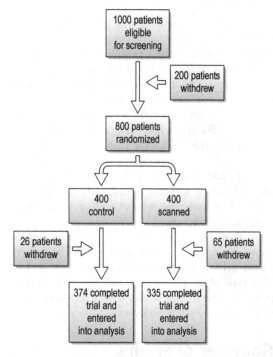

**Figure 8.13** • (Flow chart) Example of a clinical trial patient flow chart.

effectiveness of different diagnostic tests where there is a value that can be measured[16], such as blood glucose level.[17]

ROC methodology and analysis can be complex, but the references below should provide the starting point for a fuller understanding. However, a simple example of where ROC curves might be used in medical imaging is in assessing the ability of observers to discriminate between normal and abnormal images.

So, following this example, when interpreting images the decisions made can be categorised as:

- True positive (TP) – correctly interpreted as abnormal.
- True negative (TN) – correctly interpreted as normal.
- False positive (FP) – incorrectly interpreted as abnormal.
- False negative (FN) – incorrectly interpreted as normal.[15,18,19,20]

Observers are asked to record their confidence as to whether an image is normal or abnormal using a scale.[15,16,21] This allows several sensitivities (percentage of abnormal images that are identified as abnormal – the true positive fraction) and specificities (percentage of normal images that are identified as normal – the true negative fraction)[16,20] to be calculated by varying the confidence point used to identify an image as normal or abnormal.[17] If this point is set low, only a few abnormal images might be missed (high sensitivity) but many normal images might be identified as abnormal (low specificity). If this point is set high, the sensitivity will be lower and the specificity higher.[14,17,18,20,22]

ROC curves display the trade off between sensitivity and specificity[14,22] as a graph[16,20], where the

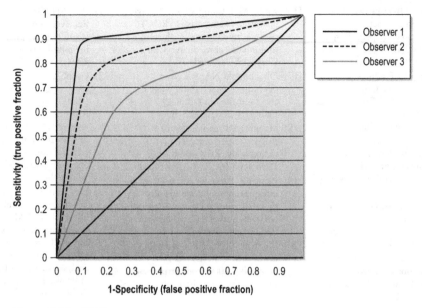

**Figure 8.14** • ROC curve.

true positive fraction (sensitivity) is plotted against the false positive fraction (1 – specificity) for the calculated points.[14,16,17] These figures are often plotted on a scale of 0–1.[16,17,18,19]

Consider the example of three different observers (see Figure 8.14 below). Observer 1 is able to discriminate at a high level between normal and abnormal images and the ROC curve will pass near to the upper left corner of the graph. Observer 2 might be considered as good and observer 3 as satisfactory. Note that the straight line represents an observer who is doing no better than guessing.[14,17,18,21,22] As this example demonstrates, a higher accuracy will result in the curve passing nearer to the upper left corner.[16,17,18,20]

Several measures derived from ROC curves have been suggested[16,17,21], one being the area under the curve.[16,17,18,19,21] In general terms, the greater the area under the curve, the better the observer(s) or test is at deciding between normal and abnormal.[17,19,20,21,22] However, when comparing ROC curves, the shape of the curves themselves might also be important.[16,17,21]

Other examples of the use of the ROC curve in medical imaging might be comparing the diagnostic performance of different modalities[23] or procedures.[14,17] For more complex image interpretation tasks, such as identifying the location of abnormalities, a number of modified ROC techniques can be used.[18,19]

# References

[1] Bowling A. Research Methods in Health: Investigating Health and Health Services. 2nd ed. Buckingham: Open University Press; 2002.

[2] Bell J. Doing Your Research Project. 4th ed. Buckingham: Open University Press; 2005.

[3] Denscombe M. The Good Research Guide: For Small-scale Social Research Projects. 2nd ed. Buckingham: Open University Press; 2003.

[4] Bailey DM. Research for the Health Professional: A Practical Guide. Philadelphia: FA Davis; 1997.

[5] Finlay L, Ballinger C, editors. Qualitative Research for Allied Health Professionals: Challenging Choices. Chichester: Wiley; 2006.

[6] Hesse-Biber S, Leavy P, editors. Approaches to Qualitative Research: A Reader on Theory and Practice. New York: Oxford University Press; 2003.

[7] Silverman D. Interpreting Qualitative Data. 3rd ed. London: Sage; 2006.

[8] Glaser B, Strauss A. The Discovery of Grounded Theory: Strategies for Qualitative Research. Chicago: Aldine; 1999.

[9] Burnard P. A method of analysing interview transcripts in qualitative research. Nurse Educ Today 1991;11:461–6.

[10] Gilbert N. Researching Social Life. 3rd ed. London: Sage; 2008.

[11] Durbin CG. Effective use of tables and figures in abstracts, presentations and papers. Respir Care 2004;49(10):1233–8.

[12] Nicol AAM, Pexman PM. Displaying your Findings: A Practical Guide for Creating Figures, Posters and Presentations. Washington: American Psychological Association; 2003.

[13] Polgar S, Thomas SA. Introduction to Research in the Health Sciences. 5th ed. Edinburgh: Churchill Livingstone; 2007.

[14] Vining DJ, Gladish GW. Receiver operating characteristic curves: a basic understanding. Radiographics 1992;12:1147–54.

[15] Gunn C. Radiographic Imaging: a practical approach. 3rd ed. Edinburgh: Churchill Livingstone; 2002.

[16] Zweig MH, Campbell G. Receiver-operating characteristic (ROC) plots: a fundamental evaluation tool in clinical medicine. Clin Chem 1993;39:561–77.

[17] Obuchowski NA. Receiver operating characteristic curves and their uses in radiology. Radiology 2003;229:3–8.

[18] Manning DJ. Evaluation of diagnostic performance in radiography. Radiography 1998;4:49–60.

[19] Piper KJ, Paterson A. Initial image interpretation of appendicular skeletal radiographs: a comparison between nurses and radiographers. Radiography 2009;15:40–8.

[20] MedCalc. ROC curve analysis: introduction. Retrieved 26 November 2009 from http://www.medcalc.be/manual/roc.php.

[21] Park SH, Goo JM, Jo C-H. Receiver operating characteristic (ROC) curve: practical review for radiologists. Kor J Radiol 2004;5(1):11–8.

[22] GraphPad Software. Key concepts: receiver-operator characteristic (ROC) curves. Retrieved 26 November 2009 from http://www.graphpad.com/help/Prism5/prism5help.html?introduction_to_receiver_operator_characteristic_(roc)_curves.htm.

[23] Weatherburn GC, Ridout D, Strickland NH, Robins P, Glastonbury CM, Curati W, et al. A comparison of conventional film, CR hard copy and PACS soft copy images of the chest: analyses of ROC curves and inter-observer agreement. Eur J Radiol 2003;47:206–14.

# Epidemiological research methods

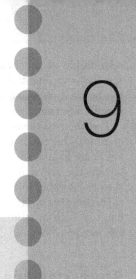

9

## David M Flinton

## Introduction

Epidemiology is the systematic study of the distribution of health and illness, or the investigation of factors affecting the health of populations. This chapter aims to describe these types of studies, which are usually undertaken to inform health professionals, allowing them to establish links between health and specific causes in order to try and prevent illness and disease through effective health strategies and campaigns.

Measuring the disease frequency usually requires the study to define a case, which is someone with the condition of interest. This can be simple. For example, consider six subjects, one of whom has cancer while the others do not. In this instance we have one case of cancer. If, however, we needed to measure cholesterol levels, there would be a continuum of severity rather than a binary outcome. When a continuum occurs we could define a case as someone outside of two standard deviations from the norm, or perhaps base the cut-off on clinical importance, i.e. at a level where the risk of heart disease increases significantly. In the UK the healthy cholesterol level is considered to be $\leq 5$ mmol/L, so for defining cases of high cholesterol this figure could be used as the starting point.

## Disease occurrence

As well as defining what a case is, it is also important to understand how disease occurrence is measured. Two common measures of a disease's occurrence are *incidence* and *prevalence*.

*Incidence* is the rate at which new cases occur in a given time period. When the risk is roughly constant incidence is measured as:

$$\frac{\text{the number of new cases}}{\text{population at risk} \times \text{time during which cases were collected}}$$

There were approximately 37 000 new cases of breast cancer in England in 2004. If the population was 50 million this would give an annual incidence of approximately 74 per 100 000. The information this figure gives, called the crude rate, is quite basic and it can mask important information such as the different rates in males and females or the relationship of the incidence of breast cancer with age. To overcome this problem, standardized rates can be used, breaking the data down into rates for specific age ranges and by sex.

*Prevalence* is the number of cases at a given point in time. The two measures, incidence and prevalence, are linked; when a new case (incident) occurs it joins the prevalence figures and stays there until the person either recovers or dies. If the time period to recovery or death is long, as it often is with chronic illnesses such as asthma, then even diseases with a low incidence rate can give rise to a high prevalence.

## Study designs

A number of different designs can be utilized in epidemiological studies. The three most commonly used designs are discussed in this section:

## Cohort studies

Cohort studies track people forward in time. In their simplest form they follow two groups (cohorts) from the point of exposure to the outcome of interest. The difference between the two groups is that one has been exposed to a risk factor whereas the other group has not. If on analysis a difference exists in the rate of the outcome of interest between the two groups it can suggest an association between the exposure and the outcome.

For example; if we were interested in investigating the effect of lens irradiation in childhood on cataract formation we could identify a suitable population to study such as children who have a condition/illness that requires two or more CT scans of the head, establish a control group such as children attending outpatients who do not require any radiological examinations, then follow both the cohorts for a number of years. At the end of the period we could then compare the number of cataracts in the two groups.

The main advantage of this type of study is that there is no recall bias; it also avoids survivor bias (see Chapter 10). It can be used to study uncommon exposures, and also to estimate the incidence rate. A weakness of this type of study is that if the outcome or event takes a long time to develop the study will take a long time to complete and therefore will be expensive. Also, maintaining contact with individuals over long periods can sometimes be difficult and the study may have a high drop-out rate.

## Case-control studies

Case-control studies are usually retrospective in nature. The study starts by recruiting a sample of subjects with a particular health disorder (cases) and a group of subjects without the health outcomes (controls). We can then assess and compare both the cases' and controls' exposure to the risk factor in question. If we were interested in looking at lung cancer and smoking we could identify a group of subjects with lung cancer and a group of controls, patients without lung cancer. A questionnaire could then be given to the subjects in both groups asking them about their smoking history. Matching the two groups allows the researcher to control for factors that might distort or confound the relationship that is being studied. Two variables that are often matched in case-control studies are age and gender.

This type of study has the ability to study rare diseases and is cheap and relatively quick to conduct. Such studies are, however, more prone to bias than cohort studies, particularly recall bias (see Chapter 10).

## Cross-sectional studies

Cross-sectional studies determine exposure and disease at the same time. They are literally a 'snapshot', as all information on both the outcome and the exposure are collected at the same point in time. If we were interested in the prevalence of back pain in radiographers a questionnaire could be sent to a representative sample. Depending on how detailed the questionnaire was, we might be able to look at the prevalence in different groups such as therapeutic practitioners and diagnostic practitioners, ultrasonographers, or try and link the prevalence to an exposure, such as the frequent wearing of a lead apron.

These are simple studies and as such are prone to bias, and not suited to rare conditions, but they are the quickest and cheapest of the studies detailed in this section.

## Bradford Hill criteria

Austin Bradford Hill proposed a set of criteria as a means of judging whether a causal relationship between a factor and a condition exists. The criteria are still widely used as a benchmark in determining a causal relationship:

## Temporal relationship

The exposure to the factor in question must always precede the outcome. If wearing a lead apron causes back pain, the wearing of the lead apron must precede the back pain. This is the only criterion that must always be met.

## Strength of association

This is defined by the size of the risk as described in the following sections. The stronger the association, the more likely it is that the relationship is causal.

## Dose–response

The greater the degree of exposure the greater the risk of the outcome. The more you smoke, the greater your risk of cancer and heart disease. If a dose–response relationship is present, it is strong evidence for a causal relationship.

## Consistency

The association is consistent across different studies; if a relationship is causal, we would expect the finding to be reproduced in the different studies.

## Plausibility

Does the association make sense? Is there a sound theoretical basis or one that can be postulated for making an association between a risk factor and the outcome being measured?

## Specificity

This is established when a single cause leads to a specific effect. This is considered by some to be a weak criterion as causality can be multiple; consider lung cancer and smoking, for example – not all lung cancer victims smoke.

## Coherence

The association should not contradict existing theory and knowledge.

## Experiment

Causation is more likely if there is evidence from randomized experiments.

## Analogy

In some circumstances the effect of similar factors and their actions may be considered. In other words, if we know that one type of causal agent produces an effect, a second similar agent may cause a similar effect.

# Odds and risk

Cohort studies often report findings as a relative risk whereas odds ratios are used for case-control studies. To understand relative risk and odds ratios better, we must first look at what risk and odds are. Risk and odds are slightly different, as shown by the formulae below, but both are strongly linked with probability which is looked at in Chapters 10 and 15.

$$\text{Risk} = \frac{\text{Number of outcomes resulting in the event}}{\text{Total number of possible outcomes}}$$

$$\text{Odds} = \frac{\text{Number of outcomes resulting in the event}}{\text{Number of outcomes NOT resulting in the event}}$$

If in a group of 200 subjects, 1 patient had presented with cancer, the risk of cancer within the group would be $1/200 = 0.005$. If we report the odds on the same group we could say that the odds were $1/199 = 0.005025$. A small difference, and for rare events we can say that the odds and risk approximate each other. However, this difference becomes greater for common events. For example, if in a group of 200 patients, 50 had cancer, the risk of cancer within the group would be $50/200 = 0.25$; the odds $50/150 = 0.33$, so the risk of getting cancer is 25%, the odds 33%. Odds and risk only approximate each other for rare events; the more common the event, the greater the difference. Risk has the advantage of presenting the data in a way that is understood by most people.

Odds and risk contain the same information, so it is possible to calculate one value if the other is known:

$$\text{Odds} = \frac{\text{Risk}}{(1 - \text{Risk})} \quad \text{Risk} = \frac{\text{Odds}}{(1 + \text{Odds})}$$

In the above example the risk was $0.25$ therefore the odds are $0.25/(1 - 0.25) = 0.33$.

# Relative risk or risk ratio (RR)

The relative risk is a ratio of two risks and describes the risk in one group as a multiple of the risk in a second group. If we have two groups, one that is exposed to a possible carcinogen and one that is not exposed, we can work out the relative risk by

**Table 9.1  2 × 2 Data table**

|           | Disease | No disease |       |
|-----------|---------|------------|-------|
| Exposed   | A       | B          | A+B   |
| Unexposed | C       | D          | C+D   |
|           | A+C     | B+D        |       |

**Table 9.2  Example data**

|           | Cancer | Disease free | Total |
|-----------|--------|--------------|-------|
| Smokers   | 288    | 257          | 545   |
| Ex-smokers| 364    | 742          | 1106  |
| Total     | 652    | 999          |       |

looking at the ratio of disease occurrence in both groups. Using Table 9.1, the relative risk would be calculated by dividing the risk in the exposed group, called the experimental event rate (EER) [A/A+B], by the risk in the unexposed group, the control event rate (CER) [C/C+D].

A resulting value of 1·0 would mean that the risk between the groups is identical values above 1 represents a positive association and values below 1 a negative association. The further a value is away from 1 the stronger the association between exposure and outcome.

If we look at some hypothetical data on subjects who are smokers and ex-smokers shown in Table 9.2, it is possible to calculate the relative risk of cancer associated with this lifestyle activity.

We first need to calculate the risk or experimental event rate, which is 288/545 = 0·53, 53%. Next the risk in the comparison or control group, the ex-smokers population, 364/1106 = 0·33 or 33%. The relative risk of cancer is calculated by dividing the EER by the CER, 0·53/0·33 = 1·6. In this

sample, the risk of cancer for smokers is 1·6 that of ex-smokers or conversely that the risk for ex-smokers is 1/1·6 = 0·63 that of smokers.

## Odds ratio (OR)

To calculate the odds ratio from Figure 9.1, first we have to calculate the odds of getting cancer in the smoking group A/B, which is 288/257 = 1·12. The odds of getting cancer in the ex-smoking group is C/D, 364/742 = 0·49. The ratio of these odds is 1·12/0·49 = 2·29. As you can see, the odds ratio has produced a figure in the same direction as the relative risk but further away from 1 compared to the relative risk.

The interpretation of odds ratios follow the same guidelines as for relative risks, a value less than 1 being a negative association, more than 1 a positive association, and 1 no association between the exposed group and the unexposed group. As with risk and odds, the relative risk and odds ratio approximate each other

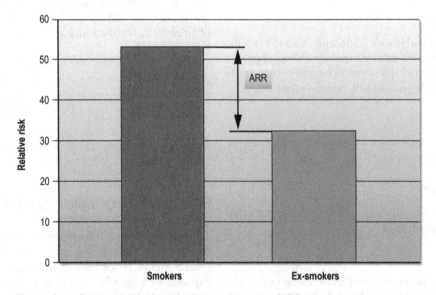

**Figure 9.1** • Relative risk for hypothetical smoking data (ARR, absolute risk reduction).

when an event is rare. For common events the odds ratio always follows the same direction as the relative risk, but may not be an accurate estimate of the risk, the odds always being overestimated, as in the above example.

With these differences between relative risk and odds ratio, why is there a need to calculate the odds ratio when we can calculate the relative risk or vice versa? Both relative risk and odds ratio are equally valid, but different measurements. Most people are more familiar with probability (risk) than odds and often the odds ratio is interpreted as relative risk. The answer is that it has to do with study design; relative risk cannot be calculated from a case-control as the design of the study involves the selection of research subjects on the basis of the outcome measurement rather than on the basis of the exposure. Also, when we are dealing with confounding variables in the analysis we use a procedure called logistic regression which calculates odds.

Small samples may give rise to a large relative risk or odds ratio which might be interpreted as being linked to causality. This is not necessarily correct as it could have occurred by chance if the sample size were small. Some studies do quote p-values for relative risk/odds ratios but it is more common when looking at papers to see confidence intervals (CI) being quoted.

Together with the risk ratio or odds ratio, the CI gives information on the size and the precision of the study results; a wider confidence interval means less precise results. It is usual to see the 95% confidence interval being used, rather than a p-value to indicate evidence of an effect. For example, a study looking at the protective effect of exercise on breast cancer reported that women who were inactive in early life but later became active had an OR of 0·60 (0·33–1·11) whereas lifelong exercisers had an OR of 0·58 (0·41–0·83). In this instance although there is a risk reduction for late-life exercisers, it is not considered significant as the confidence intervals include the value 1 (no difference), whereas the effect of exercise on the reduction in breast cancer

was significant for lifelong exercisers (confidence interval did not include the value 1).

What we see from this is that data on risk and odds are presented in various forms of grey. The study may be significant or not, but it is the degree of risk and the associated confidence intervals reported that become the main focus.

## Other terms used

Another useful figure is the *absolute risk reduction* (ARR). This can be calculated by subtracting the CER from the EER [ARR = (EER − CER)], $0·53 − 0·33 × 100 = 20\%$. Absolute risk reduction is just the absolute difference in outcome rates between the control and treatment groups. For the above data the absolute risk reduction is 20% which means that for ex-smokers the incidence of cancer is 20% less than for smokers, see Figure 9.1.

The final figure we can calculate is the *number needed to treat* (NNT). It is basically another way to express the absolute risk reduction, being the reciprocal of the ARR, and it can be thought of as the number of patients that would need to be treated to prevent one additional bad outcome. For the above data the NNT is $1/0·2 = 5$. So, for every 5 subjects who quit smoking, approximately one case of cancer would be prevented. NNTs are very easy to understand and are easy to calculate and so have gained popularity in recent publications. NNT data are especially useful in comparing the results of trials in which the relative effectiveness of the treatments are of interest. For example, the NNT for long-term survival following treatment using radiotherapy alone for breast cancer might be 10 whereas for radiotherapy and drug A it is 4. Clearly the use of drug A is beneficial as is radiotherapy alone. For every 10 treatments one death would be avoided whereas for combined treatment every 4 treatments would result in a life being saved. An ideal NNT would be 1, where everyone who receives the treatment gets better.

## Further reading

Bruce N, Pope D, Stanistreet D. Quantitative Methods for Health Research: A Practical Interactive Guide to Epidemiology and Statistics. Chichester: Wiley; 2008.

Kirkwood B, Sterne J. Essential Medical Statistics. 2nd ed. Malden: Wiley; 2003.

Hulley SB, Cummings SR, Browner WS, et al. Designing Clinical Research. 3rd ed. Philadelphia: Lippincott Williams and Wilkins; 2006.

# Sampling errors, bias and objectivity

# 10

David M Flinton   Andrew Owens

## CHAPTER POINTS

- Statistics are created when describing/investigating samples. Sampling relies on being able to define the population precisely and use an appropriate technique to avoid sampling error, and obtain an unbiased sample. There are many types of sampling, some of which are best in certain circumstances, but the best overall group of methods use probability sampling which utilizes some form of random selection. A random method of sampling gives each person an equal chance of being included in the study.

- Probability is an important concept in statistics. All experiments have more than one outcome, each of which can be specified in advance. The probability of an event ranges from 0 to 1, and the sum of the probabilities for all events must equal 1. Probability events may be dependent, when one event affects the probability of another event, or independent, when one event does not affect the probability of another event.

- Bias, a systematic error, and errors may be introduced into the study if the study is designed incorrectly. Different types of bias occur depending on the study type.

- Deciding on the sample size of the study is very important – too small and it may not be representative of the population, too large and it is wasteful. It is also possible to calculate the power of the study after the study has been conducted.

- In order for a study to be deemed 'good', the results must be both valid and reliable.

This chapter covers much of what should be considered before you undertake your research: what the population is, how to get a sample, and why sampling is important, including a small section on probability.

It then considers the different types of bias that can exist in study design. Finally there is a brief section covering power and its importance in research.

One of the key issues of any research is how to choose the sample to be studied. The sample, a subset of a population, has to be representative of the population in question otherwise the results will be biased and not represent the population parameter. A parameter is a figure that is derived from the whole population. Samples are collected because it is usually not possible to collect data from the whole population, even when it is small. The population does not refer to the population as a whole but rather is the set of individuals or items from which the sample is taken. For example, if a researcher was interested in quality of life after a heart attack in the UK, the population would be all heart attack patients in the UK, and it is from this population that the sample would be taken. If we provide figures from a sample they are statistics.

Parameters are very rarely known for a number of reasons. The main issue mentioned above is the inability to include all the population due to the huge task of tracking down and collecting data on every single person in the population. Another concern is the ethical issue of using the population when we know a sample would give an efficient estimate. There are also issues relating to the identification of the subjects that could affect the ability to collect the whole population. Let us consider individuals with prostate cancer; some people die who have prostate cancer that has never been diagnosed, so how can we include them? Finally, the transient nature of the population of interest can give problems. If we look at breast cancer, in England and Wales there are roughly 110 new cases every day and 30 deaths, so the breast cancer population changes on a day-to-day basis.

Because of these issues relating to collecting data from a population we take a smaller number of cases and assume that they are representative of the population, i.e. we sample.

## Randomness and probability

In a random event each possibility is equally likely to occur, so it is impossible to predict the outcome with any degree of certainty.

The probability (likelihood an event will occur) can easily be worked out using the following formula, which is sometimes referred to as Laplace's law:

$$\text{Probability} = \frac{\text{The number of ways an event can occur}}{\text{The total number of possible outcomes}}$$

The result always gives a figure between 0, representing an impossible outcome, and 1, representing a certain outcome.

Taking the simple experiment of tossing a coin; if we want to predict the possibility of a head, then there is 1 possible way this might occur (the head landing face side up) and two possible outcomes, a head or a tail showing. Therefore the probability of a head following a coin toss is 1/2 or 0·5.

Consider the following. A coin is tossed in the air five times, and each time it comes down it is a head. So after five heads in a row, what will the next coin toss produce? We might assume that the next toss will result in a tail because the previous five outcomes were all heads, and six in a row is unlikely. However, the probability of a random event occurring does not in any way depend on what has happened previously, and so the probability is still 0·5. By definition, a random event is one where the observer does not know what the outcome will be. Despite this, it is human nature to look for patterns in totally random events. If you look at Figure 10.1 you will see that some apparent patterns have been highlighted even though the numbers are random.

Let us consider a more complicated problem. What is the probability of rolling a dice and getting a 6? Using the formula above, the probability is 1/6 or approximately 0·17, but what about the probability predicting a sequence of rolls? To work this out we use the multiplication rule. The probability of getting an even number followed by a 6 followed by an even number is $3/6 \times 1/6 \times 3/6 = 9/216$ or 1/24 (0·04). These events are termed *independent* because the result of one event does not affect the outcome of other events.

| | | | | | | | | | | | | | | |
|---|---|---|---|---|---|---|---|---|---|---|---|---|---|---|
| 58 | 06 | 96 | 03 | 51 | 50 | 09 | 96 | 67 | 74 | 08 | 97 | 06 | 71 | 22 |
| 89 | 08 | 40 | 54 | 15 | 03 | 69 | 94 | 98 | 91 | 94 | 21 | 91 | 29 | 06 |
| 91 | 88 | 08 | 83 | 54 | 54 | 13 | 04 | 94 | 67 | 70 | 01 | 31 | 25 | 18 |
| 38 | 66 | 48 | 14 | 30 | 31 | 03 | 96 | 65 | 30 | 53 | 43 | 55 | 20 | 97 |
| 24 | 35 | 69 | 21 | 18 | 55 | 71 | 78 | 54 | 94 | 80 | 58 | 47 | 46 | 48 |
| 45 | 60 | 39 | 34 | 12 | 91 | 57 | 51 | 73 | 08 | 01 | 18 | 58 | 92 | 87 |
| 74 | 04 | 28 | 68 | 68 | 60 | 67 | 37 | 34 | 48 | 22 | 86 | 73 | 51 | 53 |
| 06 | 57 | 05 | 72 | 96 | 97 | 27 | 78 | 55 | 27 | 57 | 77 | 50 | 08 | 68 |
| 24 | 74 | 76 | 86 | 46 | 82 | 64 | 38 | 07 | 30 | 42 | 09 | 48 | 15 | 05 |
| 88 | 81 | 89 | 45 | 85 | 68 | 79 | 50 | 38 | 10 | 80 | 74 | 93 | 23 | 39 |
| 55 | 96 | 15 | 31 | 08 | 60 | 04 | 04 | 98 | 24 | 21 | 81 | 45 | 12 | 83 |
| 50 | 42 | 28 | 55 | 02 | 16 | 49 | 48 | 46 | 14 | 72 | 41 | 83 | 08 | 56 |
| 50 | 72 | 79 | 30 | 45 | 88 | 47 | 51 | 44 | 73 | 31 | 99 | 76 | 80 | 18 |
| 58 | 84 | 67 | 26 | 03 | 86 | 96 | 77 | 42 | 59 | 04 | 01 | 58 | 99 | 86 |
| 48 | 07 | 34 | 94 | 44 | 45 | 14 | 79 | 40 | 72 | 48 | 14 | 01 | 05 | 92 |
| 48 | 58 | 32 | 58 | 97 | 87 | 76 | 42 | 29 | 20 | 11 | 83 | 94 | 89 | 92 |
| 48 | 94 | 21 | 60 | 13 | 93 | 48 | 44 | 82 | 39 | 74 | 85 | 68 | 11 | 13 |
| 14 | 78 | 45 | 22 | 08 | 11 | 77 | 20 | 35 | 75 | 41 | 43 | 25 | 31 | 44 |
| 35 | 67 | 95 | 35 | 86 | 02 | 03 | 29 | 35 | 42 | 87 | 53 | 10 | 18 | 46 |
| 95 | 44 | 89 | 14 | 56 | 52 | 25 | 47 | 96 | 79 | 52 | 04 | 59 | 73 | 04 |

**Figure 10.1** • Table of random numbers.

Carrying on with the gambling theme, let us move over to cards and look at the probability of picking a red card from the deck. There are 26 red cards and 52 cards in total, so the probability of picking a red card randomly from the pack is $26/52 = 1/2$ or $0.5$. If we want to predict the possibility of two people each picking a red card from the same deck the probability is $26/52 \times 25/51 = 650/2652$ or $0.245$. Note the difference here from the previous example. Because the first person picks a red card the second person has only 25 red cards left and 51 cards in total to pick from. This is because the events are *dependent*. The first event affects the outcome of subsequent events.

## Sampling

The first stage of effective sampling is to define the population precisely and then construct a sampling frame. The ideal sampling frame is a list including all of the items/people that you are trying to sample. So, for a study investigating radiography practitioners working in the UK, a comprehensive list of all UK-based practitioners would be ideal. In practice the ideal hardly ever exists. In this case the closest we could probably get is the UK Health Professions Council (HPC) register. The list, if we could get permission to access it, would not be perfect as it would include practitioners taking a sabbatical, those who have recently retired or are maintaining their registration but working abroad.

## Sample bias

If the data collected are not representative of the population, then the population estimates will not be accurate and we say that the sample is *biased*. The selected sample is in some way systematically different to the population. There are a number of reasons why a sample may be biased:

- The first and most obvious reason is if the sample size is too small. If the sample size is too small it will not produce a reliable estimate of the population. This is explained further in the section on power calculations.
- Another factor to consider is the sampling method. There are various methods of sampling, some of which are better than others at obtaining a representative sample of the population and reducing bias.

## Sampling methods

### Random sampling

The idea behind random sampling is to remove bias so every subject has an equal chance of inclusion/exclusion in the study. There are a number of ways of performing the randomization process, some practicable, some not so practicable. Some types of sampling are detailed below, but this list is not exhaustive.

### Simple random sampling

If we were interested in investigating the patients' perception of the care received during their visit to casualty, a list of all patients who had attended casualty could be obtained from the Picture Archiving and Communication (PAC) system during the timeframe in question. A random sample could be obtained by each name being written on a piece of paper, placed in a drum and then randomly drawn.

A better approach would be to use a table of random numbers. Each patient would be given a number and the patients would be selected by matching numbers generated from the table. The table is random and so it does not matter where you start or in which direction you move. Assuming there were 820 patients available to the study, we could start at the top left corner of Figure 10.1 and reading down move from right to left, so the first number generated would be 589, the next 891, then 008, 688 … and so on. Patients 589, 008 and 688 would then be approached to join the study. There was no patient 891 as there were only 820 patients in total so any number above 820 would be ignored. This process, although still time-consuming, is better than the first option proposed, but is still only really suitable for studies of relatively small size.

Another issue that it is important to consider is when we want to allocate subjects to groups, for example if we want to produce two subject groups, one to receive the intervention and the other the placebo or alternative intervention. Again we would like to remove selection bias and have a system of allocating patients to the groups which is random, and again using the random numbers table allows us to do this.

Again let us make an assumption, this time that we want 24 subjects randomly allocated into two groups. We arbitrarily pick a starting point on the random numbers table and we have decided to move down and then along each block from left to right. The data selected are shown with a shaded background in Figure 10.1.

| 60 | 04 | 04 | 96 | 24 | 16 | 49 | 48 | 46 | 14 | 88 | 47 | 51 |
|----|----|----|----|----|----|----|----|----|----|----|----|----|
| P  | P  | X  | P  | P  | P  | I  | P  | P  | P  | P  | I  | I  |

| 44 | 73 | 86 | 96 | 77 | 42 | 59 | 45 | 14 | 79 | 40 | 72 |
|----|----|----|----|----|----|----|----|----|----|----|----|
| P  | I  | P  | P  | I  | P  | I  | I  | P  | I  | P  | P  |

**Figure 10.2** • Random numbers and sample sequence.

The numbers selected are then used to code which group they will belong to; odds go in the intervention group (I) and even into the placebo group (P). The randomization using the data in the figure would mean the allocation of subjects as shown in Figure 10.2.

The method is simple and random, but can give rise to uneven sizes of the groups, particularly in small trials, which can be a problem as if you calculated the sample size for the study it would have assumed equal group size. In the example above twice as many subjects were allocated to the placebo group compared with the intervention group.

### Block randomization sampling

Block randomization overcomes the problem of the different number of subjects in different arms of the trial by keeping the subjects balanced throughout the study. The blocks can be any size, but are usually a multiple of the number of treatments. If we use blocks with a size of four we get six possible ways of assigning the two possible (placebo or intervention) treatments keeping the balance between treatments equal (Figure 10.3).

| 1 | 2 | 3 |
|---|---|---|
| I, I, P, P | I, P, I, P | I, P, P, I |
| **4** | **5** | **6** |
| P, P, I, I | P, I, P, I | P, I, I, P |

**Figure 10.3** • Block randomization.

The allocation sequence is then decided by using the random numbers table to decide the sequence of the blocks. If we read horizontally on the table starting at the top left position we get the figures 5, 8, 0, 6, 9, 6, 0, 3, 5, 1 so the selection of the 24 patients is as shown in Figure 10.4. Note how we now have 12 subjects in each arm of the trial. This method can be further refined by varying the block length.

### Stratified sampling

Stratified sampling is a further development of block randomization. It is used when it is important to achieve a balance between important characteristics in the subjects. A separate block randomization is carried out for the important characteristic. If we were comparing alternative treatments for reducing stress in radiography practitioners, for example, it might be important to stratify by gender. Each gender would have its own block randomization, so each gender would be equally distributed between the two different treatments.

### Purposeful sampling

***Snowball sampling*** is a technique for developing a research sample where existing study subjects suggest further recruits to take part in the study from among their acquaintances. It is of particular use when the researcher is studying a hidden population, a population with no sampling frame.

***Judgement sampling*** is where the researcher actively selects the subjects they believe will be

| 5 | 6 | 6 | 3 | 5 | 1 |
|---|---|---|---|---|---|
| P, I, P, I | P, I, I, P | P, I, I, P | I, P, P, I | P, I, P, I | I, I, P, P |

**Figure 10.4** • Sample sequence.

the most productive sample to answer the research question. This can be done via a framework looking at the possible variables that might influence a subject's contribution to the study.

*Convenience sampling* is where you sample subjects easiest to reach and is generally considered as being the poorest way of getting a study sample, having the lowest credibility since the subjects are selected arbitrarily.

# Error and bias

*Bias* refers to a systematic error whereas *errors* refers to a difference between the observed value and the true value. Random errors can be reduced by increasing the sample size. Systematic errors are independent of study size.

Consider the example of an ionization chamber being used to measure dose. If the chamber was incorrectly positioned for one reading we would have a random error and as the sample size is increased this value would have less effect on the mean reading. If, however, the wrong chamber factor was given to the researcher, this would affect all the readings, moving them in one direction (higher or lower), and the number of readings taken would not affect the results. With the systematic error all readings are affected to the same degree and the bias will not be apparent when looking at the data, but we might spot the random error as it might be very different to all the other readings. This is why it is important to look at the data before you start your analysis. You can simply look at the figures to see if one stands out as being different or you could do some simple plots to check the data to see if there are any outliers. This check should always be done as it also highlights errors that occur when you input the data. Another way to reduce error coming in at this stage of the process is to carry out double entry of the data.

There are various types of bias that can be introduced into a study, some of which have already been mentioned. The types of bias a study is open to will depend on the type of study and how well the study was performed.

## Recall bias

This was a problem identified with case-control studies in the epidemiology section (Chapter 9) which relies on subjects remembering an event in their past.

A subject's recall is thought to be dependent on their disease status, the exposure, even if irrelevant, being remembered better by cases than controls, so leading to exposure being under-reported by the controls. This can be exacerbated by certain issues such as the patient's preconceptions about the link between exposure and disease. These in turn can sometimes be influenced by the media which may emphasize links between certain exposure to certain factors and the related health outcome.

## Selection bias

Selection bias can occur in two ways: firstly when the researcher selects a sample or a study to support a particular argument or hypothesis, and secondly by self-selection of individuals to participate in a study. The bias can occur in the selection of both the study and the control groups.

Figure 10.5 shows an example of selection bias in an unpublished study. All patients attending for radiotherapy were asked to join the study which was in two parts: a short interview and a follow-up questionnaire. If patients decided not to join the study they were asked if they would mind giving their age. The study was looking at factors affecting age of presentation. You can clearly see that the subjects who dropped out of the study tended to be younger than those who were included in the study, and that patients refusing to take part in the study were older than those who completed all parts of the study, a pattern repeated in both arms of the study.

## Response bias

This is a type of bias that can affect the results of a survey. Because of the way the questions are asked respondents may answer in a way they think the questioner wants them to answer, rather than what they actually think. This usually occurs if the questions are leading, but can also occur due to social desirability: if a respondent knows that there is an established social norm they will tend to respond accordingly.

An example of a badly phrased question is shown below. It leads the respondent to an affirmative answer even if they disagree – the way the question is phrased makes you want to say yes.

'Don't you agree that radiography practitioners should earn more money?'

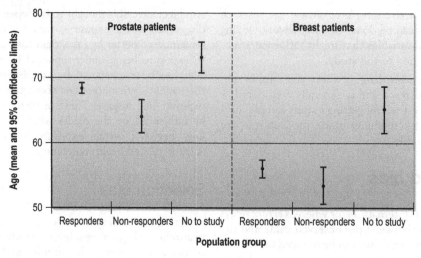

**Figure 10.5** • Age of subjects eligible for study.

## Observer bias

The bias here is with the researcher(s). This occurs when the researchers know the aim(s) of the study and allow this knowledge to influence their observations. In research the effect of observer bias can be removed by carrying out a specific type of study, a *double blind* study. This is a study where neither the researchers nor the participants know which arm of the trial the subject is in. Note that there is also something called *observer effect* which is different to observer bias. This occurs when subjects change their behaviour because they know they are being watched.

This list is not exhaustive and other types of bias occur. Another area where bias exists is in scientific publications that can be used to support or refute work. Example of bias that occur here are:

- *Publication bias*: the predisposition of journals to accept for publication studies that have a positive finding. Again this can be exacerbated by authors, who can have a tendency to only submit articles with a positive outcome.
- *Reporting bias*: the tendency of authors in studies that have multiple outcomes to only report the outcomes that are significant and ignore the non-significant outcomes.

## Power calculations

A frequently encountered problem in quantitative research is deciding how big a sample needs to be to find a 'reliable' result. The smaller a sample is,

the less likely it is that if you repeated the sampling you would find you had the same result and the less reliable it is. On the other hand you do not want to waste time and resources collecting unnecessary data when a smaller sample would give a sufficiently reliable result. In reality this only applies to instances when it is feasible to repeat the exercise (such as handing out a questionnaire) but it is possible to extend the idea to non-repeatable samples as well in an imaginary way. So how do you measure reliability? Information on reliability and validity is given later in this chapter.

When a decision is made to reject a null hypothesis it can be made on the basis that the p-value falls in a particular range of values (fixed level testing). One way to measure reliability could be to look at how often you would make the correct decision for a given significance level. This is what power calculations try to do.

There are four possible outcomes to a fixed level hypothesis test:

1. You accept the null hypothesis incorrectly.
2. You accept the null hypothesis correctly.
3. You reject the null hypothesis incorrectly.
4. You reject the null hypothesis correctly.

Power calculations work out the chance of the last possibility occurring. Notice that this does not consider all of the times that you might be correct in accepting the null hypothesis (case no. 2) so they do not consider all of the ways that you could make the correct choice, only one of them (see also Chapter 15).

There are ways in which power calculations are useful:

- They can be done before a study starts in order to predict how big a sample needs to be to give a result of a required reliability (sampling requires time so this is a way of figuring out how little you have to do in order to get a 'good' result). This is called an *a priori calculation*.
- They can be done after a sample has been performed to see how reliable it is (maybe a much smaller number of questionnaires were returned than you wanted and you want to find out how worthwhile it is to use the limited number that you have). This is called a *post hoc calculation*.

Trying to collect new data once an original sample has proved insufficient can be problematic as it involves more time and there are potential problems with dependency (i.e. one answer affecting another, for example if subjects in the group you are sampling have talked about the research before you sample the second time).

The best way to use power calculations is as an a priori tool to try to predict how effective certain sample sizes will be. When collecting data using questions with human subjects there will always be problems about compliance. When conducting studies over a period of time, subjects may also drop out (failing to complete the study). This can to some extent be corrected for by trying to predict the rates at which data might be lost and combining this with information from power calculations to find out how big a sample should be to leave data that give a reliable result. For example, a patient satisfaction survey might generate one return for every two patients in which case the sample needs to be twice the size of the sample calculated by a power calculation in order to achieve the required reliability.

It is important to realize that if you have obtained ethical approval for a study then there are ethical issues surrounding the failure to collect enough data as this may involve waste of resources and misuse of subjects (especially if the study is patient based).

The 'power' of a test is often given as a percentage. The higher the percentage is, the better the chance that your findings will be reliable. For example, the power of a test may be calculated as 80%. This means that if the sampling was repeated many times then for 80% of those occasions the null hypothesis would be correctly rejected. By now you will hopefully have spotted that this is a *probability of making the correct choice* (for 80% $P = 0.8$ – it is just two different ways of writing the same thing). A very important point

here is that because it is a probability it cannot tell you about the exact occasions when you make the right or wrong choice, only how likely it is.

In addition to a decision about what level of reliability you will accept you will also need to have an idea of what constitutes a 'significant' change or difference for your study. For example if you are trying to find out whether recovery rates following treatment are improving, at what point does a change of a significant size occur? Finally you will need to have an idea of the amount of spread in your data. If it is an a priori calculation you will need some estimate (maybe from a pilot study). This will need to be expressed in terms of standard deviation in order to perform the calculation. While it is possible to manually perform power calculations, the theory is heavily reliant on maths. In practice these calculations are performed using statistics software packages which you can do yourself or you can go to a statistician who can do them for you.

## Reliability and validity

Two other terms are often used in statistics are *reliability* and *validity*. Reliability seeks to describe the consistency or repeatability of the measurement whereas validity refers to the strength of the conclusions drawn. In order for a study to be 'good' it must be both valid and reliable – neither by itself is enough.

To illustrate this many authors refer to a metaphor of darts, as described and shown in Figure 10.6. Four

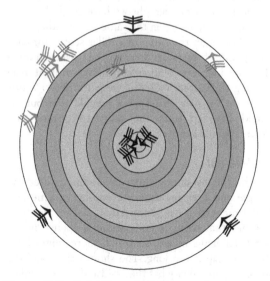

**Figure 10.6** • Reliability and validity metaphor.

people have thrown three darts each at the board, each person using a different colour, and we are interested in how far on average they are from the bull. Two people (grey and black darts) have managed to group the darts closely together, i.e. they have both been consistent and *reliable*. Two people could also be described as being accurate (black and purple darts), the average of both of these colours being the bull which equates to validity. Only one person (black darts) has been consistent and accurate, reliable and valid and this is what we should be aiming for in our research. The remaining person (mauve darts) has been neither accurate nor consistent, so is lacking both reliability and validity. But how do we know if we have a reliable and valid study?

## Reliability

There are four common types of reliability: the *inter-observer reliability*, *test–retest reliability*, *split-halves reliability* and *parallel forms reliability*. Each is briefly described below; at the end of each description there is a test quoted which is a common report of the type of reliability described.

### Inter-observer reliability

In this instance the questionnaire is tested by a number of people or judges before being given to the test population. For example, if we wanted to know if a form was good at distinguishing between good and bad radiographs we could ask three experienced practitioners to each use the tool to examine a number of different radiographs we have given them. As they are all reporting on the same set of radiographs they should get the same or similar scores for each radiograph. If the raters do not agree with each other all is not lost; we could retest the instrument after training the testers to see if we get a better score. If we do we may still have a reliable tool but we would have to train the users to ensure this. Test: Cohen's kappa.

### Test–retest

For this the test or questionnaire is administered to a sample and then re-administered after a time gap. The time gap is very important as the approach assumes that there is no substantial change in the construct being measured which there might be if the time gap is too long. Too short a time and the subjects remember what they said and try to emulate their first response. Test: Bland–Altman plot/test.

### Split halves test

The test is only given once and then the test is divided into equivalent halves; a Pearson's correlation is then calculated on between the scores from each half of the test. The closer the scores between the two halves, the better the internal consistency. Test: Correlation.

### Parallel forms reliability

This is used to assess the consistency of the results of two tests that have been constructed in the same way. A large set of questions first needs to be produced that measure the same construct. A major problem with this approach is that a lot of items that reflect the same construct have to be generated. The questions are then randomly divided into two sets and both instruments administered concurrently to the same sample. Test: Correlation.

## Validity

Again, as with reliability validity there are different types of validity. Two types are internal validity and external validity.

*Internal validity* asks the basic question, 'Did the experiment make a difference?' Another way of saying this is, 'Was the experiment carried out in such a way that we are confident that the independent variable altered the dependent variable?', i.e. how confident are we about the cause and effect? Establishing internal validity can be threatened by a number of issues, such as confounding variables, outside influences/events, regression towards the mean and attrition from the study.

Whereas internal validity is concerned with causality in the sample group studied, *external validity* is concerned with how the results can be generalized to the population. The main threats to external validity are the sample itself, sampling method and time. For example, if a study was performed looking at radiography practitioners' perception of continuing professional development and the study was conducted predominantly using newly qualified radiographers, or the data were collected during a year when the HPC audit to monitor radiographer registrants' compliance, these conditions would both affect external validity. In the first instance ensuring a random sample from all radiographers would help reduce the threat; in the latter instance a replication of the study would help eliminate the threat and demonstrate the generalizability of the results.

## Construct validity

Construct validity relates to a survey instruments, questionnaires or tests and gauges how well we might expect the tool to perform at measuring what we think it is measuring. Do not get confused here – it is not referring to how well the questionnaire is constructed. A construct is the attribute, proficiency, ability or skill that is being measured. Three variants of construct validity are briefly described below.

### Convergent validity

This relates to the degree to which the test is similar to (converges on) other tests that it theoretically should be similar to. For instance, to show the convergent validity of a questionnaire that purports to measure fatigue, we could compare the scores to a second fatigue test; high correlations would be evidence of convergent validity.

### Discriminant validity

This is almost the opposite of the above. It is validity obtained when we measure two constructs that are thought to be dissimilar and the measures can discriminate between them. For instance, to show the discriminant validity of a spatial ability test, we might compare the scores with a test that looks at intelligence. Low correlations would be evidence of discriminant validity.

### Nomological validity

This is the final criterion for construct validity and refers to the degree to which the construct fits into the existing evidence of a theory. It is a qualitative assessment that looks at both the construct in question and existing contructs for logical consistency and cannot be tested for statistically.

## Further reading

Altman DG. Practical Statistics for Medical Research. London: Chapman and Hall; 1991.

Bland M. An Introduction to Medical Statistics. 3rd ed. Oxford: Oxford University Press; 2000.

Mosteller F. Fifty Challenging Problems in Probability: With Solutions. New York: Dover Publications; 1987.

Petrie A, Sabin S. Medical Statistics at a Glance. 2nd ed. Oxford: Wiley Blackwell; 2005.

## Web resources

*There are a number of web pages that deal with sampling and probability, including some with Java applications. A nice one looks at coin tosses and shows how the percentage of heads varies with the number of tosses, but starts to approximate the true probability with more coin tosses:* http://bcs.whfreeman.com/ips4e/cat_010/applets/Probability.html.

*Another useful resource on the web is random number generators:* http://www.random.org/integers/

# Research outcome measures

11

Fiona Mellor   Karen Knapp

## CHAPTER POINTS

- Outcome measures play an integral part in evidence based clinical practice, research and patient care.
- The selection of an appropriate outcome measure will depend upon your research question.
- There is a multitude of validated and reliable outcome measures available to the researcher and practitioner; some outcome measures have data from healthy populations allowing for comparison.
- PROMs are a valuable and increasingly used tool in today's NHS.
- Care needs to be taken in the collection of appropriate data, controlling of confounders, analysis and reporting of multiple outcome measures to reduce the possibility of type 1 errors.

This chapter will describe ways of measuring the outcome of your research using existing tools, and explain why it is important to measure the outcome of your research in a universal and standardized way.

An outcome is defined by the *Oxford English Dictionary* as a consequence, or result; therefore an outcome measure is a standardized way of measuring the result. In other words, it is a way of assessing the type and amount of change of the dependent variable, or assessing the effect. The British Paediatric Association (BPA) Outcome Measures Working Group stated that outcome measures are 'measures where the change is known (or at least believed) to be attributable to an intervention',[1] or in other words, the outcome measure is the measurement of the change brought about by your manipulation of the independent variable. Outcome measures are used in both quantitative and qualitative research with many outcome measures taking the form of questionnaires. Thus outcome measures are used to:

- discriminate between patients with differing disease severity at any one point in time
- predict patient outcome
- evaluate change following an intervention.

The need for universal outcome measures in health care comes from the fact that many existing studies demonstrate wide geographic variations in the practice of medicine and research, but comparing these differences is difficult as measurements and reporting of results are different, thus direct comparisons will lead to erroneous conclusions and hinder the understanding of the appropriateness and quality of the medical intervention or diagnostic test.[2] A researcher who attempts to relate two similar studies with differing methods of measuring the result will fall foul of the popular idiom 'comparing apples with oranges'.

Wilson and Cleary[3] state that there are five types of outcomes that may be measured:

1. biological/physiological variables (e.g. ranges of motion, radiographic changes)
2. symptoms status (e.g. pain)
3. functional status (e.g. return to work)
4. general health perceptions (e.g. various aspects of global health)
5. quality of life (general well-being, patient satisfaction).

All these measures are important for a full understanding of the patient's condition. However, in practice it is not necessary to use them all; for instance, in back pain the most important outcomes are generally accepted to be symptoms and pain.[4] It is therefore important for you to determine the most important and frequently measured outcomes for the topic you intend to research by looking at previously similar studies, and include this in your research proposal.

Outcome measures are widely used in many settings including experimental research, clinical audit, clinical practice and economic assessment. As already stated, they provide a common language for reporting and allow comparisons to be made with previous results as well as nationally across sites. They are used in clinical practice by practitioners to assess their management plan and make informed decisions as to whether other directions or additional treatment should be undertaken.[5] They can also be used by patients to assess their own symptoms and function over time[6] in which case they are known as *patient reported outcome measures* (PROMs) which, as we will see, are becoming increasingly important in today's NHS. On a wider scale, outcome measures can also be used to assess quality of life and satisfaction of treatment of larger study groups which feed into providing valuable economic data on the most cost-effective methods of diagnosis and treatment.

There are a number of ways of measuring change. Some outcomes are of a very broad and widespread nature such as quality of life, which is made up of both physical and psychological components, while others are more specific, such as mortality, for which there are just two possible answers. Generally, an outcome measure will already exist for the condition that is to be measured and you are therefore advised against developing your own tool to measure your results, such as making up a questionnaire, since testing the validation and reliability is complicated. There is no need to reinvent the wheel when looking for ways to measure your results, and indeed, using an already existing outcome measure will allow you to make comparisons to previous studies and therefore make your data more valuable.

Of course the challenge in research is to ensure the selected outcome measure truly reflects the change intended to be measured. For example, a scale measuring pain may be broad enough to include both acute and chronic pain, or focused enough to measure just one aspect of pain. If you are interested purely in comparing the efficacy of one intervention to manage immediate postoperative pain, then a scale that measures both chronic and acute pain is likely to be misleading, as is a scale measuring chronic pain only.

So how do you select the most relevant outcome measure? There is a plethora of online databases that list outcome measures ranging from those which are free to use and simple to administer through to more complicated and intricate measures that require specialist analysis. It is your responsibility as the lead researcher to know whether the intended outcome measure is free to use and distribute or whether permission is needed to comply with copyright laws.

While it is important to consider outcome measures used in previous similar research, it is also essential to ensure that your selected outcome measure is acceptable to both practitioner and patient, quick and simple to use, reliable, specific to the question being investigated and cost-effective. Longer, complicated, more involved outcome measures may collect full and comprehensive data but will demand a greater input from the respondent, and correspondingly a more thorough analysis which may be beyond the scope of your research project. Conversely, basic simple analogue scales may not provide enough information to quantify the results and appropriately report differences within or between groups. Failing to detect such differences increases your risk of making a *type II error*, which means stating there is no difference and accepting the null hypothesis when there is in fact a difference. Hence, as you can see, the ideal outcome measure will provide the most comprehensive information but not induce fatigue or be so short it misses vital points. The challenge is for you to decide which outcome measure best suits your research and resources, bearing in mind that in most cases the ideal measurement may not exist.

Consequently, selecting the appropriate instrument is very important in order to reflect a comprehensive understanding of the condition and a thorough knowledge of the expected benefits and harms of the proposed intervention.[7] Therefore the choice of outcome measure should align itself with the aims of your study.

Outcome measures are a greatly valued tool in today's healthcare model. They are vital for setting the standards of care and thus it is essential that the right tool is selected. They provide a valuable opportunity for enhanced communication between patient and practitioner and set a standard for monitoring by allowing data to be pooled. The use of standardized outcome measures (particularly PROMs, as discussed later in this chapter) was identified as crucial by Professor Lord Darzi in his 2008 report *High Quality Care for All*[8] in an NHS which encourages patient choice and interaction and demands value for money from treatments and interventions.

# Types of outcome measure

There are various ways of detecting change: outcome measures may be objective or subjective, quantitative or qualitative; they may be used directly or indirectly, by the patient, practitioner or researcher; and measured over differing periods of time. They may be concerned with just one aspect, such as pain (uni-dimensional), or they may be multi-dimensional and look at many facets, such as physical, emotional and social well-being. They may relate to one condition only (disease-specific), or be more generic. This next section will describe the differences between all these types of outcome measure and help you choose which one is most suitable for your research.

Disease-specific outcome measures exist for most known conditions and are highly focused, relevant and appropriate; however, they do not allow data to be collected from healthy populations who do not have the disease. Therefore comparison between 'normal' and 'abnormal' is not possible. In contrast, generic outcome measures are applicable to the widest range of health interventions and conditions. Most generic measures are therefore also multi-dimensional and have the added advantage of being applicable to healthy populations, allowing comparisons to be made. It is therefore important to consider the populations on whom you intend to undertake your research and measurements as well as the condition you intend to measure as determined in your original research question.

In many cases, one outcome measure alone will be sufficient; however, in large multi-centred studies this may not have sufficient breadth even if multi-dimensional, in which case a combination of measures is needed. In the latter scenario, it is wise to utilize one outcome measure as the primary outcome, which answers the main research question, and additional measures as secondary, which allow consideration of combined outcomes, thus providing a fuller picture. However, using more than one outcome measure requires a lot of time and input from both the respondents and the practitioner, and so it is not recommended you use more than one outcome measure in your undergraduate research (see Using outcome measures in study design).

While the role of an outcome measure is to objectively answer a question, such as 'Is it getting better or worse?' The answer to the outcome measure may still be subjective. The majority of validated and reliable outcome measures (such as questionnaires) have accounted for this by cross-validation and cross-correlation with existing measures that investigate the same condition, but it is worth noting that some variables cannot be accounted for. The only true objective outcome measures are those that can be physiologically measured (such as temperature, blood pressure, etc.). These are also uni-dimensional measures, but unfortunately these do not tell us much about the wider consequences of the intervention or treatment.

For instance, it is accepted that stress can increase blood pressure; however, using blood pressure alone to measure stress will not only omit the wider aspects that are subjective (such as sensory, emotional and cognitive features), but will also be prone to confounding variables as there are many factors other than stress that also influence blood pressure. Nevertheless, in some participants/patients it is necessary to use such substitute measures as other options such as questionnaires cannot be implemented. For example, measuring the stress response of premature neonates may be done via blood pressure monitoring. Where there are many confounders it is wise to combine this with other measures that also indicate stress such as crying time, and this is one instance where you may use more than one outcome measure in your research.

Radiographic scoring methods are also uni-dimensional and are often used in the assessment of onset and progression of joint disease/degeneration, for which numerous methods exist.[9] But while the scoring methods are qualitative, it is wise to remember the completion of them is subjective. Therefore it is preferable to have more than one independent assessor if you intend to use such scales. You can then calculate agreement between observers which will add strength to your results and remove observer bias.

Many outcome measures are questionnaire based. An outcomes questionnaire may be completed by the practitioner, researcher, patient or carer, and all could give differing answers to the same question. Therefore be aware of who is answering the questions (for example, asking a clinician about a patient's recovery may result in completely different answer than asking the patient about their own recovery). To overcome this, many outcome measures are now directed specifically at patients with the aim of understanding the full impact of treatments/interventions from their perspective. These are called *patient reported outcome measures* (PROMs). PROMs are beginning to play a much more active role in today's NHS as patient assessment is a key mechanism in improving the quality of care in the NHS.[8] PROMs currently exist for a range of conditions including asthma, diabetes and stroke.

A widely used, multi-dimensional, generic, PROM is the Medical Outcomes Study Short Form 36-Item Health Survey (SF-36),[10] which measures health-related quality of life. The World Health Organization defines quality of life as the perception of the individual regarding his/her present life situation, including objectives, expectations, patterns and preoccupations.[11] Therefore, quality of life encompasses aspects related to health plus those that have an influence on it, such as social, cultural and economic facets.[12]

The SF-36 covers eight domains (physical functioning, role physical, role emotional, bodily pain, vitality, mental health, social functioning and general health), each of which are scored on an individual scale and then combined to produce an overall score. The SF-36 has been implemented to define disease conditions, determine the effect of treatment, differentiate the effect of different treatments, and compare conditions with other medical conditions.[13] The popularity of the SF-36 (and SF-12) is due in part to its widely tested validity and reliability. In addition, data from 'healthy' populations are available, allowing comparisons of the health status of patient groups to be compared with the general population.[14]

The one problem with interpreting PROMs is distinguishing how much movement on the scale equates to a clinically meaningful change. While scores on scales can be subject to rigorous statistical analysis, a statistically significant difference may not equate to a clinically meaningful change for the patient. The statistical test used to determine whether an effect is likely to be due to chance or not is based largely on sample size. Hence, with sufficient power a small change can be statistically significant but clinically meaningless, and conversely, the opposite may also be true. For many physiological measurements, such as temperature or blood pressure, experience and clinical judgement informs whether the results are clinically meaningful, but more subjective measurements, such as pain or stress, are much harder to define.[15]

The concept of the minimally clinically important difference (MCID) is defined as the smallest improvement considered worthwhile by the patient.[16] MCID, also known as a clinically significant improvement, is a relative newcomer to outcome measures and many of the well known measures do not have published MCIDs.[17] However, in the current climate of evidence-based practice, a measure of the impact of treatment of individual patients is of more benefit than a statistical measure based on group summary statistics.

The aims of your audit, research or assessment will determine which particular outcome measure you select and it is obviously recommended that you select those which are currently well known and used as well as making sure your selected outcome measure relates to your particular research question.

# Using outcome measures in study design

Consideration of outcome measures is integral to any research study design and, as already stated, it is usual to focus on just one outcome measure as the centre of the study. This is often termed the 'primary outcome measure'. While it is also possible to consider multiple secondary outcome measures, the findings of these need to be given less importance in the interpretation of the analyses, since using many measures means that statistically one may be significant just by chance. Collecting data on multiple outcome measures and then determining the primary outcome measure during the analysis, based on the most significant results of data collected, is poor practice. There is a risk that no significant outcomes will be measured by a study using such methodologies. Similarly, presenting only the significant outcome measures and ignoring those which were not significant (thus presenting your data as if you only used the significant outcome measure) is fraudulent must be avoided.[18]

By focusing on one primary outcome measure the study can be designed to maximize the possibility of clinical and statistical significance of the chosen measure. Many studies are published in which the sample size is too small to verify the hypothesis one way or the other. For example, many studies investigating the effect of depot medroxyprogesterone acetate (DMPA), a long-acting injectable contraceptive, on the bone health of adolescent girls contain small numbers. This is primarily as a result of large dropout (attrition) rates over the study period and they contain numbers so small at the end-point that the data fail to reach a significant level, making it difficult to draw robust conclusions from the findings.[19,20]

To overcome such problems, a power calculation can be utilized to ensure an adequate sample size to ensure the study is likely to provide significant results. The basic data required for a power calculation needs to be collated from previous research published in the literature. If there are no data available to support the study design, it is advisable to undertake a pilot study to achieve a better understanding of the possible differences or changes in outcome measures for the study (information on power calculation can be found in Chapter 10).

Power calculations are an important part of study design and without using a power calculation the study results may not provide statistically significant findings. Alternatively, too many subjects may be recruited or measurements taken, which results in wasted time and resources. It is for these reasons that many grant funding bodies and research ethics committees require a power calculation included in the study proposals they are considering. Different outcome measures will require differing sample sizes and it is important to focus any power calculations on the appropriate outcome measure, including the expected statistical and minimally clinically important differences between groups or levels of change. If you are designing a longitudinal study over a period of months or years, it is always a good idea to note the attrition rates in previous studies and you may wish to increase your baseline recruitment by the mean attrition rate to ensure there are sufficient subjects included in the study to provide robust data at the end-point.

## Confounders

It is important to consider extraneous, uncontrolled independent variables, or *confounders*, when designing a study and selecting your outcome measure. These often include patient demographics such as height, weight, age, sex, race, but might also include a multitude of other variables such as stage of disease, co-morbidity, signs and symptoms, duration of disease, and type of imaging equipment used.[21] For example, the baseline group characteristics for the data are displayed and outlined in Table 11.1.[22] When analysing these data it was important to note a difference in age

between the vertebral fracture cases and controls. Since bone density reduces with age in normal and osteoporotic subjects, merely calculating the odds ratio without any adjustment for age would have led to an over-estimation of the discrimination of fracture cases from controls. Therefore age adjustment was required in the analysis to correct for this problem. Consequently you must consider confounders to your selected outcome measures during the study design so the appropriate data are collected and are available for the data analysis, or analysis techniques to mitigate differences can be employed.

# Common outcome measures in diagnostic imaging and radiotherapy

Rapid advances in diagnostic imaging and therapeutic intervention require fast and efficient assessment of new technology. Common outcome measures associated with these are technical performance, diagnostic accuracy, patient quality of life (including patient satisfaction and pain), prognostic and therapeutic effects, morbidity, impact of patient care and cost-effectiveness.[21,23] In radiotherapy research patient survival times and adverse events are also important outcome measures in addition to many of the diagnostic end-points. In-depth examples or explanations of common outcome measures are outlined below.

## Example 1 – diagnostic accuracy

In medical imaging, new techniques and technologies are regularly introduced requiring research to test their ability to detect pathologies or to predict clinical outcomes, cost-effectiveness and patient-centred outcomes (see also Chapter 12). It is of utmost importance to ensure the implementation of new technologies are evidence based and not as a result of subjective perceptions.

One example of such a new technology assessment is for the prediction of future fragility facture risk using methods of bone measurement. If there is already a technique for the diagnosis of the pathology of interest, it is important where possible to directly compare the techniques. The best method is to undertake this within the same patient so they would have two imaging or diagnostic techniques rather than one. However, this is not always practicable or possible.

## Table 11.1 Patient characteristics (mean and SD)

|  | Young normals | Premenopausal | Postmenopausal | Fracture |
|---|---|---|---|---|
| Number | 106 | 236 | 173 | 109 |
| Age (years) | 31.5 (6.1) | 40.3 (9.5) | 59.9* (7.5) | 73.2** (7.5) |
| Height (cm) | 163.7 (17.4) | 163.8 (6.6) | 161.6* (6.8) | 154.2** (8.1) |
| Weight (kg) | 65.0 (14.6) | 65.6 (12.2) | 66.3 (10.5) | 60.4** (13.8) |
| BMI (kg/m$^2$) | 24.1 (4.5) | 24.4 (4.3) | 25.5 (4.1) | 25.2 (4.7) |
| YSM (years) | N/A | N/A | 9.6 (8.3) | 27.6** (11.9) |
| SOS radius (m/sec) | 4154 (106) | 4166 (98) | 4045* (125) | 3915** (144) |
| SOS tibia (m/sec) | 3917 (118) | 3908 (123) | 3810* (156) | 3728** (175) |
| SOS phalanx (m/sec) | 4080 (168) | 4070 (160) | 3886* (195) | 3662** (185) |
| SOS metatarsal (m/sec) | 3731 (225) | 3747 (204) | 3545* (179) | 3375** (240) |
| BMD spine (g/cm$^2$) | 1.037 (0.12) | 1.034 (0.12) | 0.935* (0.14) | 0.758** (0.14) |
| BMD femoral neck (g/cm$^2$) | 0.868 (0.12) | 0.847 (0.12) | 0.764* (0.12) | 0.585** (0.12) |
| BMD total hip (g/cm$^2$) | 0.969 (0.12) | 0.954 (0.13) | 0.899* (0.12) | 0.660** (0.14) |

*$P < 0.01$ vs healthy premenopausal women, **$P < 0.01$ vs healthy postmenopausal women.
SD, standard deviation; BMI, body mass index; YSM, years since menopause; SOS, speed of sound BMD, bone mineral density.

There is also the potential that a combination of the new technique and the old technique can improve the diagnostic accuracy above and beyond either one individually, in which case this needs to be included in the study design and analysis. Secondary outcome measures of such research will often include the radiation dose associated with each of the techniques, the cost of the technique in terms of duration of the technique, cost of the equipment and consumables, how invasive the technique is, and more recently, consumers' satisfaction with the treatment (PROMs). While some lower dose and cheaper techniques may be introduced, they must match or exceed the diagnostic accuracy of the existing gold standard.

For example: bone mineral density measurements of the central skeleton using dual energy X-ray absorptiometry (DXA) are widely considered to be the current gold standard for the diagnosis of osteoporosis.[24] However, there are other cheaper alternatives on the market that do not use ionizing radiation, such as quantitative ultrasound (QUS). The data in Table 11.2[22] are from a cross-sectional study to

## Table 11.2 Fracture discrimination

|  | OR | p-value | 95% CI | AUC |
|---|---|---|---|---|
| SOS |  |  |  |  |
| Radius | 1.4 | 0.03 | 1.03–1.99 | 0.60 |
| Tibia | 1.2 | 0.26 | 0.87–1.66 | 0.60 |
| Phalanx | 2.0 | <0.01 | 1.22–3.23 | 0.60 |
| Metatarsal | 1.5 | 0.05 | 1.01–2.24 | 0.61 |
| BMD |  |  |  |  |
| Spine | 2.6 | <0.01 | 1.70–4.11 | 0.66 |
| Femoral neck | 3.0 | <0.01 | 1.94–4.64 | 0.70 |
| Total hip | 4.8 | <0.01 | 2.81–8.29 | 0.82 |

OR, odds ratio; CI, confidence interval; AUC, area under the curve; SOS, speed of sound; BMD, bone mineral density.
Adapted from Knapp et al.[22]

investigate the ability of DXA and multi-site QUS to discriminate postmenopausal women with one or more vertebral fractures from postmenopausal women without any fragility fractures. The sensitivity (proportion of positives that are correctly identified by the test) and specificity (proportion of negatives that are correctly identified by the test) of a technique can be plotted on a receiver operator characteristic (ROC) curve.[18] The graphs and area under the curve (AUC) can be used to compare two or more techniques, which is where ROC curves prove to be most useful.[3] Other methods of comparing two diagnostic techniques are available and the analysis should be tailored to the type of data collected (see Chapter 8).

The data in Table 11.2 demonstrate the AUC to be greater for DXA compared to the newer QUS, which indicates that QUS is less able than DXA to discriminate those patients with a vertebral fracture from those without. This study indicated that while the QUS did not use ionizing radiation and was cheaper than the DXA scan, its diagnostic ability was inferior and therefore would not be a diagnostic technique of choice if DXA is available. However, the technique may be of use if DXA is not available, since it still demonstrated an ability to identify fracture cases from controls. This study used a cross-sectional design, but prospective studies with measures of many hundreds of patients using fracture as the outcome measure are a more powerful method of performing such technology evaluations. However, these require many more patients and are therefore more costly and time-consuming to undertake. They also require a period of follow-up to see which individuals have fractured and are therefore beyond the scope of an individual undergraduate research project.

## Example 2 – pain

Pain is the primary symptom that prompts people to seek treatment; therefore pain is a common primary outcome measure particularly in musculoskeletal, oncological and orthopaedic diagnosis and treatment. However, pain cannot objectively be detected by biological or physiological means in humans and is further influenced by physiological, psychological, social, cultural and economic factors. Attempts have been made can be made to objectively quantify and measure pain by assessing the amount and time of analgesic consumption, but this method is too crude and sensitivity is affected by memory of time and amount taken, or by availability of nurse/ward round. Therefore attempts to objectively measure pain depend on observations and reports, but there are well known discrepancies between patients, physicians and carers when reporting pain, with carers typically overestimating the amount of pain relief[25] and physicians underestimating the intensity of the pain felt by patients.[26]

Consequently, the measurement of pain as an outcome measure uses subjective scales which are often divided into acute or chronic. Different instruments are used for each aspect, commonly centred on either pain intensity or pain relief. Measurement of pain relief is easier to compare and more convenient as the baseline score is always zero; additionally they are also seen as more sensitive than intensity scales.[27,28]

Despite these inherent problems, a wide variety of tools now exist with which to measure pain, the most familiar being the visual analogue scale (VAS), popularized by Huskisson in the 1970s.[29] This consists of a horizontal (or sometimes vertical) line with 1–10 (or 1–100) points. Zero typically denotes 'no pain', whereas 10 signifies 'worst pain imaginable'. A variation of the VAS for pain relief has zero as the mid-point with end-points being 'maximum improvement' and 'maximum deterioration'. The major advantage of the VAS scale is that they are simple to complete; however, they are more difficult to understand than other measures of pain, particularly in those with impaired cognition such as children, and those taking opioid analgesics. VAS is also a highly subjective scale and is frequently dependent on how much pain a person has experienced in the past. A study of nursing students asked to identify pain, hurt and ache using imagined pain on a VAS reported a wide range of perceptions of the three terms, demonstrating the highly subjective nature of this scale and of the different terminology associated with pain.[30]

Verbal rating scales (VRS) are categorical scales with five points (no pain, mild, moderate, severe, worst possible pain) and were initially developed to assess respondents with impaired cognition or for those who prefer verbal ratings to numerical ratings. Although test–retest reliability for the VRS is high, it cannot be interchanged with the VAS owing to low interscale agreement.[31] However, both scales are valid measures and the choice should depend on the setting, the aims of your study, and the patient's level of education.[32]

Pain drawings are standardized measurements of the locality and quality of the pain and consist of line drawings representing the anterior and posterior body. Patients are asked to shade in the areas where they feel pain and indicate by the use of symbols the type of pain they feel. These kinds of drawings remove any ambiguity between physician and patient and have no language barriers. A variation of the pain drawing is the Faces Pain Scale,[33] originally developed for children but now used across a wide cohort of cognitively impaired patients. This scale is a set of 6–7 faces depicting expressions ranging from happy to crying. Pain drawings show good correlation with other types of pain scales.[4]

As well as simple scales, there are questionnaires intended to provide a more encompassing view of the dimensions of pain, the most popular of these being the McGill Pain Questionnaire (MPQ).[34] This questionnaire was originally used to evaluate pain therapies but has become increasingly used as a diagnostic tool. This questionnaire consists of 78 adjectives arranged in 20 subsets that describe sensory, affective and evaluative aspects of pain. For this reason it is seen as the leading instrument for describing the various dimensions of pain; however, it does require good cognitive skills and takes longer to administer than the scales mentioned above.

Finally, pain may be measured as one dimension in a multi-dimensional outcome measure, such as the SF-36. In this case, the score can be taken alone or combined with the other scores to obtain a quality of life measurement.

## Example 3 – patient satisfaction

The increasing importance of patient focused care recognizes patients' active role in the decision-making process and the notion that clinical decisions should take patients' views and perceptions into account.[35] As already mentioned, medicine is turning away from fully objective assessments of disease and medicine towards more subjective assessments that include the views of patients (PROMs).[36] Of these PROMs, satisfaction and quality of life are very often used.[37]

Satisfaction as an outcome measure focuses more on the patient's judgement of success, acceptability and value of health care received, often with bias towards non-clinical aspects such as communication and convenience. This has become increasingly important to policy makers in the NHS who incorporate such views when designing service delivery. Hence measuring satisfaction is essential to the quality

assurance process. Furthermore, satisfied patients have better health outcomes as they are more positive about their situation and more likely to adhere to treatment regimens.[38]

There are inherent problems with measuring satisfaction, however, not least the inability to control for respondents' expectations, prior experiences and desires. In addition, it is well documented that older respondents report higher levels of satisfaction, though the evidence for differences between other demographics is equivocal. Most studies of how health service features affect satisfaction are observational as it is unethical to manipulate the variables that contribute to quality of care.[38]

Satisfaction may be measured as a uni-dimensional outcome, but it is more often a feature of patient reported multi-dimensional outcome measures, i.e. quality adjusted life years (QALYs), or used as a secondary outcome measure in conjunction with clinical primary outcome measures. There are a number of ways of measuring satisfaction, ranging from observational methods through to direct surveys including questionnaires, interviews and focus groups. These methods all have advantages and disadvantages, and all have issues with validation as no gold standard currently exists. In fact the use of satisfaction as an outcome measure has been contested,[39] but nevertheless remains an important feature of a value-based healthcare system.

For further in depth information on satisfaction as an outcome measure refer to 'The measurement of satisfaction with healthcare: implications for practice from a systematic review of the literature'.[38]

## Example 4 – quality adjusted life years and their use in health care

Resources in the National Health Service (NHS) are finite with increasing technology resulting in greater diagnosis of disease and more diseases being treated. With life expectancy greater than when the NHS was first introduced, the funds are becoming ever more stretched. Therefore, there is a need to provide measurable benefits to patients, in terms of both quality of life and extension of life. With finite resources, the results from outcome measures are used to target the best therapies or preventive measures where they are most likely to make a difference.

QALYs are one method for such evaluation and are based on quality of life changes and/or life expectancy outcomes following healthcare interventions.[40]

QALYs are central to many healthcare decisions and widely used by health economists to evaluate the benefit of treatments versus costs. In the calculation of QALYs, a year of perfect health is equal to 1, and death is equal to zero. A year of less than perfect health is awarded a mark of less than 1, while some outcomes are considered to be worse than death and may be allocated negative values. When these are combined with the cost of treatment, the QALY indicates the cost to provide an additional year of perfect health.

QALYs are used in models to evaluate the cost/benefit of treatment in certain groups, comparing outcomes in patients not treated with those who are treated. If the costs outweigh the benefits then the treatment is not recommended for the population in question. For example, Schousboe et al[41] reviewed the cost-effectiveness of using aledronate,

an anti-resorptive drug currently used in osteoporosis, in postmenopausal women with osteopenia (low bone mass) but who were not considered to have osteoporosis. Costs, quality adjusted life years, and incremental cost-effectiveness ratios were calculated. They found that for women aged 55–75 years, with no additional fracture risk factors, the cost per quality adjusted life year gained ranged from 70 000 to 332 000 dollars. From these results they concluded that alendronate treatment in women falling into this group was not cost-effective.

Equally, with advances in imaging, the ability to diagnose disease earlier is increasing, along with the cost. For example, in diagnosing breast cancer, the cost of a contrast enhanced MRI is 10 times that of a mammogram. This increased cost must bring with it increased diagnostic abilities to be worthwhile.[42]

# References

[1] British Paediatric Association. Outcome Measures for Child Health. London: British Paediatric Association; 1992.

[2] Gerszten P. Outcomes research: a review. Neurosurgery 1998;43 (5):1146–55.

[3] Wilson IB, Cleary PD. Linking clinical variables with health-related quality of life: a conceptual model of patient outcomes. JAMA 1995;273:59–65.

[4] Maire JA. Evaluating the effectiveness of care in neck and back pain: pain and functional status as outcome measures. Australas Chiropr Osteopathy 2002;10 (1):16–20.

[5] Hayes C. The use of patient based outcome measures in clinical decision making. Community Dent Health 1998;15 (1):19–21.

[6] Johnson C. Outcome measures for research and clinical practice. J Manipulative Physiol Ther 2008;31 (5):329–30.

[7] Bryant D, Schünemann H, Brozek J, et al. Patient reported outcomes: general principles of development and interpretability. Pol Arch Med Wewn 2007;117(4):5–11.

[8] Darzi A. High quality care for all: NHS next stage review final report.

London: Department of Health; 2008. p. 92.

[9] Boini S, Guillemin F. Radiographic scoring methods as outcome measures in rheumatoid arthritis: properties and advantages. Ann Rheum Dis 2001;60(9):817–27.

[10] Ware JE, Kosinski M, Gandek B. SF-36. Health Survey: Manual and Interpretation Guide. Rhode Island: Quality Metric Inc; 2000.

[11] World Health Organization. Quality of Life assessment (WHOQOL): position paper from the World Health Organization. Soc Sci Med 1995;41(10):1403–9.

[12] Guyatt G, Feeny D, Patrick D. Measuring health-related quality of life. Ann Intern Med 1993;118 (8):622–9.

[13] Patel A, Donegan D, Albert T. The 36-item short form. J Am Acad Orthop Surg 2007;15(2):126–34.

[14] Busija L, Osborne RH, Nilsdotter A, et al. Magnitude and meaningfulness of change in SF-36 scores in four types of orthopedic surgery. Health Qual Life Outcomes 2008;6:55.

[15] Bolton JE. Sensitivity and specificity of outcome measures in patients with neck pain: detecting clinically significant improvement. Spine 2004;29(21):2410–7.

[16] Stratford PW, Binkley JM, Riddle DL, et al. Sensitivity to change of the Roland-Morris Back Pain Questionnaire: part 1. Phys Ther 1998;78(11):1186–96.

[17] Copay A, Subach BR, Glassman SD, et al. Understanding the minimum clinically important difference: a review of concepts and methods. Spine J 2007;7(5):541–6.

[18] Altman DG. Practical Statistics for Medical Research. London: Chapman and Hall; 1991.

[19] Naessen T, Olsson SE, Gudmundson J. Differential effects on bone density of progestogen-only methods for contraception in premenopausal women. Contraception 1995;52(1):35–9.

[20] Busen NH, Britt RB, Rianon N. Bone mineral density in a cohort of adolescent women using depot medroxyprogesterone acetate for one to two years. J Adolesc Health 2003;32(4):257–9.

[21] Crewson PE, Applegate KE. Data collection in radiology research. Am J Roentgenol 2001;177:755–61.

[22] Knapp KM, Blake GM, Spector TD, et al. Multisite quantitative ultrasound: precision, age- and menopause-related changes, fracture discrimination, and T-score equivalence with

dual-energy X-ray absorptiometry. Osteoporos Int 2001;12(6):456–64.

[23] Hunink MG, Krestin GP. Study design for concurrent development, assessment, and implementation of new diagnostic imaging technology. Radiology 2002;222:604–14.

[24] Blake GM. Fogelman I. The role of DXA bone density scans in the diagnosis and treatment of osteoporosis. Postgrad Med J 2007;83(982):509–17.

[25] Rundshagen I, Schnabel K, Standl T, et al. Patients' vs nurses' assessments of post operative pain and anxiety during nurse controlled analgesia. Br J Anaesth 1999;82:374–8.

[26] Cleeland CS, Gonin R, Hatfield A. Pain and its treatment in outpatients with metastatic cancer. N Engl J Med 1994;330:592–6.

[27] Littman G, Walker B, Schneider B. Reassessment of visual and verbal analogue ratings in analgesic studies. Clin Pharm Ther 1985;38:16–23.

[28] Sriwatanakul K, Kelvie W, Lasagna L. The quantification of pain: an analysis of words used to describe pain and analgesia in clinical trials. Clin Pharm Ther 1982;32:141–8.

[29] Huskisson EC. Measurement of pain. Lancet 1974;9(2):1127–31.

[30] Bergh I, Sjostrom B. Quantification of the pain terms hurt, ache and pain among nursing students. Scand J Caring Sci 2007;21(2):163–8.

[31] Lund I, Lundeberg T, Sandberg L, et al. Lack of interchangeability between visual analogue and verbal rating pain scales: a cross-sectional description of pain etiology groups. BMC Med Res Methodol 2005;5:31.

[32] Clark P, Lavielle P, Martinez H. Learning from pain scales: patient perspective. J Rheumatol 2003;30(7):1584–8.

[33] Hicks CL, von Baeyer CL, Spafford PA, et al. The Faces Pain Scale-Revised: toward a common metric in pediatric pain measurement. Pain 2001;93(2):173–83.

[34] Melzack R. The McGill Pain Questionnaire: major properties and scoring methods. Pain 1975;1:277–99.

[35] Mira JJ, Aranaz J. Patient satisfaction as an outcome measure in health care. Med Clin (Barc) 2000;114(Suppl. 3):26–33.

[36] Sullivan M. The new subjective medicine: taking the patient's point of view on health care and health. Soc Sci Med 2003;56(7):1595–604.

[37] Meredith P. But was the operation worth it? The limitations of quality of life and patient satisfaction research in health-care outcome assessment. J Qual Clin Pract 1996;16(2):75–85.

[38] Crow R, Gage H, Hampson S, et al. The measurement of satisfaction with healthcare: implications for practice from a systematic review of the literature. Health Technol Assess 2002;6(32):1–244.

[39] Howie JG, Heaney DJ, Maxwell M, et al. A comparison of a patient enablement instrument (PEI) against two established satisfaction scales as an outcome measure of primary care consultations. Fam Pract 1998;15(2):165–71.

[40] Bravo VY, Sculpher M. Quality-adjusted life years. Pract Neurol 2008;8(3):175–82.

[41] Schousboe JT, Nyman JA, Kane RL, et al. Cost-effectiveness of alendronate therapy for osteopenic postmenopausal women. Ann Intern Med 2005;142(9):734–41.

[42] Shih YC, Halpern MT. Economic evaluations of medical care interventions for cancer patients: how, why, and what does it mean? CA Cancer J Clin 2008;58(4):231–44.

# Section 3

## Health technology assessment

# Health technology assessment

12

Heidi Probst   Stephen Brealey

CHAPTER POINTS

- Randomization is important for ensuring balance in characteristics of patients between groups and should be performed remote from clinical practice to help ensure adequate concealment in treatment allocation.
- Sample size calculations should be conducted based on clinically significant improvements in the primary outcome measure.
- Recruitment of patients is a major challenge to trials. Methods to facilitate recruitment include careful consideration of the participant consent process, inclusion of important members of the multidisciplinary team to encourage recruiting participants, a realistic timeframe to recruit sufficient sample size and adequate funding.
- Attrition in the follow-up of patients should be limited by considering methods to reduce participant burden such as questionnaire length and minimizing the collection of missing data.
- With increasing emphasis on resource allocation it is important to consider the economic implications of any new technology or new process. In HTA a cost-effectiveness analysis maybe appropriate and can be considered alongside the design of the RCT.
- Systematic reviews differ from the conventional type of review in that they adhere to strict scientific design to make them more comprehensive, to minimize bias and errors thus providing more reliable results to support evidence-based decision making in policy and practice.
- Whereas a systematic review qualitatively synthesizes the evidence from scientific studies, a meta-analysis is a statistical analysis of the results of two or more scientific studies to synthesize their findings. An advantage of meta-analysis is

increasing the effective sample size together with confidence in the estimated effect.
- It is important to examine variation or heterogeneity across studies to inform the choice of statistical model ('fixed effects' or 'random effects') for pooling the results of studies. 'Healthcare technology' is a broad term and encompasses a variety of instruments and techniques which promote health, prevent and treat disease, and enhance rehabilitation. Although in diagnostic imaging or radiotherapy this technology tends to be complex, many healthcare approaches can rely on quite simple devices. The use of healthcare technology has medical, social, ethical and economic considerations.

Health technology assessment (HTA) is the investigation of the effectiveness and efficiency of these tools and techniques, which include diagnostic services such as MRI and therapies such as radiotherapy for breast cancer. Effectiveness refers to the extent to which benefits are brought to patients in routine circumstances, and efficiency refers to the extent to which acceptable effectiveness is achieved with the best use of resources.

In this chapter we will discuss the following research methods used to assess health technologies in medical imaging and radiotherapy. In order to give each of these areas their deserved attention, each will be covered within a separate sub-chapter, as follows:

1. Researching diagnostic tests
2. Researching therapies using randomized controlled trials (RCTs)
3. Health economic assessment and RCTs
4. Systematic reviews and meta-analyses of RCTs.

12

# 12.1 Researching diagnostic tests

Diagnostic testing can be seen as the collection of information which will clarify a patient's clinical condition and help to determine prognosis. This information can include:

- patient characteristics
- signs and symptoms
- history
- physical examination
- tests using laboratory or other technical facilities.[1]

Practitioners working in diagnostic imaging are particularly interested in providing high quality images which will permit an accurate medical diagnosis. Diagnostic imaging is a rapidly evolving speciality, and has seen technologies such as lymphangiography and myelography being replaced by ultrasound, computed tomography (CT) and magnetic resonance imaging (MRI).[2] New technologies, however, are complex and expensive and research is therefore required to evaluate them, in order to decide if and when they should be introduced into clinical practice.

The purpose of this section of the sub-chapter is twofold. Firstly, we shall broadly discuss what we mean by evaluation of diagnostic technologies. Secondly, we shall focus on research that measures the diagnostic performance (or accuracy) of an imaging modality and provides estimates of observer variability.

## Evaluative hierarchy of diagnostic technologies

Choices between alternative healthcare policies may be explored within healthcare evaluation, which, in its widest sense, includes investigation of the net value of available diagnostic technologies in terms of effectiveness and efficiency.[3]

It is not always apparent how the diagnostic technology itself brings about improvements in the prognosis or physical health of a patient. An imaging examination provides information from which a trained observer makes a report. This is then used by the clinician in combination with clinical findings and other tests to make or refine diagnosis and plan therapy which ultimately might affect patient outcome.[4] Therefore, to evaluate the effectiveness of imaging requires the measurement of a chain of events between the application of the technology

and any potential influence on disease. With the development of CT in the 1970s, Fineberg and colleagues[5] suggested that a hierarchy could be used to evaluate the effectiveness of diagnostic technologies. This has subsequently been extended to include whether the costs for a given examination are acceptable, providing an efficient use of resources.[6] Figure 12.1 presents the evaluative hierarchy as applied to the assessment of MRI.[4]

*Technical performance* is the first level of the evaluative hierarchy and is concerned with whether, for example, MRI produces good quality images from which diagnostic and therapeutic decisions may be made.[7]

The next level is *diagnostic performance*, which is concerned with whether imaging, such as MRI of the knee, correctly or incorrectly assesses the presence or

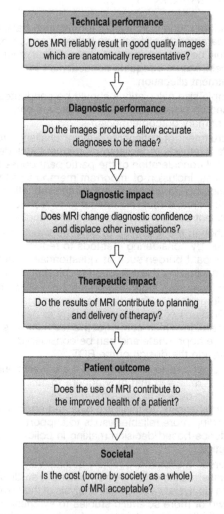

**Figure 12.1 •** The hierarchy used to evaluate MRI.

absence of disease, such as meniscal or ligamentous injury, as corroborated by a 'gold standard' test (such as arthroscopy in this instance). Assessment of diagnostic performance is expressed using statistics such as sensitivity and specificity. Sensitivity is the percentage of correct *abnormal* diagnoses in patients *with* disease; and specificity is the percentage of correct *normal* diagnoses in patients *without* disease. Furthermore, observer variation in the interpretation of medical images is substantial and has been described as radiology's 'Achilles' heel'.[8] Thus it is important to estimate observer variability, since the accuracy of the diagnostic test can be a joint function of the images produced and the performance of the observers.[6] This level in the evaluation of a diagnostic technology is discussed further in the next section.

The following three levels of the evaluative hierarchy are concerned with:

- *diagnostic impact*, e.g. does MRI replace existing technologies?
- *therapeutic impact*, e.g. do MRI findings lead clinicians to make changes in treatments?
- *patient outcome*, e.g. does MRI improve patients' prognoses?

These levels of the hierarchy are often assessed using observational research designs. In these the technologies are simply observed and compared, without the experimental intervention that would take place in a randomized controlled trial. An example might be recording pre-imaging diagnosis and management plans and comparing this with post-imaging plans. Such studies assume that any change in diagnosis and management plan, or change in patient outcome, is attributable to MRI. The effectiveness of MRI, however, might be explained by the influence of other variables. One possibility is that there is a tendency for measured outcomes to 'average out' (possibly for the better) over time following the introduction of a new policy, due to random fluctuations in performance results, if enough results are taken. This is referred to statistically as 'regression towards the mean'. Another reason could be the Hawthorne or 'guinea pig' effect, which is the tendency for data to be biased because research subjects become aware they are being observed.[9]

The best method for evaluating the effectiveness of technologies such as MRI is the randomized controlled trial (RCT), which will, in a controlled way, randomly allocate patients to receive either one diagnostic test or an alternative. Although there are logistical and financial implications to using this design,

this method helps to eliminate the threats to study validity described and provides a good basis for making statistical inferences.[10] The randomized controlled trial design is discussed later in the chapter.

The final level of the evaluative hierarchy moves beyond merely measuring the clinical effects of a technology to determining whether the cost of that technology is acceptable to society. For the policy maker entrusted with making resource allocations, it is necessary to assess the extent to which MRI is an efficient use of resources to provide benefits to society.[6] This could take the form of, for example, a cost-effectiveness study which involves computing a cost per unit of output for a medical technology such as cost per arthroscopy avoided by using MRI of the knee. The different methods of economic evaluation are discussed later in the chapter.

# Studies of diagnostic test accuracy

When diagnosing a patient, clinicians seldom have access to the gold standard or reference standard test for the disorders they suspect since these tests can be expensive, painful, invasive, or not even possible to perform on the living.[11] There are many alternative tests that can be used for patient diagnosis, such as taking a patient's history, physical examination, laboratory tests and diagnostic imaging. Diagnostic accuracy studies, which comprise the second level of the evaluative hierarchy, are vital to the assessment of imaging technologies, since they help to understand how they should be best used in clinical practice.

## The research question

Sackett and Haynes[12] identified four types of question that can be used to assess the real value of a diagnostic test such as an imaging modality:

- Do diagnostic test results in patients with the target disorder differ from those in normal people (a *phase I question*)?
- Are patients with certain diagnostic test results more likely to have the target disorder than patients with other test results (a *phase II question*)?
- Does the diagnostic test result distinguish patients with and without the target disorder among patients in whom it is clinically reasonable to suspect the disease is present (a *phase III question*)?

- Do patients who undergo this diagnostic test have better health outcomes than similar patients who are not tested?

Phase III questions are the most frequently asked in studies of diagnostic test performance and are concerned with the validity of the diagnostic test, i.e. does it measure what it proposes to measure?[13] To evaluate whether a test can distinguish normal from abnormal patients during routine clinical practice requires the results of the test to be compared against the gold or reference standard that is acknowledged as being the best available test to accurately diagnose the patient's true disease status. To compare measurements, i.e. the diagnostic test and reference standard results, is to assess *validity* and this will be the main focus of this section. Studies of the diagnostic accuracy, or validity of a test, particularly for imaging modalities, should also consider whether the different observers responsible for interpreting medical images are doing this consistently – this provides an assessment of *reliability*. The design and analysis of reliability studies will also be briefly discussed.

## Design of a study of validity

As described above, a diagnostic accuracy study involves the assessment of whether a diagnostic test can distinguish patients with and without the target disorder, as corroborated by gold or reference standard, among patients in whom it is clinically reasonable to suspect the presence of disease. If the study design is inadequate, there is experimental evidence that the performance of diagnostic tests might be exaggerated.[14] The STARD (Standards for the Reporting of Diagnostic accuracy studies) statement, which is a checklist used to guide the reporting of studies of accuracy,[15] and the QUADAS (Quality Assessment for Diagnostic Accuracy Studies), which is a generic tool used to appraise the quality of primary studies in systematic reviews of diagnostic accuracy,[16] provide thorough descriptions of the relevant design issues when considering the validity of a diagnostic test. These design issues are also discussed in Chapter 10. In summary then, when designing a diagnostic accuracy study it is important to consider the following threats to study validity which have been described as biases related to: patient selection, reference standard, measurement of results, and independence of interpretation:[17]

- Patient selection – a consecutive series of patients suspected (but not known) to have the target

disorder should be prospectively selected as a cohort of patients for inclusion in the study. There should be a clear description of the selection criteria and the setting, e.g. primary, secondary or tertiary care.

- Choice and application of the reference standard – the reference standard chosen should produce results close to the truth, or the performance of the diagnostic test will be poorly estimated. The reference standard should be applied within a clinically acceptable timeframe after the diagnostic test and preferably to the whole or at least a random sample of patients to avoid partial verification of patients. Nor should the index test form part of the reference standard.

- Measurement of results – a study should fully report indeterminate test results that occur due to factors such as technical faults or inferior image quality, and withdrawals that may occur due to patient death, move in residency, or no longer wanting to cooperate. It is important to consider whether they are non-random exclusions and the affect on generalizability.

- Independence of interpretation – the reference standard should be interpreted blind, i.e. in total ignorance of the diagnostic test result and vice versa.

## Analysis of a study of validity

Various measures can be used to assess how well a diagnostic test discriminates between patients with disease from those without disease. The diagnostic test will detect the presence of a disease, such as a lesion on a digital mammogram, and then be correctly classified as being present or absent by biopsy, as the reference standard. This 'binary' classification of results allows individuals to be classified either as true positives (TP) or true negatives (TN), which means that the test results are correct; or false positives (FP) and false negatives (FN), which means that the test results are incorrect (Figure 12.2). Positive and negative refer to the presence or absence of the target disorder.

The number of individuals classified as TP, TN, FP and FN permits the calculation of sensitivity and specificity, predictive values and likelihood ratios to answer different questions as described below:

*Sensitivity* is the proportion of patients with disease who have a positive test result, i.e. how good is my diagnostic test in detecting patients with disease?

**Test results**    **Patients**

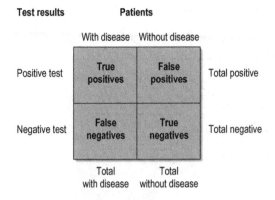

**Figure 12.2** • Binary classification of results.

Sensitivity = TP/total with disease (TP + FN)

**Specificity** is the proportion of patients without disease who have negative test results, i.e. how good is my diagnostic test in detecting patients without disease?

Specificity = TN/total with disease (FP + TN)

**Positive predictive value** is the proportion of patients with positive test results who have the disease, i.e. how well does a positive test result predict the presence of disease?

Positive predictive value = TP/total positive (TP + FP)

**Negative predictive value** is the proportion of patients with negative test results who do not have the disease, i.e. how well does a negative test result predict the absence of disease?

Negative predictive value = TN/total negative (FN + TN)

**Positive likelihood ratio** is the ratio of the true positive rate to the false positive rate, i.e. how much are the odds of the disease increased when a test is positive?

LR + ve = sensitivity/(1 − specificity)

**Negative likelihood ratio** is the ratio of the false negative rate to the true negative rate, i.e. how much are the odds of the disease decreased when a test is negative?

LR − ve = (1 − sensitivity)/specificity

Likelihood ratios can be applied to clinical practice to estimate the chances of disease in a patient according to their test result using Bayes' theorem.[18] In order to calculate the post-test odds of disease, you need to specify the pre-test odds, i.e. the likelihood that the patient would have a specific disease prior to testing. The pre-test odds are usually related to the prevalence of the disease, though you might adjust it depending on characteristics of the individual patient. Once you have specified the pre-test odds, you multiply them by the likelihood ratio. This gives you the post-test odds. Suppose a woman had a negative mammogram when screening for breast cancer and the local prevalence of cancer among women is 5% and the negative likelihood ratio for a mammogram is 0.20. Using Bayes' theorem we can estimate that the woman's probability of breast cancer prior to screening will be reduced after a negative mammogram from 5% to 1%:

- pre-test odds = prevalence/(1 − prevalence) = 0.05/0.95 = 0.05
- post-test odds = pre-test odds * LR−ve = 0.05 * 0.20 = 0.01
- post-test probability = post-test odds/(1 + post-test odds) = 0.01/1.01 = 0.01 (or 1%)

Sometimes, however, the test under evaluation might yield results as a continuous measurement or ordered categories. The images from MRI of the knee, for example, might be used to describe some anatomical feature such as degenerative changes in the menisci as definitely, probably, or possibly present, and probably or definitely absent, and then confirmed as present or absent by arthroscopy. Sensitivity and specificity could still be calculated by combining categories above and below a threshold, such as combining definitely, probably, or possibly present compared to combining probably or definitely absent.

Changing the threshold will alter the estimates of sensitivity and specificity. A more useful method, however, of measuring the performance of MRI across a range of thresholds, or 'cut-offs', is the receiver operating characteristic (ROC) curve (see also Chapter 8). The ROC curve, as shown in Figure 12.3, shows graphically the trade-offs at each cut-off for any diagnostic test that uses an ordinal or continuous variable. Ideally, the best cut-off value provides both the highest sensitivity and the highest specificity. This can be located on the ROC curve by finding the highest point on the vertical axis and the furthest to the left on the horizontal axis. Alternatively, depending on the target disorder, it might be more important to exclude disease so a higher sensitivity is chosen at the cost of lower specificity.[19] Furthermore, it is possible to calculate the area under the ROC curve. When this is 0.5 (i.e. 50% sensitive

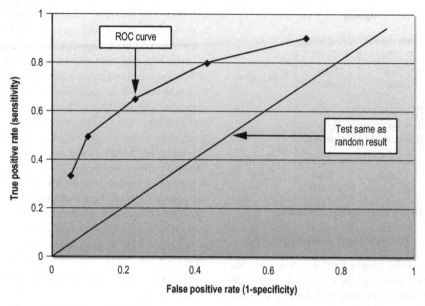

**Figure 12.3** • Example ROC curve for an imaging procedure with ordinal categories.

and 50% specific) it represents a totally uninformative test, as shown in Figure 12.3 by a straight diagonal line extending from the lower left corner to the upper right. A test that perfectly separates diseased from non-diseased patients would have an area under the curve of 1.0 (i.e. 100% sensitive and 100% specific). If the area under the curve of MRI of the menisci of the knee is 0.85, then the interpretation of the value is as follows. If two patients are drawn randomly from a sample of patients, in whom degeneration of menisci is present and absent respectively, and are both subjected to MRI to determine which patient had degeneration of the menisci, then MRI will be correct 85% of the time.[20]

## Assessment of reliability

Diagnostic performance studies of imaging modalities require observers to interpret images and it is observer variability in this task that is considered to be the weakest aspect of clinical imaging.[8] It is important to estimate the variability of observers' performance, or the reproducibility with which an observer interprets an image, as this will influence the decisions made by clinicians and could ultimately affect patient outcome. The assessment of reliability involves different observers interpreting the same sample of images, known as an inter-observer test, or the same observers interpreting the same images on separate occasions,

known as an intra-observer test.[21] We shall restrict our discussion of reliability to inter-observer variability as the principles of study design and analyses also apply to an assessment of intra-observer variability as well. In addition, inter-observer variability demonstrates observer consistencies within and between both sets of observers in the interpretation of images. Only when inter-observer variability is poor may we wish to investigate whether this arises from within and/or between observers and to use an intra-observer variability study to locate the source of unreliability.[22]

As with studies of validity, similar principles apply to the design of a reliability study such as the need for a representative sample of patients and blinding in the interpretation of images.[23] Selection bias is less likely when a consecutive or random sample of images is included and blinding avoids the knowledge of one observer's interpretation influencing the interpretation of another observer. Availability of clinical data to observers should also be considered. There is disagreement between studies which show that access to clinical details improves performance[24] or is unhelpful in lesion detection.[25] In routine clinical practice, knowledge of patients' age, sex and symptoms is required to ensure the most appropriate procedure is carried out and to avoid spending time and effort in searching for findings that would be irrelevant in the clinical context.[8] From a pragmatic perspective, providing clinical data should not be considered a bias as this reflects the context in which the images are interpreted during clinical practice. It is also important in a reliability study to carefully choose which observers are involved in the interpretation of images. For example, a study that includes highly specialist observers is likely to produce less generalizable results but in contrast could help to produce the best estimates of observer variability. Characteristics of observers that have been considered important in the assessment of reliability include: number, experience, profession and training.[26]

In studies of inter-observer variability it is not assumed that one particular observer produces the correct report, but rather there is a genuine difference in interpretation of images between observers. The measure of performance used to analyse whether observers' reports agree is called the Kappa statistic.[27] It can be calculated when the classification of an image by an observer is binary, e.g. the presence or absence of a fracture on a plain radiograph, or ordinal, e.g. a normal mammogram, one which shows benign disease, the suspicion of cancer, or the presence of cancer.

Kappa is defined as $K = (P_o - P_e)/(1 - P_e)$, where $P_o$ is the observed proportion of agreement, and $P_e$ is the proportion expected by chance. Kappa has a maximum of 1.0 when there is perfect agreement between observers and a value of zero indicates no better than chance. Kappa can be calculated for agreement between:

- a single observer interpreting the same image on two separate occasions
- two different observers on the same occasion
- comparisons of multiple observers.[8]

When considering Kappa for ordinal categories, it might be preferable to use weighted Kappa which gives different weighting to disagreements according to the magnitude of the discrepancy.[28]

## 12.2 Researching therapies using randomized controlled trials (RCTs)

## Introduction

Diagnostic imaging and radiotherapy practitioners will be aware of the pace of technological change. However, the introduction of a new technology should be accompanied by a careful assessment of its value over existing methods. Meticulous assessment

of any new technology should involve a controlled analysis of the new technology compared with the current approach.[29] The aim of this section is to provide an overview of randomized controlled trials (RCTs) and how they can be used within radiation therapy and imaging. By the end of this section practitioners should understand how to apply RCT designs for their own investigations as well as appraise RCTs published within the literature for applying evidence in practice. This section will start with a brief review of the benefits of RCTs and why they are considered a powerful research tool within HTA. Following this the specific characteristics and types of RCTs will be presented with examples of how the design characteristics could be used to investigate topics of relevance to clinical practitioners and those working in healthcare education.

The quality of a RCT, i.e. how stringent the design of the study is in limiting opportunities for bias, can influence potential outcomes by either overestimating or underestimating the benefit of the intervention. Such distortions have the potential to lead to ineffective treatments or interventions being employed and effective treatments being discarded.[30] Quality can be affected at many different stages of design and implementation and so throughout the following section attention will be paid to limitations of RCTs and the factors that may affect internal validity. The final part of this section will focus on the use of economic evaluations alongside RCTs as part of HTA utilizing a case study from a radiotherapy trial as an example of how this can be undertaken.

## Benefits of randomized controlled trials

RCTs are a true quantitative research method. For example, there is an emphasis on neutrality with an attempt to keep researcher and research participants remote from each other to avoid any influence on the study results. Characteristically RCTs seek to explain the whole by a study of one aspect or parts. RCTs are based on a science model in which there is a belief in universal laws measuring and analysing relationships using numbers to quantify effects or behaviour.[31] Objectivity is a primary aim and specific aspects of the approach are designed to provide neutrality and to avoid personal biases. Control over potential biases or confounding variables is integral to this approach. Owing to the strict controls and

**Table 12.1 The Scottish Intercollegiate Guidelines Network (SIGN) hierarchy of evidence**[32]

| Levels of evidence | |
|---|---|
| 1++ | High quality meta-analyses, or systematic reviews of RCTs, or RCTs with a very low risk of bias |
| 1+ | Well conducted meta-analyses, or systematic reviews of RCTs, or RCTs with low risk of bias |
| 1− | Meta-analyses, systematic reviews of RCTs or RCTs with high risk of bias |
| 2++ | High quality systematic reviews of case-control or cohort studies. High quality case-control or cohort studies with a very low risk of confounding, bias, or chance and a high probability that the relationship is causal |
| 2+ | Well conducted case control or cohort studies with a low risk of confounding, bias, or chance and a moderate probability that the relationship is causal |
| 2− | Case-control or cohort studies with a high risk of confounding, bias, or chance and a significant risk that the relationship is not causal |
| 3 | Non-analytic studies, e.g. case reports, case series |
| 4 | Expert opinion |

statistical strengths of RCTs, this design sits high within the hierarchy of evidence used to assess the quality of research used as the basis of radiotherapy techniques or to implement a novel imaging technique. Table 12.1 shows the Scottish Intercollegiate Guidelines Network (SIGN) hierarchy of evidence.[32]

## Why are RCTs so useful?

Consider the following scenario:

Post-operative radiotherapy for breast cancer is the accepted treatment for the majority of women who have undergone breast conserving surgery for a primary breast lesion. Radiation treatment to the breast can lead to a mild skin reaction (erythema)

which increases as the treatment course progresses. Traditionally skin care advice has been to undertake a variety of practices with limited evidence base to support the advice given which may include:

1. washing with mild soap
2. use of baby powder on the skin
3. allowing air to get to the skin
4. avoiding deodorants on the treated areas.

Recently aloe vera has been used to treat many skin conditions, including burns, because of its anti-inflammatory, antibacterial and wound healing properties. If investigators wanted to study the benefits of using aloe vera on radiotherapy patients to identify its usefulness in treating erythema they might formulate a research question as follows:

'Does the use of aloe vera on the irradiated skin during breast cancer irradiation reduce the skin reactions experienced by patients?'

Here it would be useful to take a few minutes to consider some of the different research approaches that can be used to answer this question. For the research question above, what would be the strengths and limitations of the research methods posed in Box 12.1?

As method 1 has no comparison group it is not possible to place the results in any context, so we

 **Box 12.1**

**Different approaches that can be used for research on the use of aloe vera on irradiated skin**

**Method 1**

A prospective evaluation of skin reactions on all patients irradiated for breast carcinoma using aloe vera on the affected skin during treatment.

**Method 2**

A prospective evaluation of skin reactions on all patients irradiated for breast carcinoma using aloe vera on the affected skin during treatment compared with the results of a previous study to evaluate skin reactions in irradiated breast patients using conventional skin care instructions.

**Method 3**

A prospective evaluation of skin reactions on all patients irradiated for breast carcinoma using aloe vera on the affected skin during treatment, compared with a control group of irradiated patients who are given the conventional skin care instructions. Patients can opt for either the current skin care approach or the aloe vera gel.

would still be unsure which skin-care regimen was most effective.

In method 2 a comparison group is available to provide some way of assessing the performance of the new intervention. However, using a historical control group as the comparator has a number of problems and would mean any results obtained could be viewed as unsound. For example, if we assume the results identified a statistically significant reduction in erythema in patients using aloe vera, it is possible that this result may have occurred not because of the intervention but due to other extraneous factors including:

1. A difference in patient characteristics between the two study groups. If the historical control group contained a higher proportion of larger patients than in the aloe vera group it is possible that this might account for the difference in skin reactions seen as it is known that breast size influences skin reaction.[33]

2. Technological differences between the two periods of study. As time passes changes in technology may mean application of treatment is no longer the same. The introduction of a new planning technique or a change to the immobilization device between the two data collection periods could account for differences in skin reactions observed.

In method 3 the use of a comparison group treated in parallel with the intervention group eliminates potential confounding variables associated with a historical control group. However, patients choosing between treatments could mean that patient numbers might be unbalanced between the two skin-care interventions and it is likely that patient characteristics would be unbalanced between the two study arms. Furthermore, where there is the option for choice it is possible that any patient reports of symptoms may be underplayed, especially where patients have read favourable information about a specific intervention, e.g. the healing properties of aloe vera, again limiting any confidence the researchers can have in the results obtained. Those interested in some of the research undertaken to investigate the benefits of aloe vera should view the resources available in Appendix 12.1 where practitioners can evaluate the differing research methods employed by researchers in this field.

Using the above scenario it is possible to see the need for strict control of possible confounding variables as well as the benefits of blinding participants to the

intervention, and the use of methods to ensure a balance of patient characteristics between the intervention arms. RCTs allow rigorous evaluation of a single variable in a defined patient group. Within the RCT design it is possible to eradicate potential bias by comparing two or more groups with balance in patient characteristics. Where RCTs are used this also allows the opportunity for meta-analysis comparing studies of the same investigation across different populations or geographical areas to provide a larger overall sample size and a potentially powerful analysis (see later in this section). In the next section the specific design characteristics of RCTs will be presented and some of the terminology associated with RCT design will be explained so practitioners can evaluate different RCTs presented in the literature.

## Design characteristics of RCTs

As the name indicates, RCTs involve random allocation of participants to treatment or control groups. Both groups are generally followed for a specific period and measurements taken at the same time points for both groups. The groups are analysed in terms of an outcome that is defined at the outset. For example, in the previous scenario a patient's skin reactions may be measured using a standard skin toxicity score such as the Radiation Induced Skin Reaction Assessment Scale (RISRAS)[34,35] or the Radiation Therapy Oncology Group (RTOG) scoring system at specific points throughout the treatment course. A pre-treatment assessment of skin colouration should be undertaken to ensure patients do not have erythema, perhaps associated with sun exposure, prior to the start of radiotherapy that would alter any post-treatment results. This baseline measure would also be used to ensure parity between the two groups at the outset. Measurements may be taken weekly during the course of radiotherapy and also at 4 weeks post irradiation when skin reactions may be at their peak. The timing of outcome measurements is crucial to the accuracy of the study and thought needs to be given to this aspect of the study design.

Within the RCT design controlling bias is a main focus so researchers need to consider any potential confounding variables that may influence the outcome and control for these within the analysis. For example, using the skin study scenario we have already identified that patient size can influence the skin reactions experienced so it would be important to record patient size, either chest separation or bra cup size, at the outset and test the two treatment arms for equality of this characteristic. Researchers would need to consider all possible confounding variables so other factors may include the level of homogeneity of the dose distribution[36] within the planning target volume (PTV). In the next few sections we will consider in a little more detail some of the specific design characteristics of RCTs.

## Types of RCTs

RCTs are often defined by:

- the purpose of the study, i.e. explanatory, efficacy or pragmatic trials
- how participants are exposed to the intervention, i.e. parallel, cross-over or factorial designs
- number of participants
- how the intervention is assessed.[37]

When assessing health technology, RCTs are usually pragmatic trials where the study is designed to reflect normal clinical activities. The aim of a pragmatic trial is to determine if the intervention works but also to describe any consequences of implementation of the technology. Pragmatic trials often have wider inclusion criteria to ensure the sample studied represents the normal group of patients that are likely to be seen in everyday practice. The comparison group in a pragmatic trial is often the current treatment or current imaging technique. Effectiveness trials aim to assess whether an intervention works in people who are offered the intervention. They tend to be pragmatic studies as the aim is to assess the effects under normal daily practice. They have simpler designs with less strict inclusion criteria than efficacy studies allowing participants to accept or reject the intervention offered. An example of an effectiveness study would be the early evaluation of breast cancer screening where RCTs were used to identify the impact of a screening intervention. Patients would be called for screening but may opt not to attend. Follow-up of this arm would include all patients offered screening irrespective of whether they attended the screen or not and compared with patients in a control group (who were not offered any intervention).[38,39] An efficacy study is where the aim is to identify if an intervention works in those that receive it. Figure 12.4 shows a pictorial presentation of different RCT designs.[37]

In its simplest form an RCT has two arms, an intervention arm, that may be a new process or technology being tested, compared with either a control arm, that receives no intervention, or a second intervention arm, which in HTA is usually the current treatment or current imaging modality. Cross-over designs can be a powerful way to study the impact of a new technology (see design b in Figure 12.4). Here patients or subjects are used as their own control and this avoids the need for matching characteristics across groups with different subjects that occurs with the simple parallel design. However, cross-over or repeated measures designs can only be used in HTA where the first intervention has no lasting effect on the primary outcome measure. So in the scenario used above it would not be appropriate to use aloe vera gel for the first 2 weeks of treatment and then apply traditional skin care for the remainder of the treatment course as the effect of the first skin care regimen would impact on subsequent skin reactions measured during application of the second regimen. In educational studies this design could not be used where subjects would learn through the first phase of the study. For example, in an RCT used to test the effectiveness of immersive visualization environments (IVE) for teaching complex brain anatomy to students, their test scores following exposure to the IVE would influence future test scores if they were then exposed to a traditional plastic model as the learning tool. However, this design can be used successfully when testing application of a radiographic technique in a test situation. For example, it has been used to assess the impact of work speed on the accuracy of setting up a patient for a complex technique using a phantom.[40] In this study each pair of staff were asked to set up the phantom as they would for a normal treatment, twice, under two different conditions. In condition 1, participants were given a scenario whereby they could take as much time as they needed and a radiographic image was taken of the final set-up position to assess positional accuracy. In condition 2, participants were given the same technique to apply but the scenario was that they were treating a child that was distressed and so it was important to work fast but accurately, in order to assess the impact that a time pressure might have on treatment accuracy. It was important that groups alternated in the order in which they undertook the test, i.e. condition 1, then condition 2, for one group and condition 2, then condition 1 for another group, to ensure any learning effects did not affect the overall results.

Factorial trials offer the opportunity to test individual interventions as well as studying the impact

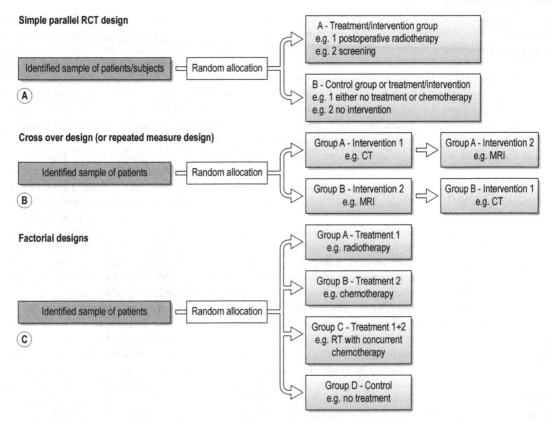

**Figure 12.4** • Different RCT designs. From Jadad, A (2003). Randomised controlled trials: a user's guide. With permission from John Wiley & Sons Ltd.

of two or more interventions applied together. In imaging the factorial design has been used in experimental conditions to test the factors that influence image quality and radiation dose.[41]

In addition, trials can be described as being single-blind, double-blind or triple-blind. Blinding refers to either the participants being blind to the intervention, i.e. they are unaware of which intervention they have been allocated to, or the investigators, such as the statistician. The purpose of blinding is to minimize opportunities for bias as a direct result of knowledge of the intervention received either by the participants or the investigators applying the treatment or collecting the data.

For example, where the participants have knowledge of the intervention they are to receive there is a possibility any patient self-reports may be influenced by this knowledge. Where possible patients should be blind to the intervention; this is not always possible as it may often be obvious which of the interventions participants have received. For example, in an educational study to evaluate the effectiveness of

an immersive visualization environment for teaching radiography students about complex brain anatomy students were randomized to have either the new intervention, the immersive visualization environment, or the standard 3-D plastic model. In this study it was not possible to blind students to the intervention due to the obvious differences in the teaching methods.[42]

Further opportunities for bias can occur during the assessment of the study outcomes. Researcher knowledge of the intervention arm can influence interpretation of key outcome measures especially where the researcher has a hypothesis to test. For example, in a study to evaluate the effectiveness of using tattoos to improve radiotherapy treatment accuracy during breast irradiation compared with gentian violet pen for marking the skin, it was necessary to blind the researcher undertaking the analysis to the intervention each subject was allocated to during the measurement of the treatment images that were used to establish treatment accuracy.[43] Knowledge of the intervention could have resulted in the favourable measurement of some images in order to prove the hypothesis being tested. To completely reduce the opportunity for any bias researchers, where possible, should aim to blind the patient, the researchers undertaking measurement of the outcomes, and the researchers undertaking the statistical analysis (i.e. single-, double- or triple-blinding).[37] Treatment effects may be overestimated by approximately 17% where double-blinding is not employed as compared with studies where double-blinding is used.[30]

## Randomization

The rationale for using randomization is to prevent bias occurring as a result of inequalities between the treatment options or intervention arms. For example, when looking at the effectiveness of breast cancer screening, it would be important for researchers to ensure equity of characteristics between the screening group and the control arm, such as age at time of entry into the study, as incidence of breast cancer is known to increase with age.[44]

There are a number of methods available to researchers for achieving random allocation. The simplest way is by tossing a coin, throwing a die or use of a table of random numbers. For example, it can be agreed at the start of the study that heads on a coin will indicate treatment arm A and tails treatment arm B or the control group. However, simple randomization methods such as this may still result in unequal numbers or unbalanced characteristics between the groups,[37] especially in small trials.[45] To overcome this one method is the use of block randomization. Generally blocks of four are used for a simple RCT design with two intervention arms, A and B, as follows: AABB, ABBA, BBAA, BABA, BAAB, and ABAB. One of the six possible combinations is selected and participants allocated to an intervention arm based on the sequence of four; the process is repeated as required depending on the sample size.

Even with block randomization some inequalities may still arise simply by chance, hence researchers need to be aware of this possibility and test baseline characteristics between the groups for equality. Where differences occur it may be necessary to control for imbalances in subsequent analyses of the outcome data. Alternatively, stratifying randomization by an important characteristic may reduce the potential for inequality. When considering the study to look at the impact of aloe vera discussed above, it may

help to stratify on patient size, i.e. large or small patients, as this is a contributing factor to skin reactions during breast irradiation. In this case a separate list of block sequences would be produced for each stratum, although as you increase the number of strata the risk of errors in application also increases.[45]

A further alternative is the use of a technique called minimization. This method is successful at obtaining equality between groups for a set of relevant characteristics even in trials with small samples.[45] Here for the characteristics that require balance, e.g. age, patient size, menopausal status, etc., a running total of how many participants have been allocated with each characteristic to each intervention arm is kept. Following random allocation of the first participant, subsequent participant randomizations are weighted to the intervention arm that would maximize balance, i.e. minimize inequalities, with totals for each arm updated after each participant is entered into the study.

A further option for researchers is the use of cluster randomization. In contrast to most randomized trials where the individual is randomized, with cluster randomization groups of participants are randomized;[37,46] clusters can be either general practitioner practices or imaging/oncology departments. The benefit of cluster randomization is a possible reduction in contamination of the control arm. For example, if you wanted to investigate the impact of a new electronic information service for patients, it is possible that those in the experimental arm might pass on to patients in the control arm, simply by chatting while in the waiting room, useful information they have gleaned as a result of the intervention. Cluster randomization may not be necessary for the majority of trial designs and therefore individual randomization should be used where possible to avoid some of the limitations of cluster randomization (see Box 12.2 for details[46]).

## Concealment of randomization

Randomization is generally accepted as the best way of removing opportunities for selection bias by removing any predictability in the assignment process. Yet the process of randomization itself can be fraught with opportunities for bias that may invalidate or reduce the quality of the subsequent results. A common approach adopted by novice researchers to the issue of randomization is to alternate participants to interventions as they are referred to the clinic or department, as they consider referral to be in its self, a random process (Figure 12.5).

**Box 12.2**

**Limitations of cluster randomization**

1. Selection bias – different types of participants maybe recruited into different arms of the study due to the geographical locations of the clusters which may result in differences, for example, in socio-economic status between arms.
2. Selection bias – in cluster trials participants are not asked to consent to the study but to consent to being included in the study analysis; if a substantial proportion of the cluster participants refuse then an imbalance will occur between the trial arms.

Cluster trials need larger sample sizes than trials that use individual randomization to ensure sufficient statistical power. If there is not full uptake of the intervention within the cluster then a dilution effect may further influence the power of the study.

Looking at the process in Figure 12.5, can you foresee any problems with this approach? Primarily there is an identifiable pattern that may introduce bias. For example, where the pattern is known, there is the opportunity for researchers to selectively change the detail of the information given to potential participants. This is done to discourage entry into the trial where that patient has co-morbid disease or any potential characteristic that the researcher considers may influence or skew the results in an unfavourable direction. Inadequate concealment of this nature can result in overestimation of the potential effect of the intervention in the order of 40% when compared with trials with adequate concealment of randomization.[30]

One method used to reduce the opportunity for bias during randomization is to use sealed opaque envelopes containing random allocations. However, this system may be prone to interference. Clinicians can open envelopes in advance, view allocations by holding the envelope up to a bright light, or when block randomization of four is used, if three of the previous participant allocations are known, the fourth can be predicted allowing the clinician to reserve entering patients into a trial until specific participants present with desired characteristics. For lone researchers undertaking a simple RCT as part of perhaps an undergraduate or postgraduate course of study the use of sealed opaque envelopes may be the only practical solution on offer; in these circumstances researchers should be aware of the potential for interference and subsequent effects on the study quality. In most cases attempts should be made to use a system that removes the randomization process from the researchers, such as a central randomization service available through local trials units.[47]

## Sample size requirements

As well as randomization of patients into the control or intervention arms, RCTs rely on statistical analysis of the primary outcome to demonstrate effectiveness of the intervention. In order to demonstrate a statistically significant difference in treatments between the study groups it is important that an adequate sample is studied to demonstrate an effect. In HTA improvements in outcomes may be small and therefore where studies have small sample sizes it may not be possible to demonstrate a difference even where a difference exists.[48] For this reason, researchers undertaking RCTs must consider at the outset what improvement in the primary outcome would be appropriate for a clinically significant improvement or benefit and then calculate the sample size required to establish this statistically. This calculation is referred to as a power calculation. For example, in a study to establish the effectiveness of a radiotherapy protocol to reduce lung morbidity for patients undergoing chest wall irradiation following surgery for breast cancer, it was calculated that a sample of 200 patients in each group would be sufficient to detect a 7% difference in respiratory symptoms, equivalent to a standardized difference 0.3 with 5% significance and 80% power[49] (see Chapter 10 for more information on power calculations).

## Recruitment of subjects

Recruitment of patients into clinical trials is often problematic. In the study of the effectiveness of a radiotherapy protocol to reduce patient reports

| Patient number | Treatment allocation |
|---|---|
| 1 | Treatment or imaging intervention A |
| 2 | Intervention B |
| 3 | Intervention A |
| 4 | Intervention B |
| 5 | Intervention A |
| 6 | Intervention B |
| 7 | Intervention A |
| 8 | Intervention B |

**Figure 12.5 •** Inappropriate method of randomization often adopted by novice researchers.

of lung morbidity mentioned above,[50] recruitment of subjects to the study was slow despite a feasibility study indicating sufficient eligible patients were available in the host centre. Recruitment was hampered by:

- clinicians forgetting to mention the study to eligible patients
- patients refusing to participate partly due to poor information about the possible side-effects of treatment at the early referral stage. Within the patient information sheet for the study details of lung morbidity were highlighted, and patients unknowing of this aspect of their treatment feared that inclusion in the study would cause unwanted respiratory side-effects, even though this was a possible corollary of treatment regardless of inclusion in the study
- limited patient awareness of clinical trials during the early stages of the study
- a strong preference for one of the intervention arms with patients not wishing to take a chance of receiving the alternative option through randomization.

Of 452 patients assessed as eligible for inclusion in the study, 92 (20%) refused to participate,[49] which is similar to reports from other cancer trials.[51] As well as an effect on the overall sample size this loss of potential participants can have an effect on the generalizability of the results as the sample recruited may not fully represent the population of patients as intended. Where studies include a placebo arm it is possible that a reduction in acceptance to randomization may also occur.[52] Generally factors reported as influential in a patient's decision to join a study include the belief that they may help future patients, or that they may benefit from inclusion;[52] hence researchers should ensure potential participants are aware of the benefits of the study during the recruitment stage. In many cancer trials a lack of participants can be reflective of strict inclusion criteria excluding a substantial proportion of patients, perhaps in the region of 30%.[51,53] Hence more pragmatic trials with less strict inclusion criteria may enhance the proportion of patients eligible for study and thus increase the potential for recruitment and generalizability.[51,54]

A comparison study of two community-based RCTs undertaking similar palliative care interventions identified a number of positive recruitment strategies. The more successful of the two trials, studied in terms of reaching an adequate sample size, employed the following strategies to maximize recruitment[54]:

- use of an inflated sample size to account for expected high attrition from early withdrawal or death
- maximal inclusion criteria and minimal exclusion criteria
- dedicated recruitment nurse
- triage process to screen for eligible patients
- recruitment interview included key messages
- patients approached for consent before GP consent was requested
- extensive marketing to raise the profile of the study topic
- effort was placed on ensuring clinician input to the study to encourage feelings of inclusion and reduce concerns
- realistic timeframe to recruit sufficient sample size
- adequate funding to support an extensive recruitment strategy.

Recruitment may be hampered where potential participants or referring clinicians have strong preferences for one of the intervention arms that leads to a refusal to be randomized. Again where these patients refuse consent to randomization, a reduction in generalizability of the results may be a consequence. Furthermore, where patients with a strong preference accept being randomized, subsequent results may be biased by strong beliefs about the treatment received where blinding of the patient is not possible.[55] A solution to this dilemma is the use of patient preference trials and there are a number of different designs currently being used (Figure 12.6).[37,55,56]

While patient preference designs may allow a greater proportion of patients to be included in a study, the disadvantage of such designs is the resultant unknown or uncontrolled confounding variables in the preference arms.[55] It is suggested that the analysis for these studies includes comparison of the two randomized arms alone and perhaps an analysis using randomization status as a co-variate.[55] A concern of using the Zelen design, where participants are randomized before giving consent, and where those randomized to the standard treatment only consent to treatment and not to participation in a study, is the possible ethical implications in therapeutic scenarios.[56] However, it has been suggested that this design is specifically helpful for population-based screening studies.[56]

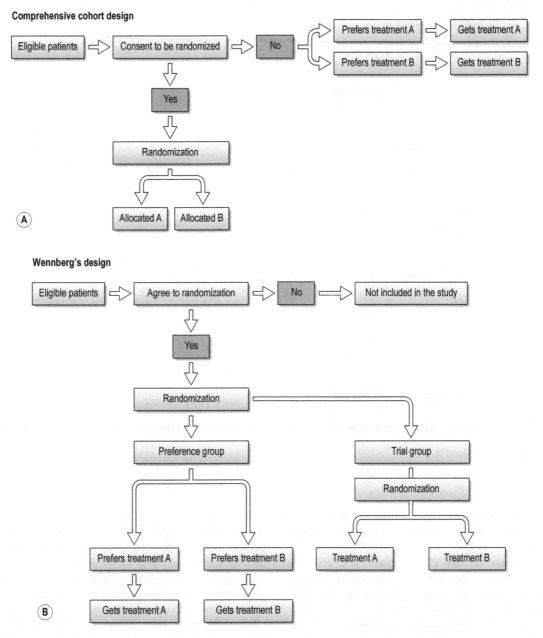

**Figure 12.6** • Patient preference study designs.

*Continued*

## Attrition

Even when researchers manage to recruit sufficient numbers to their trials problems with attrition can lead to a reduction in the strength of the reported findings. It is common for participants to fail to completely finish the allocated treatment or intervention for a number of reasons: the patient may move to a different geographical area, the intervention may cause adverse side-effects and the participant opts to withdraw leaving an incomplete data set. In addition, there may be missing data as a result of

**Zelen's design (single consent version)***

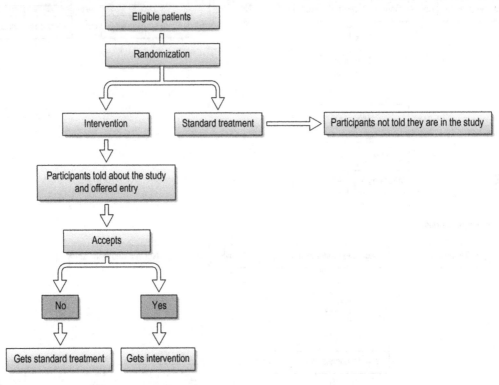

(C)   * In the double consent version participants are told which intervention they have been randomized to and offered the opportunity to switch to the alternative treatment[56]

**Figure 12.6—Cont'd**

incomplete collection, perhaps due to staff absence at the time of collection, or participants not adhering to the protocol.

Attrition through a loss of patients to follow-up or incomplete data sets can bias results when the characteristics of those with missing data differ between the randomized groups.[57] It is therefore advised that missing data be presented by researchers by providing normal baseline characteristics data for the whole study sample, and also separate data on those lost to follow-up from those remaining in the analysis so that readers can judge any imbalances between the intervention arms as a result of the missing data.[57] Using strategies to minimize attrition is beneficial and these may include minimizing patient burden by attention to the data collection methods.[54] For example, reducing the need for patients to attend clinics by visiting them at home may increase cooperation and reduce missing data; although more

costly than other approaches this method was successful in the comparison of two community-based palliative care trials.[54] Ensuring all staff involved in data collection are fully informed and included in the trial process may ensure adequate data recording and protocol compliance. In addition, regular assessment of data accrual may highlight the need for a change in strategy where rising missing data becomes apparent.

## Protocol deviations

In circumstances where there have been protocol deviations it is appropriate to use an 'intention to treat' (ITT) analysis where participants are analysed as part of the group they were assigned to irrespective of whether they competed their allocated treatment/intervention or not.[37,58] The ITT analysis should be applied to a full data set[59] but frequently protocol deviations are accompanied by missing data. Failure to include participants with missing data can result in an overestimation of the benefit of the intervention.[37] Consider the aloe vera example used previously, if patients stopped using the aloe vera because of exacerbation of the skin reaction, or left the study due to adverse reactions, this would result in missing data for some patients. If these data are excluded from the analysis the assumed benefit of this preparation may be exaggerated.[37]

When considering missing data it may be appropriate to use a 'sensitivity analysis'[37] or imputation.[60] Here it is proposed that either a worst case scenario is used, or a value is chosen that is credible given the rest of the patient's data set.[60] Sometimes it may be appropriate to use the last recorded response or to assume that responses remained constant.[59] For example, in the study of the effectiveness of a radiotherapy protocol to reduce patient reports of lung morbidity mentioned previously, 'no symptoms' were used for missing data in both groups as this was a plausible outcome given the rest of the data set.[50] However, imputations of this nature are provided to give some estimation of treatment effect and should be considered carefully; producing a range of potential outcomes for readers using different imputation methods may be the most beneficial policy.[59]

It is suggested that the use of the ITT analysis is the most cautious approach to take when handling protocol deviations.[61] However, it is proposed that using an ITT approach can lead to type II errors and there may be justified circumstances when patients with specific criteria could be excluded from the analysis.[61] These would include participants that were randomized for inclusion in a study but who were in fact ineligible, i.e. they did not meet the eligibility criteria for the study.[61] Even in these cases it is prudent to consider individual exclusions with care. In addition, the ITT approach is appropriate for effectiveness or pragmatic studies where the aim of the study is to evaluate the impact of an intervention under normal clinical circumstances where it is likely that some deviations from protocol would also occur.[59] Hollis and Campbell suggest a strategy for the full implementation of the ITT approach that researchers designing RCTs may find helpful.[59]

When evaluating RCTs presented in the literature it is important to consider how protocol deviations were handled by the researchers. In a study of RCTs published in a number of high impact journals, Hollis and Campbell discovered only 50% of RCTs published in 1 year stated explicitly that results were analysed on an ITT basis.[59] Of those stating they used an ITT analysis 13% did not actually analyse patients as randomized (which is the criteria for the ITT approach). Furthermore, the handling of missing data was variable across the studies, emphasizing the need for practitioners to undertake rigorous appraisals of published RCT study results before considering applying the evidence to practice.

# Drug trials

When a new drug is developed the development process can be time-consuming. Initially safety and efficacy of the drug will be tested through animal studies. The first human studies of cancer drugs (Phase I trials) are usually tested on volunteers with incurable diseases and are generally not tested on healthy volunteers. There is no randomization and incremental doses of the drug are administered so that side-effects can be monitored. Once safety of the drug has been established in humans the drug can then be administered to a small group of patients (approximately 20) with the condition to establish efficacy, i.e. where the aim is to establish if the drug works in people who receive it, with different doses and frequencies. There are very strict inclusion criteria to exclude patients with coexisting disease. These Phase II studies may involve randomization if the outcome measure is appropriate, i.e. pain. Where the end-point is reduction in number of deaths there may not be randomization. Phase III trials are conducted once the drug has been shown to be effective and safe in Phase II studies. Usually Phase III trials are randomized effectiveness studies.

The most recent and most well publicised cancer drug trials have been those evaluating the effectiveness of trastuzumab (Herceptin®) for the adjuvant treatment of early breast cancer in HER2-positive breast cancer. This monoclonal antibody against HER2 had proven efficacy in advanced breast cancer and the first interim analysis to be published in early breast cancer trials showed such promising results[62] that there was a desire for clinicians to consider its use in HER2-positive patients with early stages of the disease. The primary outcome in this study was disease free survival with early results showing 92.5% of patients in the trastuzumab arm free from disease at year 1; as compared with 87.1% in the control arm.[63] These results led to acceptance of the drug for treatment in early stage cancer by the National Institute for Clinical Excellence (NICE) in the UK despite a relatively short follow-up period (median follow up 2 years).[64]

## 12.3 Health economic assessment and RCTs

Economic assessments in conjunction with RCTs have become increasingly important due to the need to allocate scarce health resources in the most efficient and beneficial way. Economic evaluations deal with both costs and outcomes of activities and the basic purpose of an economic evaluation is to 'identify, measure, value and compare the costs and consequences of the alternatives being considered'.[65] Economic evaluations are comparable in the way they measure costs but differ in the way outcomes or consequences are derived. Essentially evaluations can be divided into three main types:[66]

• cost-benefit analysis
• cost-utility analysis and
• cost-effectiveness analysis.

Cost-benefit analysis involves the measurement of costs and benefits in comparable monetary terms. An example of the use of a cost-benefit analysis is the evaluation of an intensive follow-up regimen. This involves oral history, physical examination, blood tests including biological markers, annual hepatic echography, chest X-ray and a bone scan as compared with a standard clinical follow-up in breast cancer patients to identify early signs of relapse.[67] In this study the authors undertook a simple RCT comparing the two follow-up methods for number of relapses identified during scheduled follow-up appointments. The results identified no difference in the early detection of relapse between the two methods, so no benefit cost but a substantial increase in costs for the intensive follow-up schedule that was three times the cost of the less intensive follow-up regimen.[67]

Cost-utility analysis involves the use of a utility based measure such as Quality Adjusted Life Years (QALYs). By using a single measure of benefit (QALYs) across RCTs, it is possible to compare the effectiveness of different interventions and hence this type of analysis allows the assessment of the benefit of employing a particular treatment or intervention in one area against the loss in benefit caused by redirecting resources from other programmes, i.e. productive efficiency and allocative efficiency, and is considered as a variation of cost-effectiveness analysis.[66]

Cost-effectiveness analysis measures outcomes or benefits in units such as quality of life or improvements in function; in radiotherapy this may be measured as improvements in accuracy of treatment. To illustrate how an economic evaluation can be undertaken, a case study of a cost-effectiveness analysis undertaken in a radiotherapy RCT, comparing two methods for marking patients' skin in the adjuvant treatment of breast cancer, will be presented. The two skin marking methods compared were:

• traditional semi-permanent gentian skin marks
• gentian skin marks and permanent tattoos.

The aim of this study was to identify the efficiency and effectiveness differences between the two skin marking methods. There had been concern at the time that patients who did not have tattoos would take longer to set up due to uncertainty of the skin mark positions caused by the smudging effect that occurs when semi-permanent markers are used. In addition, it was felt that as some patients lost their marks as treatment progressed there would be a greater need for re-planning or re-simulation in these patients compared with those that had permanent tattoos, and this would have associated resource implications. Furthermore, therapists at the host centre were concerned about possible decreased treatment accuracy that might result from using semi-permanent marks.

The cost-effectiveness evaluation was undertaken from an NHS perspective and included staffing, and equipment running costs as described by Greene and Williams[68] utilizing more recent costs based on the equipment used at the host centre. Individual staffing costs for each patient exposure was calculated based on the procedure time and the pay rate for the highest staff grade performing the procedure. Although two therapists perform each set up, the speed of the set up may be determined by the seniority of the therapist. In our experience the greater the skill of the staff leading the procedure the quicker the procedure is completed. Similarly for simulation procedures the highest staff grade was used to estimate individual procedure costs. For cases where re-simulation occurred the cost of the procedure was calculated using the procedure time and the pay rate for the grade of staff most frequently expected to undertake the procedure (mid-scale). An additional sensitivity analysis was performed using the highest pay rate for a clinical member of staff to determine any cost differences between the two groups if a higher grade staff member was to lead the re-simulation procedure.

# Calculation of costs

The treatment time for each treatment episode, for each patient, was multiplied by the wage rate for the highest grade of staff involved in the treatment set up. To determine the wage rate the middle salary scale for each grade was used and a rate per minute was calculated. This wage rate per minute for the appropriate staff grade multiplied by the procedure time gave the initial staff cost per session. The total treatment course costs for each individual patient was then calculated by summing the individual session costs. In addition the linear accelerators (linac) running costs were calculated by multiplying each session procedure time by the running cost per minute.

The linac running costs were based on the:

- equipment purchase price (including VAT) plus interest charges on the equipment
- cost of replacement parts
- building costs plus interest charges on the building
- cost of an initial stock of parts
- energy to operate the machine and building maintenance costs
- cost of three therapists to run the unit (which must also include a proportion of a clinical manager grade that is required to supervise and manage a team of therapists).

In addition, to run a linear accelerator it is necessary to have a simulator and a treatment planning system with all the associated costs, including staffing.

This approach to costing is based on the model used by Greene.[68,69] Costs for a new 6MV Clinac (Varian) linear accelerator and Simulux (Varian) simulator were used. For building maintenance and the treatment planning system costs used by Greene and Williams[68] were adopted and were based on more recent figures. See Appendix 12.2 for a breakdown of the costs.

The interest charges on the equipment costs were based on depreciation of the equipment over the lifetime of the machine, i.e. 10 years. This was calculated at 6% per year on the diminishing capital assuming the value is depreciated in equal increments over the 10 year period.[68]

The total cost for each individual patient was calculated by summing all the costs included in Table 12.2.

Table 12.3 shows the mean calculated costs for the two skin marking methods, including a sensitivity analysis with costs for a higher grade staff to identify how much average costs would change when a higher grade staff member led the procedure.

# Treatment effectiveness

Treatment effectiveness for the purposes of the cost analysis was defined as the number of treatments with a central lung depth error between −0.3 and +0.3 cm. The magnitude of the error was selected at 3 mm as this was the mid-point of the range of random errors that were reported within the literature

**Table 12.2 Procedure costs included in the analysis**

| Costs | Scale |
|---|---|
| Staff costs | Procedure time × cost/min for staff grade |
| Linac running costs | Cost/min |
| Re-simulation costs | Procedure time × cost/min for staff grade |
| Cost of extra imaging prints | No. of extra prints × cost of prints |
| Physics re-plan time | No. of re-plans × (procedure time × cost/min for staff grade) |
| Clinician time to prescribe re-plans | No. of re-plans × (procedure time × cost/min for consultant clinical oncologist) |
| Radiographer time to check re-plans | No. of re-plans × (procedure time × cost/min for staff grade) |
| Cost of a sterile needle | Cost of one sterile needle/patient (tattoo patients only) |

Linac, linear accelerators.

Table 12.3 Mean treatment costs for the two skin marking options (based on costs for the year 1999–2000)

| Therapist scale used for re-simulation and re-plan | Average cost/pt category A (skin marks and tattoos) (£) | Average cost/pt category B (skin marks only) (£) | Difference in mean (£) | 95% CI for difference in mean costs (£) |
|---|---|---|---|---|
| Grade I | 388.02 | 403.91 | 15.89 | −1.73 to 33.51 |
| Grade II | 388.17 | 404.11 | 15.94 | −1.74 to 33.62 |

at the time. Central lung depth (CLD) was measured from 3 on treatment images taken over the course of treatment and compared with the planned CLD for each patient. Random errors in the CLD was then calculated for each patient.[43] A total of 104 patients (out of 168) within the tattoo group had treatment errors within this range (62%), compared with 88 (out of 152) in the skin marks only category (58%). The difference between these two groups was not statistically significant (chi square $P > 0.2$).[49]

## Cost-effectiveness ratio

It was calculated that the category A patients, i.e. those that had both skin marks and tattoos, incurred a cost saving per patient of £15.89 for 4% extra accuracy. To establish the influence of the skin marking category on the total procedure costs a linear regression analysis was performed. The linear regression for total procedure costs demonstrated the importance of individual characteristics such as the patient's age and size, as well as the extent of the area treated. When these other factors were considered the influence of the skin marking category had no significant impact on the total procedure costs calculated. It was apparent that older patients and patients with a larger separation took longer to treat and hence incur a greater total cost; serving to emphasize the need to evaluate economic data carefully.

## 12.4 Systematic reviews and meta-analyses of RCTs

During clinical activities practitioners may come across questions about practice that they do not know the answer to. They may choose to ask an expert who may or may not know the answer; or they may turn to the published literature for an answer. In Chapter 3 and 4, literature reviews were discussed

and the method for searching for literature was presented as an important aspect of the research process. This section will focus on the method for undertaking a systematic review of published literature in relation to HTA and will start with a discussion of the differences between discussion papers (or narratives), systematic reviews and meta analyses. Following clarification of the different types of reviews the discussion will concentrate on the method for undertaking systematic reviews with particular attention paid to the review process and aspects of the search strategy including the assessment of study quality. The final subsections will describe the common principles of meta-analyses and standards required for the presentation of systematic reviews.

## Types of reviews

Literature *reviews or discussion papers* found in journals are an informal collection of literature on a specific topic and are often invited papers from experts in the field. They are common in journals as they are easy to read and synthesize by practitioners and are often quick to produce. One of the main disadvantages is the variability in the level of detail that is presented about the search strategy employed, making replication of the review difficult. In addition, they may lack rigour and objectivity, with conclusions and recommendations based on a narrow examination of the available data. However, they can provide an opportunity for debate and allow the authors to provide an interesting perspective on a topic of current interest.

A *systematic review* is a formal review of the evidence on a particular topic with a specific research question that is to be addressed and a detailed search strategy that would allow replication. The search strategy includes details about inclusion and exclusion criteria, databases used, and the method used to assess the quality of the studies identified by the search, the process for selecting research, and the method used for data extraction and synthesis. There is also an attempt to reduce potential bias by using standardized tools for the assessment of study quality as well as using more than one assessor to evaluate selected studies and blinding of reviewers to the authors and journal names of selected studies.

A *meta-analysis* is a review where the results of RCTs undertaken independently are combined and a statistical analysis produced, usually graphically, to provide an estimate of the effect of an intervention. By combining a number of individual studies it is possible to essentially increase the overall sample size and hence increase the strengths of the conclusions that can be drawn about an intervention, making meta-analyses a major asset for practitioners needing to make decisions about clinical interventions. However, meta-analyses do have some limitations and these will be covered in more detail below.

## Systematic reviews

Planning a systematic review is crucial to its success and subsequent quality. Figure 12.7 provides a schematic presentation of the process required to plan and execute a systematic review.

## Planning the review

Before embarking on a systematic review it is important to be clear about the clinical question that needs to be answered. The research question will be used to define facets of the search strategy and any lack of clarity may reduce the effectiveness of the search. In addition, before any detailed work is undertaken in preparation of the review it is important to identify if:

- a systematic review already exists on the topic area
- sufficient data are available to undertake a systematic review.

Therefore, being clear about the question and the topic of interest is important. Once this has been clarified it is beneficial to undertake a scoping exercise to identify how much literature exists in the field. This takes the form of a small search using the main electronic databases relevant to the topic area; for example, this might include MEDLINE, CIHAHL and the Cochrane databases, using key terms. A simple search should allow the opportunity to identify whether any up-to-date systematic reviews already

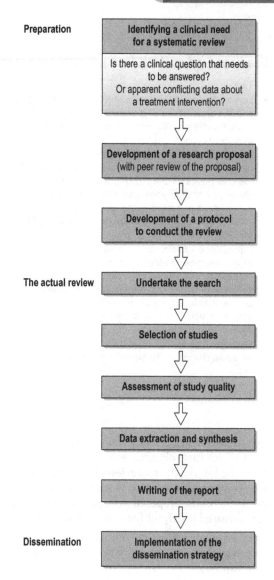

**Figure 12.7** • The process for undertaking a systematic review.

exist and indicate the amount of literature available to answer the proposed question.[70] Once the need for a systematic review in the field has been established a research proposal should be prepared. Box 12.3 highlights the key subheadings that practitioners may find useful to incorporate in a proposal for a systematic review.[71]

Once the proposal has been written it is important to gain an independent scientific review (ISR) of the proposal prior to a protocol being implemented, replicating the process undertaken for a primary

> **Box 12.3**
>
> ### Headings (and content) for a proposal for a systematic review
>
> - Title.
> - Summary – a brief synopsis of the aims of the review and the significance of the work will give readers an instant understanding of the importance of the proposed project.
> - Aims – detail of the study aims and the research questions that the review is aiming to answer as well as the end-points for the study. End-points may include development of key research questions that remain unanswered and need further primary study or identification of a specific intervention to apply in practice.
> - Background – this section should include a brief review of the literature to place the proposed work in some context, it might focus on the political, economic or social drivers for the project or give a historical perspective to current treatment or imaging rationales. Evidence identified from the scoping exercise may be beneficial in this section.
> - Method – this section should include the search strategy, databases to be used, key terms, inclusion/
> exclusion criteria, search limits, data extraction method, approach to be taken to quality assessment of the individual studies, how data will be synthesized (including information on any quantitative analysis), how reliability of the review will be determined, and how bias will be minimized.
> - Timeline – a detailed breakdown of the key milestones for the study.
> - Project management – how the study will be managed and the key roles of members of the project team.
> - Dissemination strategy – details of how the results will be disseminated should be multifaceted and practitioners may find the approach suggested by Lavis et al[71] helpful.
> - Costs – identified costs including time for researchers undertaking the review, costs of searching databases (there may be a cost for access to some databases), costs of retrieving articles as well as costs to disseminate the results.
> - References.

study. Whereas in a primary study there is a need to gain the relevant research ethics and governance approvals, for systematic reviews there may not be such stringent requirements. However, gaining some peer review of the proposed work prior to the project being initiated is helpful for a number of reasons:

- Reviewers may identify additions to the search strategy that could improve the overall quality of the study.
- Poorly designed reviews will be ineffective and may produce results that are biased or inaccurate leading potentially to an inappropriate technology or treatment being implemented. ISR can identify potentially poor quality reviews and prevent resources being wasted on projects that may not be effective.

Funding bodies provide ISR during the application approval process but practitioners may wish to seek peer review prior to a funding application and this may be available locally through a university or via the local research and development department of the employing organization. Undergraduate and postgraduate students can use the experience of their supervisors to review the quality of their proposal.

## The search strategy

Developing a multifaceted search strategy should ensure the review identifies as much of the available evidence as possible. The search strategy should detail the databases to be searched, the key terms for the search, inclusion and exclusion criteria, and any limits placed on the search. Box 12.4 provides an example of a search strategy with common databases, websites and other strategies that may be useful for those working in imaging or radiation therapy. The Cochrane Collaboration provides a useful starting point for a search strategy along with the other major electronic databases. The Cochrane Library contains a number of databases housed together:

- The Cochrane Database of Systematic Reviews (CDSR)
- Database of Abstracts of Reviews of Effects (DARE)
- Cochrane Central Register of Controlled Trials (CENTRAL)
- Cochrane Methodology Register (CMR)
- Health Technology Assessment Database (HTA)
- NHS Economic Evaluations Database (NHSEED).

## Box 12.4

### A sample search strategy

1. Databases
   a. MEDLINE
   b. CINAHL
   c. EMBASE
   d. Cochrane Reviews database including Database of Abstracts and Reviews (DARE)
   e. National Research Register including the ongoing reviews database (CRD Register of reviews)
   f. LILACS Latin American and Caribbean Literature in Health Sciences
   g. ISI Web of Knowledge to search Science Citation Index to follow citations from key papers
   h. ScienceDirect to search for articles from journals not listed on MEDLINE
2. Websites – to identify professional reports
   a. National Institute for Clinical Excellence (NICE)
   b. National Library for Health
   c. TRIP (Turning Research into Practice)
   d. Intute: Health and Life Sciences Medicine (www.intute.ac.uk/healthandlifesciences/medicine/)
   e. UK Society and College of Radiographers (www.sor.org)
   f. UK Royal College of Radiologist (www.rcr.ac.uk)
3. Key journal hand searches – these will vary according to the topic area but common journals of relevance may include:
   a. Radiation therapy
      i. *Radiotherapy and Oncology*
      ii. *International Journal of Radiation Oncology Biology Physics*
      iii. *Journal of Radiotherapy in Practice*
      iv. *European Journal of Cancer*
      v. *Clinical Oncology*
   b. Imaging
      i. *British Journal of Radiology*
      ii. *Clinical Radiology*
      iii. *Radiology*
   c. Imaging and radiation therapy
      i. *Radiography*
4. Author searching – searching databases by author may be beneficial where an author is known to publish or is a known expert in the topic area; this may be identified from literature retrieved in the original scoping exercise.
5. Grey literature
   a. Index to Theses
   b. Index to Scientific and technical proceedings (via ISI web of knowledge)
   c. Conference papers Index
   d. British Library integrated catalogue
   e. COPAC – merged online catalogue of major university and national libraries in the UK and Ireland
6. Key words – for each facet of the research question key words and MEDLINE subject headings should be identified, for example if a facet of the question included 'patients with cancer' then keywords might include:
   a. carcinoma, tumour, tumor, cancer, invasive carcinoma
   b. MEDLINE subject heading – neoplasms
7. Inclusion/exclusion criteria – these may be specific to the topic area, for example factors in a review to identify the effectiveness of partial breast irradiation inclusion criteria may be studies that consider external beam methods as well as brachytherapy (including balloon catheter methods). Alternatively the focus for inclusion may be on the types of studies to be included, for example in effectiveness reviews it may be relevant to include RCTs or quasi-experimental studies (trials without randomization).

### Search limits

For studies in HTA it is sensible to limit the review to data produced once the technology under question was implemented. For practical reasons undergraduate and postgraduate students often choose to limit studies to those published in the English language but possible bias needs to be considered where this is adopted.

The Cochrane databases can be searched together through a single search making this a useful tool for researchers planning a systematic review.

A detailed protocol using the main databases listed in Box 12.4 will go some way to helping retrieve as many of the relevant research studies as possible. However, in complex reviews it is possible that the protocol itself may only identify a proportion of the available data, and researchers should try to broaden their approach to include a range of strategies that develop as the review progresses.

For example, use of snowballing, which is using the reference lists of retrieved articles and forward tracking from a selected article to identify articles that have subsequently cited this paper – citation tracking, can increase the yield of relevant articles, and has been shown to account for approximately 53% of articles used in a complex systematic review.[72]

Other strategies to consider include using personal networks to contact individuals who may know of relevant research. This type of informal approach has been found to increase the proportion of relevant articles for a review by approximately 60%.[72]

Searching the grey literature is also of importance as this may limit the effect of publication bias.[73] In a systematic review of studies including grey literature as well as published trials, it was identified that published trials tended to show a greater treatment effect than grey literature. This may be due to differences between published and unpublished trials such as sample size differences, and grey literature studies finding the intervention has no effect, which is a less interesting result and less likely to be published.[73] Grey literature refers to studies not yet formally published and may be found in conference proceedings, indexes to theses or on trial registers.

A common problem with using electronic databases as the primary search strategy is their lack of sensitivity in some cases to identify all the relevant RCTs that have been published. The Cochrane Collaboration has developed a sensitive search strategy that should allow greater search precision and using this database to identify effectiveness trials should be a fundamental part of the search strategy. Other strategies to maximize retrieval of all relevant trials is the use of electronic databases searches that contain journals not registered with Medline. Some new journals may not be registered with electronic databases such as MEDLINE or CINAHL so individual hand searching of these journals and other key journals known to publish research in the field of interest should be considered. Hand searching has been shown to identify between 92% and 100% of the total number of trials identified from both hand searching and electronic searching,[74] with MEDLINE identifying 55% of the total trials identified.[74] While hand searching is a useful additional strategy it is time-consuming, involving review of each article, review and letter published in each issue of the chosen journal to identify relevant work.

Another aspect of the search strategy that practitioners need to consider is the restriction of the search to English language journals. This is often undertaken for simplicity in undergraduate and postgraduate studies and where funding is not available for translation. There is a possibility that limiting the search in this way may bias the outcome of the review, but evidence about the impact of such a strategy is unclear. It has been identified that the quality of English language versus non-English language articles is the same,[75,76] but it is possible that research published in non-English journals is less likely to demonstrate a significant result,[75] so by their exclusion may alter the outcome of any meta-analysis. However, in a review of language-restricted and language-inclusive meta-analyses, no difference in estimates of benefit were identified.[77,78] It is therefore difficult to predict the overall impact of excluding non-English language studies.

## Quality assessment

Chapter 4 highlighted the importance of critical appraisal of the published literature and identified a range of tools that can be used to help in the appraisal process. A number of tools are reported in the literature and these include checklists, as well as scales, with around 60 different quality assessment tools available.[79] Quality is a difficult construct to define for the range of research that a practitioner is likely to come across and no one tool may be appropriate for a range of topic areas. The QUADAS tool for the assessment of the quality of studies of diagnostic accuracy is a validated tool that is based on the results of a consensus Delphi study.[80] All quality assessment tools should be developed using formalized methods of development with assessments of face, content and construct validity and tested for reliability across different raters.[37] A tool developed initially to assess the quality of RCTs in pain research (the Jadad scale) was also based on a Delphi consensus method of agreement of experts and has been proposed for use across a range of clinical trials.[81] This tool uses a scale from 0 to 5 with reviewers scoring the answers to three questions as either yes (scores 1 point) or no (scores no points), with additional points awarded where blinding and randomization were appropriate.[81]

In contrast the Cochrane Collaboration recommends a domain-based approach to quality assessment of RCTs including assessment of the following:[82]

- sequence generation
- allocation concealment
- blinding of participants, personnel and assessors
- incomplete outcome data
- selective outcome reporting
- other sources of bias.

Assessment tools often consider the internal validity of the study as reported but published trials judged by assessment tools to be low quality may actually reflect poor reporting rather than poor design quality, resulting from a lack of understanding on how to report a clinical trial, a problem of under-reporting.[79] To overcome problems associated with publication bias, journals such as *The Lancet* and the *British Medical Journal* now hold a register of clinical trials and it has been suggested that these registers could also allow comparison of original trial reports with actual manuscripts to reduce potential problems with over- or under-reporting.[79]

A quality assessment threshold should be identified to exclude weak studies from the review and can be achieved by applying a cut-off level for study selection. This may be based on quality assessment criteria identified above, as well as using a hierarchy of study designs. For example, in effectiveness studies the primary research question is based on an assessment of one intervention over another, which is best studied using a RCT with concealment of allocation. Where these are not available the next best design should be chosen, i.e. quasi-experimental studies where there is no randomization or cohort studies.[70] For reviews considering test accuracy the hierarchy of study designs differs and the method at the top of the hierarchy is a blind comparison where there is a reference standard and a broadly defined sample of consecutive patients. Similarly, where these do not exist or are limited for the test under review it may be necessary to include studies where there is a narrow population or differential use of a reference standard.[70]

When attempting to assess trial quality it is helpful to use a data collection/extraction form that includes details of the bibliographic reference, description of study characteristics and the quality assessment. This can then be used to develop a table of evidence comprising all the included trials. Examples of such forms can be found on the SIGN website which is in the public domain (http://www.sign.ac.uk/guidelines/fulltext/50/compevidence.html).

Regardless of the chosen assessment tool or threshold level chosen it is important that the quality assessment is not only integrated into the selection of studies for inclusion in the review but also incorporated within the results that are presented. However, in many published systematic reviews, while quality assessment is apparent in the selection of included trials, the quality of the selected studies is not always transparent in the final reporting of the results.[83] Quality assessment should be incorporated into the systematic review process at the selection of studies phase, in the interpretation of conflicting trial results, in the weight apportioned to trials within a meta-analysis and in the conclusions and recommendations of the review.[70] This can be achieved in its simplest form by a description of the results with a review of any risks of bias within the individual studies included. It can also be achieved by listing the quality score, or using the method adopted by SIGN where 1++ refers to high quality and 1− refers to RCTs with risk of bias (see Table 12.1) against the tabulation of the individual trial characteristics so that readers can instantly see how the study quality may influence the overall outcomes of the review.

## Meta-analysis

Where individual studies allow, a formal quantitative analysis of the results may be undertaken in the form of a meta-analysis. This quantitative analysis provides a precise estimation of intervention effects and can indicate heterogeneity between studies where this exists. Including inappropriate studies in the meta-analysis can lead to misleading results, hence care needs to be taken in the execution of the analysis. For systematic reviews that include meta-analysis inclusion criteria need to prescribe the characteristics of studies that allow them to be combined in the meta-analysis; this may be trials studying the same intervention with the same outcome measures, undertaken on patients with similar characteristics (such as age or disease type).

The meta-analysis itself involves combining the results of all included studies that are combinable, i.e. have the same outcome measure. The individual trial results are weighted according to trial size although weighting based on trial quality has been proposed.[79] The methods used to combine the data are defined by two models, 'fixed effects' and 'random effects'. The choice of model depends on the presence of heterogeneity or variability between studies. Variability across studies, i.e. between-studies heterogeneity, can be assessed using either a Q statistic or an $I^2$ index.[85] The Q statistic produces a binary outcome identifying whether heterogeneity is present or absent. The $I^2$ index has been proposed as it gives a better indication of the level of heterogeneity that is present. Studies with an $I^2$ index of 25%, 50% and 75% would be classified as having low, medium or high variability respectively.[85]

The 'fixed effects' model combines the results of studies assuming that the effect of the intervention is constant across studies so only within-study variation is included in the analysis. In contrast, the 'random effects' model is based on the premise that the true treatment effect is different across individual studies[86] and this method is preferred when variability across studies is high.[84,85]

The results of combining data is often presented in graphical form; traditionally this has been using a forest plot like the one in Figure 12.8.

Figure 12.8 depicts the forest plot from the Early Breast Cancer Trialists Collaborative Group meta-analysis of randomized trials to establish the impact of radiotherapy on breast cancer mortality.[87] Each trial is described by one line. Black squares indicate the ratio of death rates for radiotherapy versus the control group, the size of the square is proportional to the weight of the trial within the analysis. The horizontal line on forest plots usually defines the 95% confidence intervals. The solid vertical line indicates a ratio of 1.0 (i.e. 1.0 indicates no difference between radiotherapy and the control group). For each category of trial the total ratio and the 95% CI are shown as a diamond. The overall results of this meta-analysis identified a small benefit from additional radiotherapy that was translated as a non-significant reduction in the annual death rate (3.9%). There was heterogeneity between the trials which would be expected given 40 trials were combined, including trials running over a 20 year period covering a range of different radiotherapy techniques and dose fractionation schedules. This meta-analysis serves to highlight an important dilemma in HTA primarily, that when mature data are available for analysis, the technology and treatment options may have moved on substantially, making the outcomes difficult to interpret within a new context. However, what this meta-analysis did highlight was an increase in the radiotherapy trials in non-cancer related (vascular) deaths which served to draw awareness of the need to consider the dose to cardiac tissue within radiotherapy chest wall fields for this group of patients.

Meta-analyses do have limitations which may be ascribed to the quality of the original RCTs available for analysis. As described in the previous section, inadequate sample sizes or opportunities for bias, such as inadequate concealment, may reduce the quality of the research which may then lead to inaccuracies in subsequent meta-analysis. Furthermore, research with a positive result is more likely to be published than a study showing no treatment or intervention benefit. Therefore, meta-analyses may suffer the effects of publication bias if search strategies to identify eligible studies exclude the grey literature. In addition, meta-analyses suffer the risk of bias that may occur from the process of undertaking a systematic review including bias in the selection of studies, the assessment of study quality by the reviewers and problems with poor reporting of study results or errors in the data of the published reports.[88] A method proposed to identify publication bias in meta-analyses is the use of a simple graphical presentation of the individual trials estimate of treatment effect plotted against the trial sample size (funnel plot). If there is no bias the plot should be symmetrical, depicting an inverted funnel with greatest dispersion of effects among trials of small sample sizes and a less marked dispersion in trials with larger sample sizes,[86,88] with meta-analyses that contain bias demonstrating asymmetrical funnel plots.[86]

## Reporting the results of a systematic review

In a review of the methods of reporting of systematic reviews of diagnostic tests in cancer, Mallett et al[89] identified significant variability in reporting of critical criteria such as defining the target condition where 51% failed to report if tumours were primary, recurrent or metastatic, with equal failings when it came to reporting tumour stage.

To improve the quality of reporting of systematic reviews a consensus report (by the QUOROM group) proposed a checklist of items and a flow diagram that should be included in systematic reviews and meta-analyses.[90] The checklist and flow diagram can be downloaded from the author section of most leading journal websites and consists of 21 headings and subheadings to guide authors in the reporting of this type of research.[90] The standard proposed by the QUOROM group covers the detail that is needed in the reporting of the search strategy, selection of studies for inclusion in the review, quality assessment of the selected trials, method of data extraction, details of the study characteristics, the quantitative data analysis (including assessment of publication bias) and the flow diagram to indicate the number of trials identified, those included, and information about trials that were excluded.[90]

## Assessing the quality of a systematic review

Now that the process of undertaking and reporting a systematic review has been discussed we can consider how to assess the quality of a systematic review;

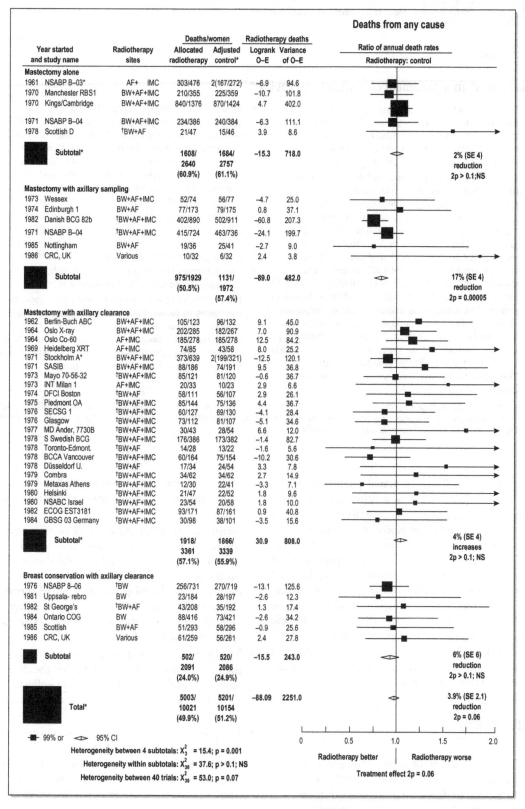

**Figure 12.8** • An example of a forest plot. Reprinted from The Lancet, vol. 355, Early Breast Cancer Trialists' Collaborative Group, Favourable and unfavourable effects on longterm survival of radiotherapy for early breast cancer: an overview of the randomised trials:1757–70, copyright (2000), with permission from Elsevier.

## Box 12.5

### Example of an assessment of a systematic review*[91]

- Does the study address an appropriate and clearly focused question? Yes – incremental accuracy of breast MRI in addition to annual mammography with or without breast ultrasound and clinical breast examination in screening women ≤50 years.
- Is the search strategy extensive? The databases and key terms used were appropriate, additional website searching was undertaken (although actual sites not explicitly stated so difficult to replicate), other strategies were used to maximize accuracy of yield including using experts and reference lists of retrieved articles. It is not clear if hand searching was employed or how extensive the use of grey literature was. A large number of potentially relevant articles were identified ($n=3367$) reflecting an extensive search. The search was limited to articles published in the English language and this may introduce bias but data is contradictory on the impact of excluding non-English trials and for this specific topic it is unclear how much this would have altered the results. The inclusion and exclusion criteria for trials were explicit.

- Assessment of study quality – the authors used a validated tool (QUADAS) to assess the quality of selected articles. Retrieved abstracts were reviewed by two independent assessors to reduce bias in the selection process. However, it is unclear whether there was blinding of reviewers to the authors and journal of the trials, possibly introducing some bias. A clear quality standard was used for included trials.
- Data extraction and analysis – detailed information is provided on the data extracted and methods used for further statistical analysis including assessment of heterogeneity which is detailed in the results section.
- Presentation of the results – detailed data are presented in tables for all five eligible studies.
- Minimization of bias – authors used two independent assessors to review abstracts for agreement with eligibility criteria, used validated tool for quality assessment of included studies, and present a flow-chart depicting selection and rejection of research from the original 3367 hits of potentially relevant publications.

*Reprinted from the European Journal of Cancer, 43: 13, Lord SJ, Lei W, Craft P, et al. A systematic review of the effectiveness of magnetic resonance imaging (MRI) as an addition to mammography and ultrasound in screening young women at high risk of breast cancer, 2007, with permission from Elsevier.

to do this we will use an actual published article. The work by Lord et al[91] is a systematic review of effectiveness studies comparing MRI in addition to mammography and ultrasound in young women considered at increased risk of developing breast cancer. You can read this article directly from a paper copy of the journal or electronically through Science Direct if your employing institution subscribes to this service. You can refer back to Chapter 4 where critical appraisal of the literature was discussed and some tools and checklists were proposed to help in the process. In Box 12.5 some key questions and answers about the quality of the review are proposed in order to demonstrate the process.

## Summary

- The full evaluation of a diagnostic test requires assessment at every level of the evaluative framework to demonstrate how good quality images contribute to accurate diagnoses,

beneficial changes to diagnoses and management plans, improved patient outcomes, at acceptable costs.
- Diagnostic accuracy studies that compare the results of the test under evaluation with a reference standard to establish whether it can distinguish patients with and without the target disorder are vulnerable to a plethora of threats to validity, but can be addressed by the conscientious and judicious application of tools and design issues referred to in this chapter.
- The performance of a diagnostic test can be measured using a variety of statistics, the choice of which depends on the type of data collected (binary, ordinal or continuous) and the question being addressed.
- In studies of diagnostic accuracy, it is important to estimate the variability of observers' interpretation of images as the accuracy of the diagnostic test can be a joint function of the images produced and the performance of the observers.

# References

[1] Knottnerus JA, Van Weel C. General introduction: evaluation of diagnostic procedures. In: Knottnerus JA, editor. The Evidence Base of Clinical Diagnosis. London: BMJ Books; 2002. p. 1–18.

[2] Dixon AK. Evidence-based radiology. Lancet 1997;350:509–12.

[3] Russell IT. The evaluation of computerised tomography: a review of research methods. In: Culyer AJ, Horisberger B, editors. Economic and Medical Evaluation of Health Care Technologies. Berlin: Springer-Verlag; 1983. p. 298–316.

[4] Mackenzie R, Dixon AK. Measuring the effects of imaging: an evaluative framework. Clin Radiol 1995;50:513–8.

[5] Fineberg HV, Bauman R, Sosman M. Computerized cranial tomography: effect on diagnostic and therapeutic plans. JAMA 1977;238:224–7.

[6] Fryback DG, Thornbury JR. The efficacy of diagnostic imaging. Med Decis Making 1991;11:88–94.

[7] Mackenzie R, Logan BM, Shah NJ, et al. Direct anatomical-MRI correlation: the knee. Surg Radiol Anat 1994;16:183–92.

[8] Robinson PJA. Radiology's Achilles' heel: error and variation in the interpretation of the Röntgen image. Br J Radiol 1997;70:1085–98.

[9] Brealey S, Scally AJ. Methodological approaches to evaluating the practice of radiographers' interpretation of images: a review. Radiography 2008; In Press.

[10] Pocock SJ. The justification for randomised controlled trials. In: Pocock SJ, editor. Clinical Trials: A Practical Approach. Chichester: John Wiley; 1983. p. 50–65.

[11] Sackett DL, Haynes RB. The architecture of diagnostic research. In: Knottnerus JA, editor. The Evidence Base of Clinical Diagnosis. London: BMJ Books; 2002. p. 19–38.

[12] Sackett DL, Haynes RB. Evidence base of clinical diagnosis: the architecture of diagnostic research. BMJ 2002;324:539–41.

[13] Chien FW, Khan KS. Evaluation of a clinical test. II: Assessment of validity. BJOG 2001;108:568–72.

[14] Lijmer JG, Mol BW, Heisterkamp S, et al. Empirical evidence of design-related bias in studies of diagnostic tests. JAMA 1999;282:1061–6.

[15] Bossuyt PM, Reitsma JB, Bruns DE, et al. The STARD Statement for reporting studies of diagnostic accuracy: explanation and elaboration. Ann Intern Med 2003; l38:1–12.

[16] Whiting P, Westwood M, Rutjes AWS, et al. Evaluation of QUADAS, a tool for the quality assessment of diagnostic accuracy studies. BMC Med Res Methodol 2006;6:9.

[17] Kelly S, Berry E, Roderick P, et al. The identification of bias in studies of the diagnostic performance of imaging modalities. Br J Radiol 1997;70:1028–35.

[18] Deeks J. Systematic reviews of evaluations of diagnostic and screening tests. In: Egger M, Smith GD, Altman G, editors. Systematic Reviews in Health Care: Meta-Analysis in Context. London: BMJ Publishing Group; 2001. p. 248–82.

[19] Fan J, Upadhye S, Worster A. Understanding receiver operating characteristic (ROC) curves. CJEM 2006;8(1):19–20.

[20] Habbema JDF, Eijkemans R, Krijnen P, et al. Analysis of data on the accuracy of diagnostic tests. In: Knottnerus JA, editor. The Evidence Base of Clinical Diagnosis. London: BMJ Books; 2002. p. 117–44.

[21] Brealey S, Scally AJ. Bias in plain film reading performance studies. Br J Radiol 2001;74:307–16.

[22] Streiner DL, Norman GR. Reliability. In: Streiner DL, Norman GR, editors. Health Measurement Scales: A Practical Guide to their Development and Use. Oxford: Oxford University Press; 2003. p. 137.

[23] Khan KS, Chien FW. Evaluation of a clinical test. I: Assessment of reliability. BJOG 2001;108:562–7.

[24] Rickett AB, Finaly DB, Jagger C. The importance of clinical details when reporting accident and emergency radiographs. Injury 1992;23:458–60.

[25] Good BC, Cooperstein LA, DeMarino GB, et al. Does knowledge of the clinical history affect the accuracy of chest radiograph interpretation? AJR 1990;154:709–12.

[26] Brealey S, Westwood M. Are you reading what we are reading? The effect of who interprets medical images on estimates of diagnostic test accuracy in systematic reviews. Br J Radiol 2007;80:674–7.

[27] Cohen J. A coefficient of agreement for nominal scales. Educ Psychol Meas 1960;20:37–46.

[28] Altman DG. Some common problems in medical research. In: Altman DG, editor. Practical Statistics for Medical Research. London: Chapman & Hall; 1991. p. 406.

[29] Lee W. Technology assessment: vigilance required. Int J Radiation Oncology Biol Phys 2008;70(3):652–3.

[30] Kunz R, Oxman AD. The unpredictability paradox: review of empirical comparisons of randomised and non-randomised clinical trials. Br Med J 1998;317:1185–90.

[31] Sapsford R, Jupp V. Validating evidence. In: Sapsford R, Jupp V, editors. Data Collection and Analysis. London: Sage, Open University; 1998. p. 1–24.

[32] Scottish Intercollegiate Guidelines Network. SIGN 50: A Guideline Developers Handbook, Available at:http://www.sign.ac.uk/guidelines/fulltext/50/index.html (accessed 4 October 2009).

[33] Fernando IN, Ford HT, Powles TJ, et al. Factors affecting acute skin toxicity in patients having breast irradiation after conservative surgery: a prospective study of treatment practice at the Royal Marsden Hospital. Clin Oncol 1996;8:226–33.

[34] Noble-Adams R. Radiation induced reactions 2: development of a

measurement tool. Br J Nurs 1996;8(18):1208–11.

[35] Noble-Adams R. Radiation induced reactions 3: evaluating the RISRAS. Br J Nurs 1999;8(19):1305–12.

[36] Neal A, Torr M, Helyer S, et al. Correlation of breast dose heterogeneity with breast size using 3D CT planning and dose volume histograms. Radiother Oncol 1995;34(34):210–8.

[37] Jadad A. Randomised controlled trials: a user's guide. London: BMJ Books, John Wiley & Sons Ltd; 2004.

[38] Moss S, Waller M, Anderson TJ, et al. Randomised controlled trial of mammographic screening in women from age 40: results of screening in the first 10 years. Br J Cancer 2005;92:949–54.

[39] Hendrick RE, Smith RA, Rutledge JH, et al. Benefit of screening mammography in women aged 40–49: a new meta-analysis of randomised controlled trials. J Natl Cancer Inst Monogr 1997;22:87–92.

[40] Probst H, Griffiths S. Increasing the work speed of radiographers: the effect on the accuracy of a set-up of a complex shaped cranial field, part of a matched cranio spinal junction. Radiother Oncol 1996;38(3):241–5.

[41] Norrman E, Persliden J. A factorial experiment on image quality and radiation dose. Radiat Prot Dosimetry 2005;114(1–3):246–52.

[42] Appleyard R, Beavis A, Bridge P, et al. Developing spatial cognition of brain anatomy using an immersive visualisation environment: a pilot study, In: Proceedings of the 7th International Educational Technology Conference, 6 pages, 3–5 May 2007, Cyprus.

[43] Probst H, Dodwell D, Gray JC, et al. An evaluation of the accuracy of semi-permanent skin marks for breast cancer irradiation. Radiography 2006;12(3):186–8.

[44] Office for National Statistics. Cancer statistics registrations 2005 MB1 no 36. National Statistics online 2007. Available at: http://www.statistics.gov.uk/statbase/Product.asp?vlnk=8843; [accessed 4 October 2009].

[45] Roberts C, Torgerson D. Understanding controlled trials:

randomisation methods in controlled trials. Br Med J 1998;317:1301.

[46] Torgerson DJ. Contamination in trials: is cluster randomisation the answer? Br Med J 2001;322:355–7.

[47] Torgerson DJ, Roberts C. Understanding controlled trials. randomisation methods: concealment. BMJ 1999;319 (7206):375–6.

[48] Pocock SJ. The size of a clinical trial. Clinical Trials: A Practical Approach. Chichester: John Wiley; 2008. p. 123–41.

[49] Probst H. Investigating Radiotherapy Protocols for Breast Carcinoma: An Evaluation of Respiratory Morbidity, Treatment Accuracy and Efficiency. Leeds: University of Teesside and Yorkshire Centre for Clinical Oncology, Leeds; 2002.

[50] Probst H, Dodwell D, Gray J, et al. Radiotherapy for breast carcinoma: an evaluation of the relationship between the central lung depth and respiratory symptoms. Radiography 2005;11(1):3–9.

[51] Pippa Corrie JSRH. Rate limiting factors in recruitment of patients to clinical trials in cancer research: descriptive study. Br Med J 2003;327:320–1.

[52] Welton A, Vickers M, Cooper J, et al. Is recruitment more difficult with a placebo arm in randomised controlled trials? A quasirandomised, interview based study. Br Med J 1999;318:1114–7.

[53] Hancock BW, Aitken M, Radstone C, et al. Why don't cancer patients get entered into clinical trials? Experience of the Sheffield Lymphoma Group's collaboration in British National Lymphoma Investigation studies. BMJ 1997;314(7073):36.

[54] Mitchell G, Abernethy A. for the Queensland Case Conferences Trial and the Palliative Care Trial. A comparison of methodologies from two longitudinal community-based randomized controlled trials of similar interventions in palliative care: what worked and what did not. J Palliat Med 2005;8(6):1226–37.

[55] Torgerson DJ, Sibbald B. Understanding controlled trials. What is a patient preference trial. BMJ 1998;316(7128):360.

[56] Torgerson DJ, Roland M. What is Zelen's design? BMJ 1998;316 (7131):606.

[57] Dumville JC, Torgerson DJ, Hewitt CE. Reporting attrition in randomised controlled trials. BMJ 2006;332(7547):969–71.

[58] Pocock SJ. Protocol deviations. Clinical Trials: A Practical Approach. Chichester: John Wiley; 2008. p. 176–86.

[59] Hollis S, Campbell F. What is meant by intention to treat analysis? Survey of published randomised controlled trials. BMJ 1999;319 (7211):670–4.

[60] Altman DG, Bland JM. Missing data. BMJ 2007;334(7590):424.

[61] Fergusson D, Aaron SD, Guyatt G, et al. Post-randomisation exclusions: the intention to treat principle and excluding patients from analysis. BMJ 2002;325 (7365):652–4.

[62] Piccart-Gebhart MJ, Procter M, Leyland-Jones B, et al. Trastuzumab after adjuvant chemotherapy in HER2-positive breast cancer. N Engl J Med 2005;353(16):1659–72.

[63] Smith I, Procter M, Gelber RD, et al. 2-year follow-up of trastuzumab after adjuvant chemotherapy in HER2-positive breast cancer: a randomised controlled trial. Lancet 2007;369 (9555):29–36.

[64] National Institute for Clinical Excellence. Trastuzumab for the adjuvant treatment of early-stage HER2-positive breast cancer. London: NHS Department of Health; 2006 NICE Technology Appraisal Guidance 107.

[65] Drummond MF, O'Brien B, Stoddart GL, et al. Basic Types of Economic Evaluation: Methods for the Economic Evaluation of Health Care Programmes. 2nd ed. Oxford: Oxford University Press; 1997. p. 6–26.

[66] Palmer S, Byford S, Raftery J. Economics notes: types of economic evaluation. BMJ 1999;318(7194):1349.

[67] Amparo O, Santaballa A, Munarriz B, et al. Cost-benefit analysis of a follow-up program in patients with breast cancer: a randomized prospective study. Breast J 2007;13(6):571–4.

[68] Greene D, Williams PC. Accelerator operation. In: Greene D, Williams PC, editors. Linear Accelerators for Radiation Therapy. 2nd ed. London: Institute of Physics Publishing Bristol and Philadelphia; 1997.

[69] Greene D. The cost of radiotherapy treatments on a linear accelerator. Br J Radiol 1983;56:189–91.

[70] Centre for Reviews and Dissemination. Undertaking systematic reviews of research on effectiveness: CRD's guidance for those carrying out or commissioning reviews. Centre for Reviews and Dissemination, University of York; 2001. Centre for Reviews and Dissemination Report 4.

[71] Lavis J, Ross S, McLeod C, et al. Measuring the impact of health research. J Health Serv Res Policy 2003;8(3):165–70.

[72] Greenhalgh T, Peacock R. Effectiveness and efficiency of search methods in systematic reviews of complex evidence: audit of primary sources. BMJ 2005;331 (7524):1064–5.

[73] Hopewell S, McDonald S, Clarke M, et al. Grey literature in meta-analyses of randomised trials of healthcare interventions. Cochrane Database Syst Rev 2007; (2) MR000010.

[74] Hopewell S, Clarke M, Lefebvre C, et al. Handsearching versus electronic searching to identify reports of randomised trials. Cochrane Database Syst Rev 2007; (2) MR000001.

[75] Egger M, Zellweger-Zahner T. Language bias in randomised controlled trials published in English and German. Lancet 1997;350(9074):326.

[76] Moher D, Fortin P. Completeness of reporting of trials published in languages other than English: Implications for … [cover story]. Lancet 1996;347(8998):363.

[77] Moher D, Pham , Klassen TP, et al. What contributions do languages other than English make on the results of meta-analyses. J Clin Epidemiol 2000;53(9):964–72.

[78] Juni P, Holenstein F, Sterne J, Bartlett C, et al. Direction and impact of language bias in meta-analyses of controlled trials: empirical study. Int J Epidemiol 2002;31(1):115–23.

[79] Verhagen AP, de Vet HCW, de Bie RA, et al. The art of quality assessment of RCTs included in systematic reviews. J Clin Epidemiol 2001;54(7):651–4.

[80] Whiting P, Rutjes A, Reitsma J, et al. The development of QUADAS: a tool for the quality assessment of studies of diagnostic accuracy included in systematic reviews. BMC Med Res Methodol 2003;3(1):25.

[81] Jadad RA, Moore D, Carroll C, et al. Assessing the quality of reports of randomized clinical trials: is blinding necessary? Control Clin Trials 1996;17:1–12.

[82] Cochrane Collaboration. Cochrane Handbook for Systematic Reviews of Interventions Version 5.0.0, [updated February 2008]. Available at:http://www.cochrane.org/resources/handbook/index.htm (accessed 2 October 2009).

[83] Moja LP, Telaro E, D'Amico R, et al. Assessment of methodological quality of primary studies by systematic reviews: results of the metaquality cross sectional study. BMJ 2005;330(7499):1053.

[84] Egger M, Smith GD, Phillips AN. Meta-analysis: principles and procedures. BMJ 1997;315 (7121):1533–7.

[85] Huedo-Medina TB, Sanchez-Mecca J, Bottela J, et al. Assessing heterogenity in meta-analysis: Q statistic or I2 index? Psychol Methods 2006;11(2):193–206.

[86] Egger M, Davey SG, Schneider M, et al. Bias in meta-analysis detected by a simple, graphical test. BMJ 1997;315(7109):629–34.

[87] Early Breast Cancer Trialists' Collaborative Group. Favourable and unfavourable effects on long-term survival of radiotherapy for early breast cancer: an overview of the randomised trials. Lancet 2000;355(9217):1757–70.

[88] Felson DT. Bias in meta-analytic research. J Clin Epidemiol 1992;45 (8):885–92.

[89] Mallett S, Deeks JJ, Halligan S, et al. Systematic reviews of diagnostic tests in cancer: review of methods and reporting. BMJ 2006;333(7565):413.

[90] David M, Cook D, Eastwood S, et al. Improving the quality of reports of meta-analyses of randomised controlled trials: the QUOROM statement. Lancet 1999;354:1896–900.

[91] Lord SJ, Lei W, Craft P, et al. A systematic review of the effectiveness of magnetic resonance imaging (MRI) as an addition to mammography and ultrasound in screening young women at high risk of breast cancer. Eur J Cancer 2007;43(13):1905–17.

## Appendix 12.1   Aloe vera articles

Richardson JE, Smith M, McIntyre R, et al. Aloe vera for preventing radiation induced skin reactions: a systematic review. Clin Oncol 2005; 17(6): 478–84.

Nystrom J, Svensk AC, Lindholm-Sethson B, et al. Comparison of three instrumental methods for the objective evaluation of radiotherapy induced erythema in breast cancer patients and a study of the effect of skin lotions. Acta Oncol 2007; 46(7): 893–9.

Maddocks-Jennings W, Wilkinson JM, Shillington D. Novel approaches to radiotherapy-induced skin reactions: a literature review. Complement Ther Clin Pract 2005; 11(4): 224–31.

# Appendix 12.2 Linear accelerator running costs (example costs are relevant to the time of the study analysis in 2000)

| | Detail | Annual cost (£) |
|---|---|---|
| Linac staffing | Senior I | 23 095 |
| | Radiographers × 2 | 34 250 |
| | Superintendent III (10%) | 2549 |
| *Total linac staffing* | | *59 894* |
| Simulator staffing | Superintendent III | 25 490 |
| | Senior I | 23 095 |
| | Radiographer | 17 125 |
| *Total simulator staffing* | | *65 710* |
| Physics staffing | Based on the salary of one technical officer, for the servicing of one linac, i.e. approx 10% of total physics staffing (Greene D 1983) | *25 379* |
| | Cost of operating equipment over 10 years | Cost (£) |
| Linac equipment costs | Capital cost of a 6 MV linac | 552 250 |
| | Interest payments | 149 107.50 |
| | Building (40 year life 1/40 of building cost) | 9000 |
| | Interest payments on building | 7600 |
| | Initial stock of parts (2.5% of initial capital cost) | 13 806 |
| | Replacement parts consumables | 4000 |
| | Energy to operate machine | 500 |
| | Building maintenance costs | 4700 |
| Simulator costs | Capital costs | 434 750 |
| | Interest payments on equipment | 117 382.50 |
| | Building (40 year life 1/40 of building cost) | 2500 |
| | Interest payments on building | 2100 |
| | Initial stock of parts | 10 868 |
| | Replacement parts | 7000 |
| | Energy to operate machine | 500 |
| | Building maintenance costs | 2300 |

| | Detail | Annual cost (£) |
|---|---|---|
| Treatment planning system (TPS) | Capital cost | 12 000 |
| | Interest payments on equipment | 3600 |
| | Building (10 year depreciation 40 year life) | 1200 |
| | Interest payments on building | 1000 |
| | Replacement parts | 500 |
| | Energy to operate machine | 500 |
| | Building maintenance costs | 2300 |
| **Total TPS costs** | | **21 100** |
| **Total annual running costs** | | **287 039.40** |
| | | |
| **Total running cost/min** | | **2.30** |

Linac, linear accelerator.

# Section 4

## Dosimetry and service evaluation

# Dosimetry

13

Martin Vosper

## CHAPTER POINTS

- Although dosimetry can appear off-putting at first sight, it can provide a relatively straightforward route to completing a diagnostic imaging or radiotherapy research project.
- The steady pace of change in diagnostic imaging and radiotherapy means that new dosimetry research is always valuable.
- The measuring devices and techniques used in dosimetry are not infallible and all have limitations, which can provide sources of error.
- In diagnostic imaging radiation doses are relatively small and the main role of dosimetry is to measure the stochastic risks of cancer induction. There is interest in effective doses to the whole body, measured in sieverts. These are obtained indirectly via calculations and estimates.
- In radiotherapy the radiation doses are relatively high and the main role of dosimetry is to ensure that radiation treatments to tumours are optimized. Unwanted side-effects of radiotherapy include deterministic damage such as skin erythema and stochastic risks such as cancer induction. There is interest in measuring absorbed doses to target tissues, which can sometimes be recorded directly.

The subject of radiation dosimetry could easily fill a volume in its own right and this chapter aims to provide an overview of research opportunities and issues, rather than a comprehensive text.

## Why should we undertake research in radiation dosimetry?

'Dosimetry' here refers to the recording of doses of ionizing radiation received by patients, staff and members of the public during medical imaging and radiotherapy procedures. Many practitioners feel inclined to avoid research in radiation dosimetry, perhaps because they believe it is a very 'dry' subject or that they have to be high-flying experts in physics (and maths) to manage it. But neither of these worries is really justified. In fact dosimetry can be a useful introduction to medical imaging and radiotherapy research, because:

- It is easy to argue that dosimetry research is useful and relevant, as all hospital departments of imaging or radiotherapy must keep radiation doses to patients and staff as low as reasonably practicable (ALARP) and take steps to monitor this.
- Dosimetry is a form of experimental research, giving the opportunity to control the experimental variables and leave little to chance. This is a refreshing change from the situation in many types of human research.
- The methods used are already well described and can be followed quite easily.

1

© 2010, Elsevier Ltd.

- If human subjects (such as patients or staff) are not involved, there is usually no need for formal ethics approval.
- Since every piece of clinical equipment is to some extent unique and every hospital department has individual practices, dosimetry research can readily provide original information.
- The rapid pace of technical change, for example in digital imaging, multi-slice CT and intensity modulated radiotherapy, means that new dosimetry studies are always valuable and welcome.
- There is a range of 'phantoms' available which can simulate the human body for dosimetry purposes.
- It might be possible to undertake some dosimetry research in a convenient laboratory, perhaps at your university.
- Dosimetry usually avoids the need for questionnaires (and many people you might ask to take part in radiography research already suffer from 'questionnaire fatigue').

This all sounds promising, but are there any 'down sides' to dosimetry? Well you do need access to the necessary equipment, such as radiation detectors, dose readers and possibly phantoms (if you are not using human subjects). Some of these things are expensive, or might not always be available. Remember to check and book them in advance – it is not good to find out at the last minute that the apparatus has broken down or is already on loan to another student. You will also need some training in equipment use. More will be said about equipment and techniques later in this chapter. If you are thinking about doing some dosimetry, you will need to be comfortable presenting numerical data with tables and graphs, as well as doing some fairly straightforward calculations. If you are the sort of person who is interested in human viewpoints and feelings you will probably steer away from dosimetry, but how about doing some qualitative research on the way that patients and staff feel about radiation risks?

As in any other sort of research, it is important to ask a question. This question should be clinically relevant and of interest, but it would not normally be expected that the dosimetry research method should be completely original. It is completely acceptable, and in fact necessary, that tried and tested methods are used, in order to permit comparisons between study data. This is a big help to any new researcher. Every hospital radiography environment is different,

and so fresh dosimetry readings will always be of value, both for audit purposes and for addition to existing data collected by national surveys of medical radiation protection.

The constant pace of technical and procedural change in radiography provides plenty of opportunities for original dosimetry research. There should not be any excuse for trying to ask research questions which were answered many decades ago and published in standard textbooks. An example of unoriginal and unnecessary research which would fail a 'so what?' test would be a study of whether a PA or AP technique affects patient dose in diagnostic lumbar spine radiography. The answer is 'yes – of course it does and the PA technique reduces dose'. Studies to demonstrate this were published over 30 years ago. It is not likely that the situation will be any different today. But what you *could* perhaps ask in a research project is: 'Since the PA lumbar spine projection reduces patient dose, why is this not the standard radiographic technique today?' That would identify a lot of factors: image quality issues, personal preferences, resistance to change.

# Topics for radiation dosimetry research

In medical imaging with ionizing radiations (which are mostly X-rays but also gamma rays in radionuclide imaging), there is a clear need to obtain a high quality diagnostic image while giving the lowest practicable radiation dose to patients and staff. However, the very best possible quality images tend to require larger doses of radiation; this has always been the case, ever since the discovery of X-rays in 1895, and continues to be so, despite recent improvements in technology. Given the trade-off between these two factors, image quality and dose, it is wise to consider image quality when studying the doses of radiation given during medical imaging procedures. It must be remembered that a very low dose X-ray procedure might not be of much benefit to a patient if the image is too indistinct to enable the proper diagnosis of their disease.

In medical imaging dosimetry you might be able to research:

- the effects on dose of manipulating the technique for a given procedure
- new and improved techniques for dose reduction
- the effectiveness of radiation protection measures, such as shielding and filtration

- magnitudes of doses to the 'whole body', individual organs, or to the fetus
- 'environmental doses', in areas close to radiation sources such as X-ray tubes or radioisotopes
- dose variations between imaging departments, different pieces of imaging equipment, different practices or even different operators
- dose variations over time
- doses received by staff, e.g. imaging practitioners and other groups
- the relationships between dose and image quality
- the effects of new technology, such as digital imaging or multi-slice CT
- the effects of staff training and radiation awareness
- the effects of systems of work, including administration, image archiving and patient referral.

In radiotherapy, dosimetry is very much an integral part of the work process and is an essential element of treatment planning. 'In vivo' dosimetry is playing an increasing part in providing rapid verification data during the external beam treatment itself. While in medical imaging the damaging effects of radiation are always an unwanted side-effect, in radiotherapy the damaging effects of radiation on tumours are deliberate and planned. Here the aim is to promote an adverse effect – but only on cancer cells. There is still a need to restrict the unwanted dose to normal and vulnerable tissues, both within and without the radiation field. Advances in radiotherapy have often focused on the need to deliver optimum doses to cancers, including the tumour margins, while limiting the doses to non-cancerous tissues and minimizing the risks to neighbouring vulnerable organs. Radiotherapy dosimetry involves a greater variety of ionizing radiations – not only X-rays from linear accelerators (linacs) and gamma rays from cobalt sources, but also fast-moving particles such as electrons, protons or neutrons.

In radiotherapy dosimetry you might be able to research:

- the effects of altering the technique for a given procedure, such as when using high energy beams, electrons, multiple treatment fields
- new and improved techniques for dose reduction in at-risk tissues
- the effectiveness of radiation protection measures, such as shielding, filtration, distance

- in vivo dosimetry during radiation treatments, for example using electronic portal imaging
- doses in total body irradiation prior to bone marrow transplantation
- 'environmental doses', measuring leakage radiation in areas close to radiation sources such as linacs or radioisotopes
- dose variations between different pieces of radiotherapy equipment, different practices or even different operators
- doses in the simulator suite and in the CT-simulator
- doses in brachytherapy
- doses in superficial radiotherapy
- fractionation regimes
- new developments in areas such as 3-D conformal radiotherapy, intensity modulated radiotherapy
- the effects of staff training and radiation awareness
- the effects of systems of work, including administration.

The damaging effects of ionizing radiations are well known and fall into two major categories:

- *Stochastic* effects can occur at all magnitudes of dose and are a product of chance. The end result can be the induction of cancer, or the conveyance of a genetic abnormality to future offspring. The likelihood of the effect increases with radiation dose, but is neither impossible at low doses nor inevitable at high doses. Dosimetry in medical imaging is mostly concerned with measuring small radiation doses which, although relatively low-risk, might still cause stochastic effects. In radiotherapy, although doses are much higher and stochastic effects therefore more likely, it must be remembered that the patient already has a cancer and that the risk from 'under-dosing' a malignant tumour is likely to be greater than the risk from inducing cancers in surrounding normal tissues. However, the risks of genetic damage to reproductive cells such as ova or sperm, or radiation-induced secondary cancers, are always relevant considerations. Stochastic effects tend to be 'late effects', which means that they only appear after a time period which is usually measured in years, and not immediately. Thus it is normally hard to link a stochastic effect to a single episode of previous radiation exposure with certainty.
- *Deterministic (or tissue reaction)* effects only occur at relatively high doses and are of increasing severity as dose increases. The result is extensive

cell death and tissue damage, which may manifest as erythema (skin reddening), fibrosis, cataract, reduction in blood cell count, infertility, bowel disturbances and other serious changes. Deterministic (tissue reaction) effects are largely predictable and are common side-effects of radiotherapy. They can be minimized by delivering a radiation dose over an extended period of time rather than in a single large 'burst'. This is one of the benefits of dose fractionation in radiotherapy. Dosimetry in radiotherapy is mostly involved with measuring large radiation doses, which are intended to kill tumour cells but might have unintended deterministic or stochastic effects on normal tissues. In medical imaging, deterministic effects are rare but can result from extended fluoroscopy. Some types of detriment to the developing embryo or fetus in utero can also be regarded as deterministic in nature and might result from over-use of relatively high dose diagnostic procedures such as pelvic CT in an unsuspected pregnancy. Deterministic effects tend to be 'early effects' which appear within a period of days or weeks.

There are some general principles regarding the use of ionizing radiations, which apply both in medical imaging and radiotherapy:

- Increasing the number of ionizing rays (or particles) will always increase the radiation dose.
- Increasing the size of the beam (or field) of radiation will always increase the radiation dose.
- Increasing the energy, or penetrative power, of the radiation beam will tend to reduce the skin dose where the beam enters the human body, and tend to increase the dose at depth. It will also tend to produce more 'forward scatter' of radiation and less 'back scatter'.
- Increasing the distance between the source of radiation and the human body will reduce the radiation dose. This is particularly so if we are talking about *electromagnetic* radiations such as X-rays and gamma rays and is covered by the 'inverse square law'. As an aside, we should note that the dose from *particle* radiations such as electrons and protons may actually increase in some regards as the radiations pass deeper into the human body, due to something called the Bragg effect.
- Increasing the number of radiation exposures will always increase the dose, assuming that the size of the individual exposures is unchanged.

- Shifting sensitive tissues and organs away from an incoming radiation beam, for example by turning a patient to face away, will tend to reduce the dose.
- Leaving sensitive tissues and organs outside the radiation beam, either by angling, redirecting or limiting the beam, will reduce the dose.
- A rapid radiation procedure is not necessarily a low dose one, since improvements in technology mean that large doses can be given very quickly.
- No dose of radiation is ever totally without risk, no matter how small the exposure, although the risk from very small exposures is negligible.
- The size, or weight of a patient will affect the dose they receive, since radiation absorption will be influenced by body composition and dimensions.
- Young patients, especially children and babies, are more likely than elderly patients to suffer harm from a radiation exposure.

It is important to consider physics and radiobiology principles like these, as they will help you to explain unexpected findings and interpret your results.

To give an example of the appliance of science principles to real X-ray doses, let us consider the plain and simple (postero-anterior) PA chest projection in medical imaging. Here a high kV (high kilovoltage and hence high beam energy) technique should give a lower dose to the patient's chest than a low kV technique. This seems quite reasonable, as the more penetrating rays should pass through the patient's chest without being absorbed. But increasing the kV of the exposure increases not just the energy of the X-rays, but also the number of rays produced. To maintain the image density and keep patient dose at an acceptable level, a radiographer will turn down the mAs (milliampere-second) setting to compensate for the increased kV. A general rule of thumb is that a 15% increase in kV can be compensated for in terms of image density by halving the mAs. All looks good again for our high beam energy technique as a means to reduce dose.

The next practical issue is that higher energy beams tend to produce scatter within the human body that is more energetic and more forwards in direction. Thus it is more likely to reach the imaging plate. To avoid this scatter degrading the image, the practitioner may be obliged to use a secondary radiation 'grid' in order to maintain image contrast and quality. Unfortunately such a grid typically requires a three to four factor increase in the number of X-rays produced by the X-ray tube, to compensate for the removal of X-rays by the grid. These increased rays will still strike the patient, although they will not reach the image. The increase in dose resulting from the use of the grid might outweigh any dose benefit arising from the use of the high kV technique.

Another issue is that some modern digital imaging plates may be less efficient at high beam energies, requiring a further increase in the number of X-rays produced by the tube.

Finally, tissues lying outside the beam during PA chest radiography (such as the thyroid and eye) may receive a slightly higher dose at high beam energy, since the scattered radiation will be more penetrating and more likely to reach them.

This example illustrates that patient dose is affected by a number of practical considerations in 'real world' radiography. It also shows that a dosimetry study which does not also consider image quality can often be irrelevant.

# Devices, quantities and units of measurement in radiation dosimetry

To get to grips with radiation dosimetry we need to know the meaning of the several terms used to describe 'dose', as these can be a source of misunderstanding.

We need to know what we are measuring and why. In radiation dosimetry it is much easier to take physical measurements of the amount of energy deposited by ionization in non-living materials, rather than to take biological measurements of the actual 'injury' inflicted by that ionization in living tissues. Although it is the tissue injury which most interests us, usually this can only be extrapolated or calculated indirectly from the more direct physical measurements of ionization in non-living materials. Microscopic measurement of cell injury, for example through examination of chromosomes, is not available for most student projects, although macroscopic skin damage from large radiation doses (only likely during radiotherapy) is easily visible and can appear quite quickly. Some of the non-living materials used in radiation dosimetry to record doses are summarized in Table 13.1.

None of the materials listed in the table will perfectly mimic the absorption of radiation by the human body, although some of them, such as lithium fluoride thermoluminescent dosimeters(TLDs) may be fairly similar in density and atomic number to soft tissue. But all of them will be able to give a good idea of the relative sizes of different radiation exposures. Often in radiation dosimetry it is these relative values which are used to compile local and national surveys.

**Table 13.1 A selection of non-living materials used to absorb radiation in dosimetry**

| Non-living material used to absorb radiation | Applications |
| --- | --- |
| Air in a graphite or other container | Ionization chambers such as – thimble chambers and pencil chambers<br>Dose area product (DAP) meters<br>Pocket dosimeters ('pen' meters or 'bleepers'), which are modified Geiger devices |
| Argon or helium gas in a glass/graphite container | Geiger counters |
| Phosphors such as lithium fluoride with other additives | Thermoluminescent dosimeters (TLDs) |
| Phosphors such as sodium iodide doped with thallium (scintillators) | Scintillation detectors |
| Silver halides | Film dosimeters |
| Silicon, germanium | 'Diode' type solid state semiconductor devices |
| Metal oxide and silicon | Metal oxide field effect transistors (MOSFETs), a type of solid state semiconductor device |
| Amorphous silicon | Flat panel detectors used in electronic portal imaging devices (EPIDs), for portal dosimetry |
| Ferrous sulphate solution | Fricke dosimeters |

Bulky ionization chambers might be useful for providing reference dose standards and very sensitive measurements, but are not convenient for estimating a dose within a small patient volume. Large hand-held Geiger counters are valuable for detecting radiation and for environmental monitoring, but likewise not very practical for monitoring doses to individuals. Personal monitoring of staff is usually based on compact devices such as pocket dosimeters, TLDs or film badges, none of which are perfect tools but do give an idea of relative doses.

The most accurate way to monitor doses to patients' tissues would be the direct method of placing a small dosimeter within the body. This is not normally practicable of course, although it may be possible to place a dosimeter in the body in some radiotherapy situations. As an alternative, tissue-equivalent whole body phantoms, of about 75 kg weight for an adult male or about 50 kg weight for an adult female, such as the Alderson ART phantoms, may be used to accurately simulate typical organ doses for diagnostic imaging or radiotherapy procedures. These phantoms consist of a stack of body slices which can be dismantled, with holes at regular intervals to accept TLDs. Of course these standard phantoms cannot simulate the wide range of body sizes and weights found in real patients. An entire Alderson body phantom costs over £15 000, but if you have access to one you will find it very useful and it may remove the need to involve actual patients in your research. In radiotherapy, a simple water-equivalent epoxy resin phantom with holes to accept ionization chambers can be very useful to measure absorbed doses arising from treatment fields for audit purposes and for comparisons between radiotherapy treatment devices or hospital centres.

In practice, you will often be able to attach small dosimeters, such as TLDs, MOSFETs, diode type semiconductors or thimble ionization chambers, to the patient's skin surface. This is an indirect method for judging doses to internal organs, but does give a direct measurement of entrance surface dose (ESD) and exit dose (where the radiation beam enters and exits the body). TLDs are the most convenient devices for a patient as they do not come attached to wiring. They are also better than semiconductor devices for measuring skin dose or lens of eye dose, since they are not surrounded by a radiation-attenuating cap.

The most commonly used measurement for radiation dosimetry is the gray (Gy) which refers to energy absorbed in joules (J) per unit mass of matter in kilograms (kg). It is described as a unit of *absorbed dose*. The energy deposition in the matter takes place by ionization and the irradiated matter can consist of air, water, or solids such as body tissue. The gray is a physics-based unit and does not tell us much about the biological effects of radiation on living tissues.

You will also come across the term *kerma*, which, like the absorbed dose, is measured in joules per kilogram of matter. Kerma refers to 'kinetic energy released (per unit) mass'. The process of absorption of uncharged radiation (photons such as X and gamma rays, or particles such as neutrons) in matter results in the release of 'secondary' charged particles (electrons) from the atoms in that volume of matter. These electrons may come to a halt within the volume, or pass outside it. Put simply, while the kerma only records energy deposited by electrons which arise from ionizations within the volume, the absorbed dose also records energy deposited by electrons which arise from ionizations just outside the volume but which come to a halt within it.

# How can we get an idea of the biological harm caused by ionizing radiations?

To do this we need to consider not just the absorbed dose in body tissue but also how damaging different types of radiation are to tissue. This consideration gives us a unit called the *equivalent dose*, measured in sieverts (Sv). The damaging ability of the radiation is termed the *relative biological effectiveness* (RBE), which is quantified using a *radiation weighting factor*. In some older books you might find the term 'quality factor', which means the same thing as the more recent term radiation weighting factor. In order to simplify calculations, X-rays, gamma rays and electrons of all energies are assumed to have a radiation weighting factor of 1. For these radiations, the equivalent dose in sieverts is equal to the absorbed dose in gray multiplied by 1. In reality of course we know that relatively low energy X-rays, for example in mammography or superficial radiotherapy, are absorbed more than high energy X-rays and will thus be a bit more damaging, but these slight differences are ignored for the purposes of clinical dose limitation, control and routine assessment. A different radiation weighting factor has to be used if we are measuring the damaging effects of alpha particles, protons or neutrons. These heavier particles will of course do more harm, rather like an elephant crashing around inside a china shop. Proton and neutron beam treatments may be encountered in radiotherapy. Current recommendations are that protons have a radiation weighting factor of 2, while the radiation weighting factor for neutrons varies from about 2 to 20, depending on energy. Alpha particle emitters are not nowadays much encountered in medical imaging or radiotherapy but may arise from inhaled or ingested heavy elements like radon, radium or thorium. Alpha particles do not travel far but are very ionizing and are given an estimated weighting factor of 20.

The equivalent dose concept is used in the personal dose monitoring of staff via film badges or TLD tablets. The *personal dose equivalent* is that dose in tissue at a point just below the monitoring badge. It is used as a guide to likely doses received by the whole body. It is also possible to measure an *ambient dose equivalent* when monitoring doses received in an area such as a location in a workplace.

To get a more meaningful measurement of the real damaging effects of radiation on a human body, we need to know not only the damaging power of the radiation but also a) the individual doses received by all the organs and tissues exposed to that radiation and b) the individual sensitivities of those organs and tissues. This is not easy to measure. The term *effective dose* takes account of the damaging power of radiation and its effects on all of the body's vulnerable tissues. The *tissue weighting factor* describes the relative contribution from various organs and tissues to the likely total harm that a person will receive from ionizing radiation. More vulnerable organs have a higher weighting factor and the factors are given in Table 13.2.

The effective dose to the whole body provides a dose value in sieverts and is used to calculate the risk of stochastic radiation-induced events, chiefly cancer. Thus it is widely used measure for radiation protection of staff, patients and the public. To calculate an effective dose, we need to know the equivalent doses to each organ or tissue and multiply these by their appropriate tissue weighting factors. The total effective dose is then the sum of the individual tissue-weighted equivalent doses. In most clinical situations the radiation beam will not cover the whole body and thus many organs will only receive a small dose from scattered radiation. It is those organs which lie within the primary beam which will receive the greatest equivalent doses. Stochastic effects (both whole body and to individual organs) are also of interest in radiotherapy, as dose to normal tissues may arise from beam passage through the body on the way to the target volume, from scatter

**Table 13.2 Tissue weighting factors for radiation dosimetry (revised ICRP draft recommendations 2006)**

| Organ or tissue | Individual weighting factor for each organ or tissue | Total contribution |
|---|---|---|
| Lung, stomach, colon, bone marrow, breast, remainder* | 0.12 | 0.72 |
| Gonads (mean of ♂ and ♀) | 0.08 | 0.08 |
| Thyroid, oesophagus, bladder, liver | 0.04 | 0.16 |
| Skin, brain, bone surface, salivary glands | 0.01 | 0.04 |
| Whole body | | 1.00 |

*The 'remainder', a combined contribution of 0.12, is due in equal parts to the following fourteen tissues: adrenals, gall bladder, heart wall, kidneys, lymph nodes, muscle, oral mucosa, pancreas, prostate, small intestine, spleen, thymus, uterus/cervix and extra-thoracic tissue.

and from radiation leakage via the linac treatment head. Newer intensity modulated radiotherapy techniques, although they reduce the dose to at-risk structures near the tumour, may actually increase the volume of normal tissue irradiated.

## How can effective doses be calculated in practice?

One solution would be to insert TLDs in appropriate positions to record organ doses within the slices of an anthropomorphic tissue-equivalent whole body phantom, such as the Alderson ART phantom. However, this might require a lot of measurements, looking at the long list of organs in Table 13.2. An alternative is to calculate the equivalent doses to the organs using mathematical calculations based on standardized mathematical models of the volumes, shapes, densities and atomic numbers of the structures in the human body. These are often called Monte Carlo calculations – not as exotic as that seaside resort but based on the mathematical laws of chance just like the gambling in Monte Carlo's casinos. In this way, equivalent doses to internal organs can be calculated from equivalent doses measured at the surface of a real human body. This is made possible by the fact that entrance surface doses (where the radiation beam enters the human body) will tend to be the highest equivalent doses for many types of radiation beam and thus depth doses can be estimated from these values without too much inaccuracy. Computer programmes to provide Monte Carlo calculations are now more powerful than previously and a number of software packages are available. A full discussion of Monte Carlo techniques is beyond the scope of this chapter and advice should be sought from a local medical physicist.

Effective doses can be estimated from easily measurable quantities – the dose–area product and the entrance surface dose. These quantities will now be described. They have the advantage that they can be readily reproduced using standard equipment and are a good basis for comparisons of doses between hospitals and between X-ray equipment in national surveys. Conversion coefficients have been published to give estimates of effective dose from quantities such as dose–area product and entrance surface dose. These coefficients will vary with the radiation procedure being undertaken.

The *dose–area product* or DAP reading is obtained from an ionization chamber attached directly to the source of radiation. The measurement is a dose in air, recorded in grays per square centimetre. The dose value depends not only on the radiation output of the radiation source but also on the size of the radiation field or beam. The value will increase as the tube output and radiation field increase. It is a mistake to describe DAP readings as patient doses, but this error is often made in project write-ups. The DAP reading does provide us with an indication of the relative sizes of doses given to different patients, but is not a direct measurement of patient dose. Calibration factors can be used to estimate effective doses for given procedures in a given X-ray room. One pitfall is that the recorded DAP value increases greatly with a larger beam size, whereas the beam size will not greatly affect the dose to an organ that is in the centre of the beam. DAP values are more useful if field size and radiation output factors are also recorded. One big advantage is that a DAP meter gives an immediate digital readout.

In radiotherapy, the *electronic portal imaging device* (EPID), rather like the DAP meter, acts 'in beam' during actual patient procedures. Portal imaging devices, originally used for verifying patient position, may now be used to provide 2-D dose readings during linac treatments. EPIDs are usually of an older liquid-filled ionization chamber or a newer flat panel solid state amorphous silicon design. These devices permit calculation of either dose rates or absorbed doses, by applying software to the image data. Like the DAP meter, there is some dependency on field size. There is also some over-sensitivity to relatively low energy photons, which can be reduced using a copper filter. Solid state EPIDs, due to their fine matrix of individual detectors, are likely to be useful in connection with intensity modulated radiotherapy (IMRT).

The *entrance surface dose* (ESD) is perhaps a rather more reliable measurement than the DAP as it produces equivalent dose values at the skin surface, either using TLD tablets of near tissue density or the air of a small ionization chamber, either being attached at the point where the radiation beam enters the body. The reading is only affected by beam size to a relatively small degree, assuming that the beam is large enough to cover the TLD tablet or ionization chamber and surrounding area. But entrance surface dose readings can be affected by back-scatter of radiation from the patient or phantom and thus a correction needs to be made for this. The equivalent doses of organs lying quite close to the skin surface, such as the thyroid or breast, can be easily estimated from the ESD after making a reduction for attenuation. Monte Carlo techniques, as mentioned above, can derive effective doses from ESD values. TLD tablets are useful in that they do not interfere with the diagnostic image or radiotherapy treatment field. However, their sensitivity varies, both between batches and with beam energy. Also they cannot be read directly – they need to be processed to produce a visible light output which is proportional to the radiation dose absorbed. This delay brings about the possibility of fade and experimental errors, due to the need for ancillary equipment to read the tablets.

In radiotherapy, where doses to the tumour target volume must be precise and preferably subject to less than 3% variation from the planned dose, solid state semiconductor devices (termed 'diodes') attached to the skin surface in vivo have the advantage that they provide rapid ESD readouts, permitting alteration of radiotherapy technique during the treatment if necessary to deliver the planned dose. Strict calibration of the devices is required, as there is some variation in sensitivity in response to field size, focus to skin distance (FSD) and use of a wedge. The semiconductor device is surrounded by a 'cap' whose thickness may be needed to be adjusted for different beam MV values or electron treatment. In vivo dosimetry is preferable to data transferred from the planning system, due to possible errors with the latter. ESD measurements help to check radiation output, patient positioning and the calculation of number of monitor units (MU) needed.

The *exit dose*, measured at the skin surface where the beam leaves the patient, is a very useful additional value, especially in radiotherapy, as it allows better estimation of the actual dose delivered inside the patient, when used in conjunction with the ESD. It also permits verification of the dose delivery calculation and checking of the effect of the patient's size and body composition on dose. Exit dose, like entrance surface dose, can be measured using semiconductor devices or TLDs. If semiconductors are used, the entrance and exit devices should not be positioned directly above each other as the former may interfere with the beam reaching the latter. The increased use of 3-D and conformal radiotherapy has brought about the need for a high precision in dose measurement. In intensity modulated radiotherapy (IMRT) there is a need for rapid and accurate dose readings from small volume detectors, especially when dynamic multi-leaf collimation (that moves during the actual radiation delivery) is used.

# Dosimetry in computed tomography (CT)

This is a distinct topic in radiation dosimetry with its own terms and measurements, due to the nature of tomographic process. The technique gives some of the highest effective doses to patients in medical imaging, due in part to the speed and ease with which large volumes can be scanned. Indeed many doses from spiral and multi-slice scanners have risen in recent years, making CT a very good area for dosimetry research. The dose received in CT depends on a large number of factors: kVp (peak tube voltage), mA (tube current), volume coverage, pitch (CT table distance in millimetres moved per tube rotation), slice thickness, slice spacing or overlap (or 'bed indexing') and beam collimation. Many of these parameters are

within the control of the operator. Image noise (which reduces image quality) can be suppressed if higher dose parameters such as high mA, low pitch and narrow slice spacing are used. This presents a familiar conflict between image quality and dose and there has been a tendency to over-dose, including in CT of children. A common term in CT dosimetry is the *computed tomography dose index* or CTDI, which represents the area under the CT slice profile curve in a graph of absorbed dose (Gy) versus horizontal position across the slice (mm). The CTDI is expressed in Gy divided by mAs and slice thickness. The weighed *CTDI* or $CTDI_w$ takes account of the fact that dose in a phantom (or a real human body) decreases from the edge to the centre. Doses in CT are influenced by the total width of the number of slices used (or the detector array width for a multi-slice scanner), as well as the mAs and kVp. Values of CTDI can be obtained 'free in air' simply by using a line of TLD tablets or a thin pencil ionization chamber placed along the long axis of the scan profile. This may provide useful comparisons between scanners. Readings of $CTDI_w$ can be obtained by using a pencil ionization chamber inserted into holes both at the centre and four points around the periphery of a Perspex CT phantom. Another use of a line of TLDs is to record the shape of the dose profile across a single slice, which ideally should be rectangular but is usually a curve-sided peak in practice. A further term you might encounter is the *volume weighted CTDI* or $CTDI_{vol}$. This is the $CTDI_w$ divided by the pitch of the scanner.

As can be seen from the complexity of the topic, most people would be well advised to seek the advice of a medical physicist when recording and using CTDI data. As an alternative, some straightforward readings of equivalent doses to organs could be obtained by placing TLDs in suitable holes within the slices of an anthropomorphic phantom. This is another useful way to compare doses between different scanners or between different scan parameters. Remember that the traditional concept of entrance surface dose does not really apply in CT, due to the rotation of the X-ray beam around the body. Some modern CT scanners provide digital readouts of $CTDI_{vol}$ values, although these do not always correlate totally with independent measurements. Effective doses can be obtained from $CTDI_{vol}$ values, by multiplying by the total length of the scanning volume and applying correction coefficients based on patient age and the body area being scanned.

# Some practical issues in radiation dosimetry

As in other forms of research, when doing radiation dosimetry you need to remind yourself of the following questions:

- What am I aiming to achieve with this research?
- How am I going to apply my results to clinical practice?
- Are there any errors in my data?
- What is feasible?

Complex calculations of reliable effective doses to patients are necessary if you are intending to calculate the small but real increased risk of stochastic effects such as radiation-induced cancer. But is this information vital to your department's clinical practice? Will procedures be altered as a result? Possibly yes, but realistically you are probably more interested in the relative magnitudes of equivalent doses due to different practices, decisions and equipment set-ups. For this purpose the simple application of TLDs to patients' skin surfaces will suffice. In radiotherapy, the accurate and reliable determination of equivalent doses to at-risk normal tissues and malignant cancers is vital, owing to the large sizes of the doses and their immediate impact on patients' well-being. Choosing 'horses for courses' is a clear message here.

When dealing with small doses, perhaps arising from scattered radiation outside the primary beam, we need to ask whether the values are actually measurable with the equipment we have available. It might be possible to make multiple exposures in order to give a detectable reading and then calculate the dose per individual exposure, but this will not be feasible if a patient is involved. Similarly, some changes in radiographic technique might not produce a measurable difference in dose. It is wise to do a pilot study to check if this is the case.

Many of the methods used to estimate doses have inherent margins of error, due to assumptions and approximations made in calculations. Thus it is not always justified to report results to a very high accuracy – error ranges can be usefully quoted. Also, since dosimetry is based on experimental methods, there are a number of biases which can affect our results. Let us consider the variables which can affect our experimental readings in dosimetry research:

- faults and fluctuations in the radiation detector(s)
- alterations in detector efficiency according to beam energy

- variations in the output of the radiation source
- errors in the equipment used to record dose values
- differences in size and composition between human bodies, and between phantoms and human bodies
- inconsistency in the use of parameters such as source-to-skin distance, collimated field size, detector positioning, beam energy and intensity, beam filtration
- variations in the intensity of scattered radiation, due to lead shielding, presence of nearby solid objects, human body or phantom size and composition.

As a researcher you should be aware of these variables, try to minimize them where possible and always consider them in the discussion of your results.

Data errors are a feature of dosimetry, since all of the measurement devices available have their own particular shortcomings, as can be illustrated by the following brief discussion of thermoluminescent dosimeters (TLDs). The TLD is a widely-used device and has some advantages, including small size, good sensitivity, near tissue density equivalence and a response that is not much influenced by dose rate. But it is important to be aware of the variations that can occur when using TLDs. They need a complicated 'annealing' cycle to remove past readings, and may show alterations in sensitivity due to various causes. Also they suffer from fade and their response to radiation might not be linear at large doses. The process of annealing involves heating TLDs to temperatures of up to 400°C and then allowing controlled cooling. This process removes any residual readings from absorbed radiation and affects sensitivity. The temperature in the annealing cycle must reach equilibrium and avoid variations. It is possible that TLDs can lose sensitivity after many anneal cycles and sensitivity is also affected by the cooling rate after removal from a high temperature oven.

It is important that the TLDs are handled with tweezers during the radiation dosimetry process or kept sealed in containers, as dirt contamination can affect the readings. It is always a good idea to calibrate TLDs against a reference ionization chamber placed in the same radiation beam and using a beam energy which will be used in the subsequent dosimetry experiment. This should take place no more than 2 hours or so after annealing. If there are wide variations between TLD values, 'rogue' TLDs can be removed before the actual dosimetry measurements.

It is known that TLD responses can vary by 30%, due to manufacturing variations. Another pitfall of using TLDs is that steps must be taken to identify them individually, especially when they are applied to different locations on a human body or phantom. This is not always easy when dealing with these tiny tablets. After irradiation, the TLD reader, such as those manufactured by Harshaw, pre-heats the TLDs in an inert nitrogen environment in order to eliminate some low energies (which are liable to fade) absorbed from the radiation exposure and improve accuracy at low dose levels. Heating in the reader during the 'acquire' cycle emits light which is recorded by a photomultiplier and converted to an electrical signal. Following the acquisition of signal, the TLDs are annealed in the reader device as described above.

Practical issues when using air-filled ionization chambers include the fact that sensitivity to radiation increases according to the size of the chamber. Thus large chambers are more accurate for recording small doses, including those arising from scatter or background radiation. However, a large chamber will be cumbersome and difficult to attach with much anatomical precision to a human body or phantom. Ionization chambers tend to be less effective at high beam energies, due to reduced absorption and the greater range of the secondary electrons reduced by ionization. Air ionization chambers are sensitive to changes in atmospheric pressure and temperature, and are also subject to 'drift', requiring regular accurate calibration.

Although effective doses are widely published and give an idea of the relative risks of stochastic effects, it must be remembered that derivation of effective doses from DAP or entrance surface dose values is prone to large uncertainties. The mathematical conversion values employed tend to assume an average body composition, such as the 70 kg adult male, and do not take much account of the reductions in radio-sensitivity that occur in real people from childhood to old age. While considering artificial models, we can note that the Alderson range of anthropomorphic phantoms, such as the Rando and ART, are very useful for dosimetry research but were originally designed for radiotherapy beam energies and may give overestimates of internal organ doses when used with diagnostic exposures of less than 70 kVp.

Radiation dosimetry provides much opportunity for interesting and valuable research, and is expanding due to continuous developments in medical imaging and radiotherapy. Original work can still be done with relatively modest equipment. Although the science appears to provide a firm foundation, the researcher should not take this apparent certainty for granted and should be aware of the pitfalls and possible uncertainties highlighted in this chapter.

## Further reading

Bomford CK, Kunkler IH. Walter and Miller's Textbook of Radiotherapy. 6th ed. Edinburgh: Churchill Livingstone; 2003.

Graham DT, Cloke P, Vosper M. Principles of Radiological Physics. 5th ed. Edinburgh: Churchill Livingstone; 2007.

Intensity Modulated Radiation Therapy Collaborative Working Group. Intensity-modulated radiotherapy: current status and issues of interest. Int J Radiat Oncol Biol Phys 2001; 51(4):880–914.

Stabin MG. Radiation Protection and Dosimetry: an Introduction to Health Physics. New York: Springer; 2007.

# Quality assurance and clinical audit

# 14

Elizabeth Miles    Jagdeep Kudhail    Martin Vosper

## CHAPTER POINTS

- In diagnostic imaging and radiotherapy, QA and audit are particularly concerned with radiation doses and with the accuracy of treatment or diagnosis. Other performance measures may include waiting times, patient satisfaction, cost-effectiveness, as well as broader aspects of health and safety.
- Quality assurance and audit, in addition to being a routine and necessary part of maintaining best practice in diagnostic imaging and radiotherapy, can provide valuable research evidence.
- These monitoring activities are not normally driven by a formal 'research question' or hypothesis, but do require a rigorous methodology.
- Quality assurance (QA) is the planned and systematic evaluation that takes place within the attainment of quality. Quality control (QC) involves the practical testing of processes, ensuring that these conform to a set standard. Thus QC is a practical part of the overall QA mission. QC adjusts and corrects performance to ensure that quality requirements are met.
- A quality assurance programme requires that regular, systematic and documented activities are carried out on a continual basis. It is possible to compare current data with past data and judge performance against set standards. This requires adherence to set protocols and trends in attainment should be visible. Any tests of equipment are undertaken at appropriate set frequencies and the findings will be interpreted using predetermined tolerances and action levels.
- Audit is the assessment of an activity measured against a 'gold standard' or reference. This may be in the form of, for example, guidance notes,

protocol, procedure, or trial specification. Documentation in place in clinical departments assists the workforce with their activity and ensures standardized practice.

This chapter considers aspects of quality assurance and audit that are applicable to service evaluation in both diagnostic imaging and radiotherapy practice.

## Introduction

Quality assurance (QA) and clinical audit have been regarded in some quarters as a little less than 'true' research. To such people, QA and audit might be merely the day-to-day monitoring and evaluation of routine clinical service delivery. However, quality assurance and audit permit us to ask clinical research questions and provide a ready source of fresh issues or findings worthy of enquiry. Normally a formal research hypothesis would not be expected in QA and audit, although a firm method most definitely would be. In fact QA and audit have several advantages for a student doing a BSc level research project:

- The project findings are likely to be of clear interest and value to clinical staff working in diagnostic imaging and radiotherapy.
- As a result, permission to proceed and cooperation with the project are likely to be easier to obtain.
- In many cases, if the data do not include information on human subjects (patients, staff and public), the work may be regarded as 'service evaluation' and not require ethics committee

approval. This will save time and paperwork. But do bear in mind that permission to proceed from a clinical manager will always be necessary.

- The findings will benefit the clinical service, including patients.
- Often a student can make use of existing monitoring processes, rather than designing new methods.

A fundamental requirement of any clinical department within the health sector is to deliver a quality service. Clinical governance was implemented throughout the NHS following the publication, in 1997, of the government's White Paper 'The New NHS: Modern Dependable' which placed a statutory duty of quality care upon all NHS bodies.

At this point it would be useful to state exactly what is meant by quality assurance. Quality assurance (QA) is the planned and systematic evaluation that takes place within the attainment of quality. It is broad-ranging and can cover most aspects of a clinical department's activities. Quality control (QC) involves the practical testing of processes, ensuring that the processes conform to a set standard. Thus QC is a practical part of the overall QA mission. QC adjusts and corrects performance to ensure that quality requirements are met. Minimum standards are defined with appropriate action levels set. Some standards are set by external bodies; however, in the absence of external or peer review standards, departments should set their own levels based on evidence-based practice. Individual departments will have a set of ongoing tests and surveillance procedures to monitor quality.

# What is quality?

What do we mean by 'quality' in a clinical imaging or radiotherapy department? Quality may be objective or subjective, and perceived in different ways by different people, whether they be operatives (staff), users (patients and public) or managers. You could probably jot down quite a lot of possible aspects of quality, but here are a few suggestions:

Quality can involve:

- the 'fitness for purpose' of diagnostic images, assessed in terms of resolution, contrast, signal and acceptability to reporters or clinicians
- the effectiveness of radiotherapy treatments, assessed in terms of cancer eradication, reduction or alleviation

- minimization of adverse effects or injuries to patients and staff
- justification, optimization and limitation of radiation doses, to levels that are 'as low as reasonably practicable'
- perception of the clinical service, from the patient's perspective; this may include comfort, cleanliness, friendliness, empathy, waiting times and communication
- perception of the clinical service, from the referring clinician's perspective; this may include speediness of results or treatments, waiting times, communication, patient feedback, accuracy of information, effectiveness of treatment
- the cost-effectiveness of the service
- the job satisfaction and morale of staff
- the improved quality of life and duration of life of patients (these can be hard to measure).

Clearly such a list can generate many opportunities for research. It should be mentioned also that a researcher may have the chance to obtain a larger picture and compare the quality of several clinical departments.

# Quality in radiotherapy

The following sections on quality in radiotherapy provide examples of the application of QA and QC principles to the clinical setting. Many of the general principles discussed are also relevant to diagnostic imaging departments.

Following several major radiation incidents in the 1980s, radiotherapy departments have been advised to implement a quality management system as advocated by ISO 9001. This has since been endorsed by the Health Care Commission (HCC) Inspections, the independent watchdog for health care in England. Quality management encompasses quality assurance (QA), quality control (QC) and also audit.

The overall approach to QA must be multi-disciplinary and cooperative. It is a comprehensive approach, covering an entire process. QA for radiotherapy is defined by the World Health Organization (WHO) as:

> those procedures that ensure consistency of the medical prescription and the safe fulfilment of that prescription as regards dose to the target volume, together with minimal dose to normal tissue, minimal exposure of personnel, and adequate patient monitoring aimed at determining the end result of treatment.[1]

National and international organizations provide recommendations for standards in radiotherapy; these include the Institute of Physics and Engineering in Medicine (IPEM), the European Society for Therapeutic Radiology and Oncology (ESTRO) and the American Association of Physicists in Medicine (AAPM).

This section will provide an overview of quality management and assurance for external beam radiotherapy focusing on the clinical QA programme concerned with the patient pathway and also the process of clinical audit.

## Quality standards in radiotherapy

In the UK, the standard for QA in radiotherapy is QART, a quality management system (QMS) aimed at ensuring safe delivery of radiotherapy. Hence QART and QMS are interchangeable terms. This formal system provides a comprehensive framework on which local quality manuals are based. All departments are responsible for developing a comprehensive quality programme considering the objectives and resources of their own institution and covering processes from decision to treat to patient follow-up. Quality should be ensured at each process step. The quality system framework is required to be flexible and details minimum standards to be achieved against which the integrity of an activity can be assessed.

Most radiotherapy (and indeed diagnostic) quality management systems (QMS) have three levels of documentation:

Level 1 – quality manual to provide an overview of the quality system including trust level policy statements

Level 2 – procedures manual containing all processes within the scope of the system

Level 3 – work instructions for specific activities.

All levels are interlinked and should have clear pathways linking each level to the next. The confidence of the QMS is tested by ongoing quality activities of which QA, QC and audit are integral components.

## QA programmes in radiotherapy

A QA programme is implemented to ensure each individual step of each process is within an acceptable tolerance. It looks for consistency and finds discrepancies and includes both physical and clinical components. The clinical aspect covers the radiotherapy process whereas the physical aspect covers radiotherapy equipment. These aspects are summarized but not fully explored in this text and the reader is encouraged to refer to the appropriate documentation for further details.

## Equipment QA programme

Equipment QA exists to ensure that standards of safety and performance are maintained. The term equipment includes external beam treatment units, treatment planning system, simulator and CT. The basic framework of a quality assurance programme for equipment is summarized below:

- equipment specification, acceptance testing and commissioning
- QC tests
- additional post-change quality control
- preventive maintenance.

## Equipment QC

A QC programme ensures accurate and safe working of radiotherapy and radiotherapy-related equipment by implementing recommended tests performed at appropriate set frequencies to predetermined tolerances and action levels. Tolerances are set to be clinically acceptable and technically achievable. An equipment QA programme should be developed and updated in line with national and international recommendations.

## Clinical QA programme

Clinical QA is concerned with the patient pathway. All patient activities should follow department protocol and must be clearly documented and accurately recorded. Independent checking methods are recommended at all stages, and are most rigorous when there is any transfer of data to allow early detection of potential errors. Process maps of treatment should include checking tasks at every stage where a risk of error can occur. This requires a comprehensive risk assessment of treatment techniques with work practice geared towards appropriate checks at appropriate stages. The checks required are department specific and are associated with the type of equipment in use. Data transfer, for example, is associated with high risk and the recommendations are to transfer data preferably via IT networks rather than manually, the latter being associated with transcription errors.

## Pre-treatment evaluation

After a patient history is taken investigations will be performed to determine the extent of disease. Disease stage or grade is documented according to an agreed system such as the UICC (International Union Against Cancer) TNM cancer staging system and will inform the treatment objective and intent. Clinical protocols will define the minimum data set of diagnostic information that is required to prescribe radiotherapy treatment.

## Treatment planning

The treatment planning processes include patient positioning, localization, plan design and plan verification. Each stage will have its own individually tailored QA and QC procedures:

- Patient positioning – procedures should be in place to ensure patient reproducibility and stability. Immobilization is assessed and in turn informs the planning and treatment process with respect to margins and set-up tolerances.
- Localization – the acquisition of patient contours and anatomical information to facilitate localization of target volumes and organs at risk.
- Plan design – a clinically acceptable dose distribution is produced using the treatment planning system.
- Plan verification – verification is specific to the technique in use. Complexity and associated risk of technique will inform the method used. For example IMRT (Intensity-Modulated Radiation Therapy) treatments require a far more detailed verification process compared to a standard isocentric breast treatment which does not require pre-treatment verification. Treatment units with 'On Board Imaging' (OBI) facilities are able to use kilovoltage radiation to verify treatment position prior to any megavoltage exposure.

## Treatment prescription

In its simplest form the treatment prescription must include total dose, number of fractions and overall treatment time. This is then signed and dated by the oncologist. In complex RT techniques the prescription is defined by the volume of critical structures that will also be irradiated.

## Treatment delivery

Work practices involving medical exposure to ionizing radiation in the UK are governed by the Ionizing Radiation Regulations (IRR) and the Ionizing Radiations (for Medical Exposure) Regulations (IR(ME)R).

- Patient identification – work practices need to be in place to ensure cross-referencing of correct patient with correct documentation and the correct electronic record.
- Equipment procedures – COIN observes that while record and verify (R&V) systems can improve patient treatment safety, when used as a set-up system they may lead to unintentional introduction of systematic errors.
- Patient chart/treatment record – the patient treatment record contains patient demographics, details on disease plus all information relating to the patient's prescription and treatment details and as such all data entries should be subject to QA.
- Regular chart checks should be routine throughout a patient's treatment course and particularly after any modification of treatment data or change in treatment parameters, for example a change in prescription dose. Planning data, to include patient set-up instructions, beam parameters, MU calculations, should be independently checked. Much of the data transfer through the patient pathway to treatment is electronic and as such happens automatically. Procedures should be in place to verify that data have been transferred correctly.

## Treatment verification

Portal imaging and in vivo dosimetry are systems providing an independent verification of the quality of the treatment delivered to the patient, in respect of positional aspects and dosimetric information. They are useful QA tools which in turn require QA programmes with respect to their clinical use.

- Portal imaging – verifies patient set-up with reference to field positioning and field shaping using blocks or multi-leaf collimator (MLC). Protocols for use should clarify the imaging frequency, criteria for informing acceptability and responsibility for verification/approval. Practices should be in place for ensuring competency of staff. Results of portal imaging may inform on areas for improvement such as immobilization for patient positioning. Portal imaging also has associated risk. The additional radiation exposure directly adjacent to the treatment volume carries the risk of inducing second malignancy. This risk has increased with the increased use of three-dimensional planning CT scans plus portal imaging.

- In vivo dosimetry – measures actual dose at a specific point. Used as a QA tool to verify dose delivery and hence the overall accuracy of the treatment planning process.

Errors identified should be investigated and as a result may inform a change in procedure to eradicate the possibility of the error being reproduced.

## Recording of exposure

Recording of radiation dose to the patient is governed by IR(ME)R. Relevant exposure information should be included in the treatment record to ensure an estimation of the effective dose to the patient can be made at a later date if necessary. All exposures of radiation need to be appropriately documented and are part of regular audit review.

## Technological advances

Continued development of radiotherapy technology requires dose to be delivered to a high degree of accuracy and reliability. More complex treatment techniques require more complex QA. However, to optimize outcome for any technique, simple or complex, each step of the radiotherapy process must be subject to comprehensive, multidisciplinary QA. Increased accuracy and reproducibility is key to facilitating implementation of advanced radiotherapy techniques such as IMRT (Intensity-Modulated Radiation Therapy) and IGRT (Image Guided Radiation Therapy).

A radiotherapy department should have dedicated teams tasked with technique review and improvement of treatment delivery. The necessity to keep up to date with technological advances is paramount as equipment capabilities are rapidly changing. Implementation and review of changes in work practice need to be managed subject to review.

## Clinical trials QA in radiotherapy

A QA programme is an integral part of any radiotherapy trial. Developments in the UK and Europe through the NCRI Radiotherapy Clinical Trials Quality Assurance Group, the European Organization for Research and Treatment of Cancer (EORTC) and the European Society for Therapeutic Radiology and Oncology (ESTRO) have placed increased emphasis on QA within clinical trials as has the Radiotherapy and Oncology Group (RTOG) in the USA. QA programmes aim to ensure that technical guidelines detailed in protocols have been understood by trial participants and that the dose prescription will be delivered according to protocol. This ensures that in multi-centre trials, clinical observations will reflect the trial schedules rather than deviations from protocol, and end-points can be interpreted accurately. There are a number of required elements contributing towards comprehensive QA in clinical trials. These include:

- protocol design
- questionnaires
- pre-trial outlining and planning exercises
- site visit
- individual patient QA.

## What is audit?

Audit is the assessment of an activity measured against a 'gold standard' or reference. This may be in the form of, for example, guidance notes, protocol, procedure, trial specification. Documentation in place in clinical departments assists the workforce with their activity and ensures standardized practice. All such documents require ownership and recognition of their accuracy and worth. Audit is an umbrella term. It is an effective method of measurement and analysis of processes that are already in place and also provides a means of introducing improvements that can be assessed over a specific timeframe. All aspects of a QMS can be tested for compliance through audit.

The quality system approach to quality assurance concentrates more on the process approach and requires assurances that the steps within that process are as effective and efficient as possible. This requires a systematic approach. The aim is to achieve and maintain a high quality of care through the process of setting standards, observing practice, evaluating results and as necessary implementing change. The term 'audit' is widely used in the healthcare sector and there are numerous terms associated with audit activity. In health care most audit activity is categorized under the umbrella term of 'clinical audit'.

## Clinical audit

The aim of clinical audit in the healthcare sector is to provide:

- a systematic review of the clinical practice of the whole multidisciplinary team involved in the patient's care
- a process of measuring current practice against specified standards aimed at improving patient care
- a tool to enable healthcare professionals to disseminate good practice
- a tool to demonstrate evidence-based practice (EBP)
- an organizational/management tool to assess activity
- a quality assurance (QA) tool so that action can be taken to remedy discrepancies.

There are many ways to conduct an audit and they can be categorized depending on the method in which the data is to be collected:

- *Compliance audit*: ensuring compliance with a gold standard. This could be in the form of professional guidelines, national protocols, or local policies and procedures.
- *Audit trail/process audit*: following a process through from beginning to end; for example, a patient from a radiotherapy treatment localization or diagnostic scan to provision of follow-up with a view to improve the efficiency or effectiveness of the process.
- *Improvement audit*: using either of the above to review process/procedure to identify improvements. Used primarily in an area where an issue has already been identified and a systematic approach is required to implement change.
- *Documentation audit*: a review of a specific document to ensure the content is required and relevant to current practice.

## Audit activity

The clinical governance framework and the QMS approach use audit as a major tool to measure the quality of service that is being delivered. Audit of

activity is an essential component of clinical governance. In line with this the Commission for Health Improvement (CHI) is charged by the Department of Health (DH) to carry out inspections otherwise known as clinical governance reviews. NHS Trusts will prioritize audits against specific standards, for example National Institute for Health and Clinical Excellence (NICE) guidance and National Service Frameworks (NSFs).

These form the higher level Trust audit programme and thus are required to feature heavily in some directorate clinical audit programmes. The methodology is often established centrally by the clinical audit and effectiveness departments within individual trusts. These areas are of particular interest to commissioning bodies and strategic health authorities (SHAs) as evidence of fitness to practice. Mandatory trust audits include, for example, consent, do not attempt resuscitation, incident and errors, patient complaints. These are in line with the National Patient Safety Agency (NPSA) requirements.

The directorate managed audits include activity governed by the professional bodies. Individual departments also have a local activities audit programme that covers activity around the local processes involving day-to-day activity.

For audit activity to be effective and meaningful it requires a coordinated multidisciplinary approach. There will be a named clinical governance lead for most departments performing a clinical activity. Departments with quality systems in place based on the ISO requirements will also have a named quality manager to manage the approach towards audit activity. Audit is an effective method of measurement and analysis of processes that are already in place and also provides a means of introducing improvements that can be assessed over a specific timeframe. This will ensure that the requirements of the Trust, directorate, local users and patients are continuously monitored to ensure a quality service is being delivered.

## Management of audit activity

Many Trusts will have a department dedicated to clinical governance/audit activity. These departments will play a central role in project design, project management, data collection, data analysis and report production and often hold a list of specific audit activity that has to be conducted. This is often related to the current political agenda, for example infection control audits. Diagnostic imaging or radiotherapy departments will have a named clinical governance lead. Departments with a QMS will have an audit plan for the year that ensures the system documentation is audited on a regular basis. This will be managed by the quality manager. Other departments may favour a team approach with multidisciplinary team meetings to coordinate audit activity. Whichever method is used, the audit reports and recommendation will need to be managed by named individuals to ensure the audit process is effective and efficient at implementing a quality service.

Under the clinical governance framework all clinicians are required to be involved in audit activity. For all other clinical staff, although it is not a compulsory activity, audit activity is often assessed during the performance appraisal process with managers.

## How to plan and conduct an audit

- In addition to mandatory audit topics, the choice of topic should be based on the standard criteria of areas with high volume, high cost and high risk. Audit is an effective tool for change in specific areas where compliance is weak and an improvement in practice or assessment of process is required.
- Audit activity needs to be appropriate for an individual's level of influence, ensuring results will impact on changing activity. Traditionally persons independent of the task being audited undertake audit activity, for example finance audits. This is to ensure that activity is transparent and without bias. This method would be effective if a review of services was taking place or several work areas are being compared for efficiency. However, within the healthcare sector it is common for an individual to assess an activity that relates specifically to his or her own level of work, or an activity that is having a fundamental effect on how they work. In this way the audit is more likely to influence and change current practice. Care must be taken not to conduct an audit where criticism or blame is directed at another staff group or department without their knowledge or involvement. Joint audit is far more effective where the goal is to improve the quality of care provided and not to pass on blame.
- The audit questions need to be specific and unbiased. The data collection should be transparent to present facts that accurately reflect

conclusions being made. The data collected should answer the audit question.

- The timeframe in which the audit is to be conducted has a major impact on the audit itself. If the data collection period is too long interest will be lost and data may no longer be accurate. Any enforced time constraints should be respected; hence the scope of the data collection and type of analysis required needs to be considered at original audit design. There is little point in generating 6 months' worth of data requiring analysis of thousands of samples unless you have the means by which the statistical analysis can be conducted. When designing an audit, potential seasonal fluctuations should be considered, for example patient throughput may increase following the summer vacation period hence a larger sample of data may be required to ensure data collection accurately reflects the current situation. A multidisciplinary approach will ensure that such patterns are recognized and the audit designed appropriately.
- The aim of the audit must be defined from the outset. An awareness of what is to be achieved will keep continued focus on the audit and ensure that activity is worthwhile. An accurate definition of the audit question and the defined scope are essential to evaluate results within the context of the actual data collated.

## Data collection

- The sample size needs careful consideration. Timescale will have a direct bearing on sample size.
- Retrospective data collection is reliant on old data. This type of data collection is effective if the individual collating the data understands what has previously been recorded. Therefore one can collect the data oneself. However, the sample size will need to be taken into consideration in that the data recorded may be incomplete. It is often found that the specific data required is missing in the original sample; further raw data will then be needed. It also means that historical data are collected so careful consideration needs to be given to the sample size and recognition that the activity is still current.
- Prospective data is more accurate. It allows for real time data which reflects current, rather than historic, practice. Case notes are easily assessable

and the proforma can be designed to ensure that all relevant data are collected. Again this is an activity in which time must have a bearing on sample size. If you are reliant on others to record the data for you the data collection again may be inaccurate or incomplete. Colleague cooperation will be essential. Audit should not inhibit normal clinical activity and data collection by colleagues should not be laborious.

Do not design separate data collection tools if the information is already recorded elsewhere. The sample size should be small enough to allow for rapid data collection but large enough to be representative.

## Audit report

- The audit activity needs to be recorded as a report with methodology, results and conclusion along with recommendations. Accurate recording will allow the same audit to be repeated at a later date.
- Where an audit indicates a need for improvement in practice, an action plan must be considered. The recommendations made by the audit activity need to be specific to the data collection. A hidden agenda to enforce an activity may not be acceptable if the data collection does not show that it is required. To ensure the audit activity will result in a long-term improvement, a period of informing and education is required. Results need to be reported to all the relevant stakeholders to ensure compliance. Following any change in practice a follow-up or repeat audit is required at an appropriate time interval. It is only following a repeat audit with improved results that an improvement in outcome can be proven.

## Audit recommendations

- Audit activity is more than data collection and presentation of results. The action plan that follows an audit activity is the fundamental work that ensures the activity has been worthwhile in improving practice and establishing quality.
- If action is implemented then a review/re-audit should be planned within a relevant timeframe during which the activity can be implemented. Never be afraid to reject a change if it has been found to be ineffective.

## Audit cycle

Successful audits follow the audit cycle illustrated in Figure 14.1. This involves:

- setting standards of practice – what ought to happen
- observing practice – what is actually happening
- comparing observed practice with the set standards
- disseminating results and agreeing any action with colleagues
- implementing any change necessary to meet the standards
- re-auditing to complete the cycle and see if standards are now being met.

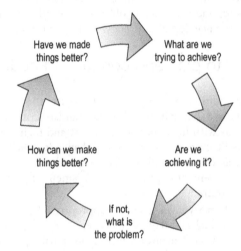

**Figure 14.1** • The audit cycle.

# Succeeding in quality assurance and clinical audit

In both diagnostic imaging and radiotherapy, someone embarking on research based on quality assurance or clinical audit needs to consider the following principles:

- DO ensure that you have the permission of clinical managers, including radiologists or oncologists if necessary, to undertake the research. It is best to obtain a written permission letter.
- DO consider the timeframe needed to undertake the research. Although a 'snapshot' of clinical activity or performance at a certain point of time may be useful in many situations, such as in ongoing quality assurance, it may be necessary to collect data over a period of several months. Is this feasible for you?

- DO remember that you may not always be present at the clinical site to collect data. In your absence, are there people who have the time and ability to undertake data collection for you? And if so, will the data be collected in the same way that you would do yourself?

- DO check that there are measuring instruments or procedures in place which are capable of gathering the data you need. Also, are you capable of using them, or will you need training?
- DON'T assume that retrospective data will always be available, or accurate.

## Reference

[1] World Health Organization. Quality Assurance in Radiotherapy. Geneva: WHO; 1988.

## Further reading

Department of Health. Quality Assurance in Radiotherapy (QART) Standard. London: Department of Health; 1991.

Department of Health. Manual for Cancer Services. London: Department of Health; 2004.

International Standards Organization. The Integrated Use of Management Systems. Geneva: International Standards Organization; 2008.

NHS Clinical Governance Support Team. A Practical Handbook for Clinical Audit. London: CGST; 2005.

NICE. Principles for Best Practice in Clinical Audit. Oxford: Radcliffe Medical Press; 2002.

Royal College of Radiologists, Society and College of Radiographers, Institute of Physics and Engineering in Medicine, National Patient Safety Agency, British Institute of

Radiology. Towards Safer Radiotherapy. London: Royal College of Radiologists; 2008.

Thwaites D, Scalliet P, Leer JW, et al. Quality assurance in radiotherapy (European Society for Therapeutic Radiology and Oncology Advisory Report to the Commission of the European Union for the 'Europe Against Cancer' Programme). Radioth Oncol 1995;35:61–73.

# Section 5

## Data analysis

# Quantitative methods and analysis

15

Andrew Owens    David M Flinton

## Introduction

This chapter focuses on the techniques of analysis that can be used when the information you have collected has been based on numbers. Interval data, which are based on an absolute scale, such as time and ordinal data, where there is a relative sense of the relationships involved between groups (for example when they are rated from best to worst), are the most suitable for this kind of treatment. For nominal or categorical data (data that are not related by a sense of order or position on a scale, for example comparisons of males and females) the possibilities become a little more restricted. Data involving ratios or proportions (where one measurement is divided by another, for example percentages) are not considered here as the tests covered use raw data not data in this form. There are methods available which allow analysis of information based on words which use pattern recognition techniques; however, this has specialized applications and is discussed in Chapter 9. The various types of research information/data are discussed in Chapter 8.

The information provided in this chapter is delivered in a basic manner as it is assumed that the reader has little prior knowledge in this area. This chapter should be consulted as a basic toolkit and although it has all the information you may require for an undergraduate project, you may wish to consult additional texts for more sophisticated data analysis. Furthermore, there are 'test your knowledge style' examples of statistical tests that have been discussed in this chapter and textbook that can be accessed online using *Evolve*.

The chapter is divided into subchapters with a summary of key points at the end of each one.

The first considers some descriptive techniques involving *summary statistics*; the second concerns itself with more analytical methods such as *hypothesis testing*; the third discusses data analysis tools and how to choose the correct one; and the fourth looks at common statistical tests. Finally there is a section examining *correlation* and *regression*. Do not worry if that sounds a little complicated at this stage, as with most things mathematical, the name is a lot worse than the actual ideas involved.

## Using summary statistics

While graphical methods give a good visual impression of what is going on, it is also useful to use characteristics of the data which are based on numbers, called summary statistics. Some of these summary statistics are commonly encountered, for example averages, while others are a little more obscure, for example standard deviation. All of them relate to aspects of what the data look like when plotted in the form of a graph, and in order to understand what they represent it is best to think of them in graphical terms. Once you understand the way that they work it is possible to see how they can then be used to analyse data in more sophisticated ways. Sometimes algebraic symbols are used to represent these values. Be aware that they can vary between textbooks and websites. The important thing is to make sure that you know what the summary describes and not just which symbol is used to represent it.

There are two things that summary statistics are concerned with. The first is trying to describe where

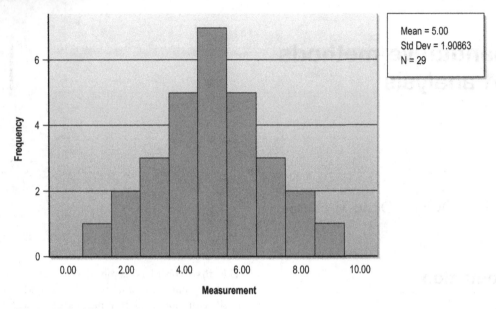

**Figure 15.1** • Histogram 1.

there are concentrations of measurements. If a lot of measurements crop up in the same position then perhaps we can describe this with a single number that is close to the other numbers in the data. The second thing is to try to describe how spread out a collection of numbers is. If lots of measurements are very closely grouped then this is a different pattern from a very loose grouping. Figure 15.1 shows a histogram which has data spread across a range of values from 1 to 10. The measurements are grouped about the value in the middle, 5, and the spread of the data tails off reasonably evenly in both directions.

Compare this with Figure 15.2 and consider the differences in the shape of each graph. They both have the same number of observations recorded on them. (Notice that the scale on the vertical axis is different.)

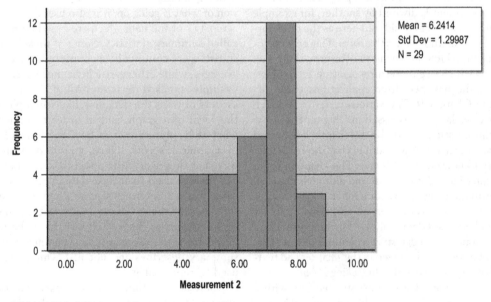

**Figure 15.2** • Histogram 2.

In Figure 15.2 the data are not as spread out and they tend to be grouped around a value of 7, compared to a value of 5 for 15.1. The two histograms are different and it is the job of summary statistics to show these differences in the form of numbers. These histograms will now be used to introduce some basic summary statistics.

## Measurement of central tendency

*The mean* – for any set of data add the values up and divide by the number of bits of data.

If you look to the right and low down next to the two histograms you will see the mean values for the numbers used to generate each histogram. There are some other values but you need not worry about these at this stage. The mean changes as the position of the peak of the histogram changes, but note that it does not track it exactly. Move the peak to the right, as for histogram B compared to histogram A, and the mean increases, moving the mean to the right on the horizontal scale. Be aware that using the method for calculating the mean given here gives the 'arithmetic' mean (there is also a variation called the geometric mean which does not concern us here.).

*The median* – if we arrange all of the bits of data in order this is the number in the middle of the list. If the middle of the list lies between two numbers, we take the mean of the two numbers, i.e. go for the mid-point between the numbers.

For the histograms above the median values were 5 for histogram A and 7 for histogram B.

As with the mean, notice that for histogram B the median is further to the right on the horizontal scale and sits in the regions where there are most measurements.

*The mode* – is the value in a range of data that occurs the most times.

For both histograms there is one mode; 5 for histogram A and 7 for histogram B. The mode corresponds to the peak of the graph. It is not always the case that there is one peak (unimodal), so the mode needs to be used with caution as a second smaller peak would not be obvious by using the mode value on its own. If there is more than one mode (peak) it is described as multimodal and each obvious peak value would be given for a better description of the shape of the plot. A good example of this in medical imaging might be when looking at the energy of events detected from a radioactive source that emits gamma rays at different energies. A source such as 67-gallium emits three distinctly different photon energies and a histogram of energies

detected would show a mode corresponding to each of the energies.

## Measures of spread

You can see from the two histograms that the two sets of data are spread over a range of values, 1–9 (although in 15.2 some of the lower parts of the range have a value of zero.) For histogram B the measurements are more tightly clumped around the peak than for histogram A. The tightness of this clumping is part of the pattern that the data make and this feature needs a different summary statistic, one that measures the spread of the data.

*Standard deviation* and *variance* – measure how spread out the data are from the mean. It is important to notice that it is the spread around the mean and not any of the other measurements of central tendency (median or mode). Look at the histograms again. Just below the values for the mean are values for standard deviation and the shape of the graph is again reflected by the values. For histogram A the data are more spread out and the standard deviation is higher than for histogram B. The greater the degree of spread in the data, the higher the standard deviation will be.

There is no mention of variance in the diagrams but it is very easy to find the variance: simply multiply the standard deviation by itself. You might wonder why we have two different ways of expressing the degree of spread when one is based on the other. You will need to get a little more mathematical to see the reasons for this, but at this level it is enough to say that there are good reasons. The important point is to make sure that you know what both of them describe.

## Symmetry

There is something else we can say about data concerning the shape of a graphical plot. This relates to the way that data are distributed either side of the mode. If the data are spread equally on either side of the mode then the pattern is symmetric, if not the pattern is asymmetric. If there is asymmetry in the pattern then it can be called *skewed*. Figure 15.3 illustrates this. It is important to identify skew as it dictates which measure of central tendency is most representative (an therefore useful) and also indicates whether it is valid to use certain statistical tests. When looking at Figure 15.3 notice what effect skew has on the position of the mean relative to the peak of the graph. The greater the degree of skew the less reliable the mean is as a way of describing where

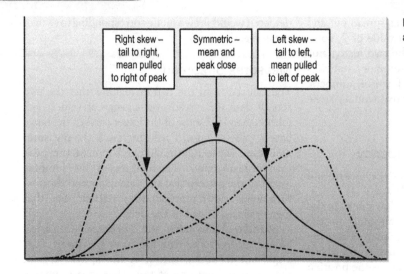

**Figure 15.3** • Symmetry and asymmetry.

the majority of the data sit. If there is no skew the mean and the peak are in the same place.

In general the median does not move from the peak as much as the mean does when the data are asymmetric, and so in these cases can be thought of as a better measure of central tendency. Remember that if one or more extra modes exist then this complicates things and may make the mean and the median redundant for measurement of central tendency. Using the example of a gamma ray emitting source such as 67-gallium, the mean or median gamma ray energies are meaningless as neither of these measures will correspond to any of the particular emitted gamma rays; they occur in the gaps between modal peaks. In this case these measures of central tendency do not relate to any real aspect of the overall pattern of distribution.

An important point at this stage is to realize that for a unimodal, symmetric set of data, the mean and the median are found at exactly the same point on the horizontal scale of the plot. This can be a very useful way of spotting whether or not data are symmetric just from the summary statistics alone, so you could figure this out without a graph.

## Key points

- Descriptive statistics can be based on graphical representations and on numbers that represent key features of the data collected.
- These techniques attempt to summarize the data in some way so that any patterns can be interpreted more easily.
- They cannot reveal anything beyond the properties of the data collected and therefore have no

predictive value. In order to start to make predictions (whether right or wrong) a different branch of statistics is used; this is called inferential statistics.

- The two techniques are of equal importance, as descriptive techniques frequently suggest ways in which data can be examined in order to perform inferential testing. A particularly important example of this would be graphical methods suggest a particular pattern to data which then suggests that a mathematical model, and hence a 'parametric' inferential test might be applicable. A commonly encountered application might be the suggestion that data are normally distributed; in which case a t-test would be applicable (this will become clearer when the normal distribution and the t-test are described).

## Distributions

As you saw in the previous section on summary statistics, one of the points of interest about a set of data is when it follows a particular pattern. Some patterns are quite complex and difficult to describe, or may even be non-existent in a set of data, while others are rather more orderly. A good example of a non-orderly pattern would be produced if you recorded the occurrence of the UK national lottery numbers. Great pains are taken to make sure that they are random and to prevent any pattern from emerging that would make it possible to predict the next set of numbers. Orderly patterns suggest ways in which we can make predictions. For this reason data in orderly patterns are of particular interest. They are of even greater interest if the patterns observed follow a mathematically predictable pattern. An example of an orderly pattern would be way in which the intensity of an X-ray beam changes as it is attenuated by thicknesses of a uniform (homogeneous) material. The mathematical pattern which is observed in this case is an exponential decrease and it can be used to ensure that the thickness of lead used in particular circumstances is enough to give a predictable level of protection.

## Mathematical distributions

Mathematical relationships can be represented graphically as patterns. These patterns are not real; they are mathematically generated patterns. Some patterns fit what we observe in the real world quite closely; we know this because when data are collected, they fit the mathematical predictions very well. You may have had met some orderly observations when you have seen graphs of exponential relationships for attenuation of X-rays and radioactive decay. In these cases the data that are collected are distributed in such a way that they fit a mathematically predicted pattern. Other sets of data are not so orderly, as in the example of the the UK national lottery draw used above.

Because predicted patterns allow us to make future predictions they are of particular interest when looking at data. Not surprisingly the predictions made by statistical testing rely heavily on predictable patterns. There are many such patterns; however, this section will focus on one particular and very special pattern. It is called the normal (or Gaussian) distribution.

## The normal distribution

This is also known as the Gaussian distribution after Karl Gauss, a German mathematician who did early work in statistics. It is special because large numbers of natural observations follow this particular pattern. Variations in the lengths of particular bones, errors in blood tests, variations in height and weight of patients all follow this pattern. (The first written description of the pattern followed a series of measurements of the chest sizes of soldiers in Scottish army regiments.) Another interesting point is that if people are given a series of related questions where they have to rate their responses on a scale (such as strongly disagree, disagree, don't know, agree, strongly agree – with each having a score of 1–5) then the total scores of their answers are normally distributed.

There are some key points about the pattern of a normal distribution.

- It is symmetric and unimodal: the mean, median and the mode have exactly the same value.
- The spread of the data follows a predictable pattern and this is best demonstrated on graph (Figure 15.4).

The graph in Figure 15.4 contains some algebra that needs explaining. The symbol μ (Greek letter 'mu') represents the mean of the data. Notice it sits at the peak and the distribution is symmetrical about it.

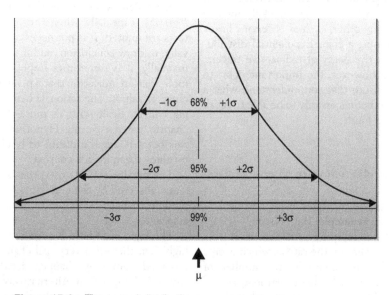

**Figure 15.4** • The normal distribution.

The symbol σ (Greek letter 'sigma') represents the standard deviation of the data. The diagram indicates regions that are one standard deviation, two standard deviations and three standard deviations either side of the mean.

The percentage of observations that fall in certain regions (when real world data follow a normal distribution) is predictable (subject to some random variation) and the numbers on the graph give some values for these percentages. It is possible to calculate the percentage value for any distance away from the mean; the values for σ, 2σ and 3σ are convenient benchmarks and it is worth committing these to memory if you can. Looking at this graph it is possible to determine how likely a measurement is to fall within a certain distance from the mean before taking it. In other words it gives a prediction of how likely an observation is. Also, the further the observation occurs away from the mean, the less likely it is that the observation belongs to the main group. It is important to realize that there is no definite prediction here; it is rather a prediction based on how likely something is. There is always room in the real world for unlikely events to happen; individual UK national lottery winners show us this on a regular basis.

## Other distributions

There are some other distributions that are useful and each one is useful in certain circumstances.

Poisson distributions tell us about the likelihood of random infrequent events such as major incidents in casualty departments. Uniform distributions tell us about occasions when it is just as likely for one thing to occur as any other, such as observing heads or tails when flipping a coin. Exponential distributions tell us about the decay of radioactive tracers. There are others; however, the important point to make here is to ensure that you understand what a distribution is, and not necessarily to be able to recall all of the different kinds.

## Key points

- Patterns can be observed when observations are made.
- Patterns can also be generated using abstract mathematics. For example, the Poisson distribution is generated by a mathematical equation which relies on the rate at which events occur. It could be used to predict the numbers of patients arriving, in an X-ray department, as casualty referrals, within a given period of time.

- When it is possible to match real world observations to theoretical mathematical patterns we can develop ways of predicting how likely it is that some event will be observed. Using the example above the number of staff required to deal with a given rate of arrivals in a department could be estimated and provide a basis for staffing levels.
- This does not give the power of absolute prediction but when likelihoods (or unlikelihoods) get very extreme then it is possible to get reasonably close to absolute prediction.
- The real world never allows us to give definite predictions from statistics and is full of unlikely events.

## Probability and p-values

In Chapter 10 the idea of probability was discussed. Probability expresses the chance that a particular result may occur when there is a choice of possible outcomes. In the context of quantitative analysis, probability is commonly expressed in the form of a 'p-value'. It is important to understand what a p-value tells you as it allows you to make judgements about your own research when you use statistical testing and also allows you to understand what other people's research has discovered, as well as when other researchers draw inappropriate conclusions from their findings.

It is common to find that p-values are not reported as exact figures but as being less than a figure (e.g. $P < 0.05$), especially when the results of statistical tests are quoted. It is not necessary to have an exact value to draw conclusions and if tests are performed manually, it is sometimes impossible to obtain any more than an indication that a p-value lies in a certain range of values. The rationale behind statistical testing will be dealt with in more detail later in the chapter when covering Hypothesis testing, but at this point it may be useful to briefly explore what p-values mean in this context.

The p-value reflects the probability that the outcome observed by the test happened as a product of random chance as opposed to being an effect or real association.

The logic used here is such that if the p-value is high then there is a very real chance that what was observed could just happen accidentally without any underlying reason. Alternatively if the associated p-value is very small then the opposite is likely to be the case, that is to say that there is some underlying reason for the observation made. This gives rise to the idea of 'significance'. If the p-value for an observation is found to be below a certain level, decided by the researcher, then it is commonly referred to as a statistically significant finding. This means that something has happened and it does not seem to be an accidental occurrence and therefore there must be an underlying reason for it. This is why, when researchers produce low p-values in papers, it should act as a flag in the readers' mind saying that there is something interesting going on. Equally when high p-values are encountered, it is good practice to check these findings against the claims of a researcher who reports that they have discovered something happening. For example a researcher claims that a significant improvement in patient recovery has been observed following a change in treatment regime. This is supported this with evidence from an inferential test with a resulting p-value of 0.11 in favour of their claim. P-values above 0.05 provide weak evidence to support the claim. Clearly, in this case the evidence is weaker and many would consider it too weak to be relied on for support.

## Key points

- 'Likelihoods' are expressed formally as p-values.
- P-values use an assumption that in the event that there are many possible outcomes for an observation, all of the possibilities add up to 1.
- It follows that if something will definitely happen $P = 1$ (so likely it must happen). For example, death is a definite event for all individuals and in statistical terms the probability of this event occurring is 1. If something is impossible then $P = 0$ (so unlikely it never will happen). For example, the chance of an X-ray exposure not involving ionising radiation is 0. A commonly encountered p-value in research papers is $P = 0.05$. This reflects a probability of 1 in 20. Many researchers consider that if their observations have this probability of occurring by chance then they have observed something significant happening, that is to say that it is not down to chance and the observation signifies that there is some real effect or association involved. This choice of what is significant is purely arbitrary. A more stringent researcher could choose a lower p-value as an indicator of significance. A lax researcher would choose a higher p-value as an indicator of significance.

# Hypothesis testing

In previous chapters and sections within this chapter you have been introduced to a number terms and ideas; hypotheses, summary statistics, mathematical and real world distributions and p-values. These form a toolkit from which it is possible to develop a way of trying to find out what information may be contained within a collection or collections of data.

Hypotheses form the backbone of the research process by giving us a *question to answer*. Summary statistics allow us to *condense key features* about data into a manageable form (although it is not always necessary to use summaries; the data can be analysed in its raw form). Distributions allow us to try and *determine the probability* of obtaining observations; and p-values give us a formal way of *expressing* them.

This section will look at how you can combine them into an analytical package which can then be used to address the purpose of your research.

## Hypotheses: asking the right kind of question

As mentioned in Chapter 2, a hypothesis is a question or idea that your research sets out to find out about. It is important at this stage to ensure that you distinguish between the two different kinds of hypotheses. An experimental or research hypothesis sets the context of your research, giving a reader an idea of what your research aims to do. This is not quite the same as the way in which the word hypothesis is used in statistics. Because statistics involves mathematical methods, a statistical hypothesis has a very different and somewhat strict meaning. Whereas in the real world the way in which we describe things can offer many different options; statistical hypotheses only consider two options. Either the observations fit a hypothesis or they do not. It is a very simplistic, rather black and white version of the world. Many people new to research experience problems because they have too much confidence in the power of statistical testing to provide answers to complex questions. The findings of your test will only be a good as the quality of the questions that you ask. Vague questions are usually very complicated when you look at them in depth. A good example would be a study where a researcher wants to 'know how to optimize a particular type of examination'. A noble endeavour no doubt, but how do you do it in practice? The following questions may arise:

- What is optimal?
- Is it dose related?
- Is it image quality related?
- Does it relate to the patient's perception?
- Is it all of these factors together?

It is critical to formulate clear hypotheses otherwise you will find yourself in the situation of setting out to investigate the problem, collecting data and then, when it comes to drawing conclusions, there will be a mass of confusion. Clearly, vague questions are to be avoided.

That is not to say that vague questions cannot be tackled, but that they are best broken down into a number of simple but related questions. Normally, unless you are a full time researcher, where the time to tackle complex problems is available, it is best to keep it simple. At this point it is worth mentioning that this approach is not without risk. The real world is complex and it is sometimes the case that when you test for an association between two variables it is really the case that your observations are the result of other influences. When this happens the results are said to be 'confounded' by the influences of these variables and this is a source of confounding bias. In strictly mathematical terms there is seen to be a 'confounding variable'. It is important to try to spot occasions when this is possibly happening and also to be alert to the possibility of confounding in other people's research. The simplest questions, and the ones most prone to confounding, are the ones with the fewest options for the answers. The obvious extreme of this is when the answers involve the use of two options; yes or no, but this is exactly the kind of approach that is necessary. Now to progress we really have to get a 'bit mathematical' because there are some statistical terms necessary for formulating these questions in order to use them for statistical testing.

*Null hypothesis* – refers to the idea that there is no difference between some particular quality concerning sets of data, perhaps a summary statistic, that you are testing. This leads to the inference that the groups of data are the same or are similar in some way, e.g. similarities between the means of the groups or patterns in the data sets, etc. The null hypothesis is commonly given the symbol $H_0$.

*Alternative or experimental hypothesis* – refers to the idea that there is a difference (the exact opposite of the null hypothesis). The alternative hypothesis is commonly given the symbol $H_1$.

Notice at this point that for the purposes of conducting a statistical test, there are only two possibilities. Questions which potentially allow more than two possible answers cannot be tackled using these techniques. The pair of hypotheses (null and alternative) that you use are also described as *one or two tailed*. If the alternative hypothesis is that there is a difference but it does not matter what the difference is then it is two tailed. If the alternative hypothesis is that one group of data has a quality that is greater than or less than another then it is one tailed. A good example would be a drug trial where the investigator is looking to see whether a new kind of drug is better than the existing one. This is a one-tailed situation. If the investigator just wanted to show that they were different to each other then this would be two tailed. In practice a two-tailed test of a drug's performance would be useless because if you saw a difference you would not be certain whether it was because the drug made the patients healthier or less healthy.

## Matching statistical hypotheses to the point of your research

Having developed the idea of a statistical hypothesis the next step is to see how you might use it to address the experimental hypotheses of your research. The process of testing relies on trying to figure out how likely it is that observations happen by chance. If there is a high probability that what you have measured could happen by chance then it will be difficult to make predictions based on these observations. Thinking of this terms of winning a lottery, the process is accidental. Because of this it is impossible to make predictions about subsequent winners based on observations of previous winners. If, on the other hand, there is a very small probability of your observations being due to chance then the opposite will be the case and your observation will allow you to make good predictions about future events. This suggests that the most useful tests will look for circumstances where chance is unlikely to have played a big part in what you have observed. So how does this work in practice?

A statistical test looks at the probability that one of the statistical hypotheses is unlikely to have happened by chance. Let us think about what this means by considering the following points:

1. If the chosen statistical hypothesis (remember there are two, null and alternative) is unlikely to have been observed by chance then the opposite must be true; something must really be going on to give the observation.

2. If the chosen hypothesis is likely to have been observed by chance (the opposite of point 1

above) then it means nothing, as it could be just a bit of random luck, so we choose to ignore it.

**3.** If we are going to ignore one hypothesis and there are only two possibilities, null or alternative, then the other hypothesis must be the case.

In practice statistical tests always look at the likelihood of the null hypothesis having occurred by chance. To see how this works it is better to construct a flow chart as given in Figure 15.5, from the points above.

Perhaps it is worth repeating that the logic used here is simplistic and therefore will only accommodate simple questions. If you try to do anything more sophisticated with a statistical test on its own, then it does not work. An example might be a patient survey which is investigating degrees of satisfaction with their X-ray examinations. A single test, used on its own, could only distinguish between one source of satisfaction between two groups of patients. Any other number of possibilities cannot be directly explored as the test only permits two possibilities, of the researcher's choice. In this case a more complex approach would be necessary to investigate the patient's feelings.

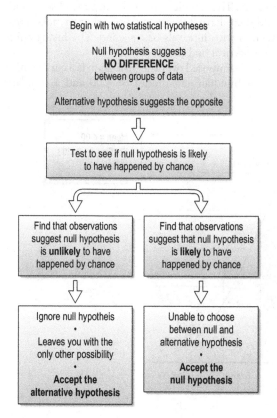

**Figure 15.5** • Process for fixed level testing.

Another important aspect to consider here is the way in which the statistical hypotheses are used in relation to experimental hypotheses. Most experimental hypotheses seek to show that something is going on, perhaps that a particular form of treatment does have an advantage. If statistical testing is used to investigate this it looks at the likelihood that there is *no benefit*, i.e. that the null hypothesis is the case, and in the event that it is found that is it is unlikely that there is no benefit then there must be a *real benefit*, the alternative hypothesis is the case. The logic here is strong if you find that there is a benefit, but weaker when the null hypothesis of no benefit is accepted. In this case you are accepting the null hypothesis because you are in a position where it is difficult to decide one way or the other. Imagine that a clinical trial is conducted and this gives no evidence that a new oncology therapy regime is more effective than its predecessor. On the basis of this evidence no change is made. But what if a repeat trial does reveal that a benefit exists? In this case a single trial was not enough to uncover the necessary evidence to arrive at the correct conclusion and the decision to err on the side of caution by accepting the null hypothesis was incorrect. It is this tendency to be cautious that provides the weakness in the logic. Using a significance level as a basis for accepting or rejecting hypotheses is an inherently conservative action.

It is worth bearing this in mind as it means that statistical testing is better at spotting differences than it is at spotting similarities.

Do not worry if you do not grasp this 'warped' logic all in one go. It is counterintuitive and sometimes it is necessary to look at it a few times before the logic makes sense. After the next section there will be an example showing how statistical testing might be used to investigate a real problem and this should help to make the logic clearer.

## Key points

- The process of hypothesis testing requires questions to be formulated in terms of hypotheses.
- The null hypothesis considers the idea that there is nothing special about what has been observed (it could be random chance that produced it).
- The alternative hypothesis usually represents what the researcher is looking for.

- The observation has to be shown to be improbable in order for the alternative hypothesis to be accepted.
- We accept the alternative hypothesis by gathering evidence that allows the rejection of the null hypothesis.
- Remember that 'absence of proof' is not 'proof of absence'.

## Choosing the correct data analysis test tool

Having figured out how you will use the process of statistical testing, the next step is to choose an appropriate test. There are many tests available and it can be a bewildering choice. The choice of a test is relatively logical as each test is a tool which has its own particular application. The way to figure out which one suits your particular job is by considering a number of key points about your research:

1. Regardless of the chosen test the data used should be random. The less random the data can claim to be, the weaker the results of a test are.
2. The choice of test is influenced by dependency in the data. Some tests do not work at all if one measurement could influence another. For other tests it is necessary that the data are dependent, matched or related (these words are used interchangeably).
3. The number of tails required to tackle the experimental hypothesis (see previous section).
4. The size or anticipated size of the groups of data and how many groups there are. Many statistical tests do not produce accurate results if the samples of data are too small. Each test has its own limits.
5. Whether the data can be tested using parametric or non-parametric methods.

Whether data are parametric or non-parametric depends upon one very simple point: whether they could fit a mathematical distribution or not. It is important to stress the word 'could' here because unless you can collect impossibly large amounts of data it is very difficult to say that that they definitely fit a theoretical distribution. Random chance always plays a part in stopping you from going this far. The idea of a mathematical distribution was covered earlier but it is worth looking at an example to make sure that it is quite clear.

Figure 15.6 shows a set of data from a fictitious sample. The sample is made up of time observations and these have been grouped together to make a histogram with intervals of 1 second. The histogram is symmetrical and unimodal.

Superimposed over the histogram is a curve with a mean (median and mode) of 4.00 and a standard

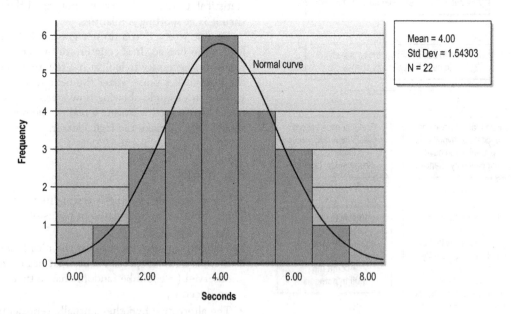

**Figure 15.6** • Data with a fitted normal curve.

deviation of about 1.54 (these figures are at the right hand side of the diagram and are true for both the histogram and the curve).

The curve is a theoretical mathematical shape placed on the same plot as the histogram and has been drawn using two 'parameters' that determine the shape of normal curves: the mean and the standard deviation. To create the curve the mean and standard deviation of the histogram data have been used, which is why they are the same for both. It looks like the shapes of the histogram and the 'fitted normal curve' are very similar so in this case the data seem to be 'parametric' in nature and the parameters relate to a normal distribution.

The distribution does not have to be 'normal'; it can be any shape (see the section on Other distributions). As long as the data seem to fit a theoretical pattern a parametric test can be used. Particular tests will relate to particular distributions, a common one being the normal distribution. An important point to remember is that theoretical mathematical distributions are made from variables on a scale, so the underlying parameters will be on an 'interval' scale. This type of test will generally only apply to interval data. A notable exception is where some types of ordinal questionnaire based data from Likert scales can be combined to give data that fit a normal curve.

The case in Figure 15.6 is artificial. Usually such small sample sizes, like this one having 22 measurements, have a great deal of random variation and it is difficult to identify a pattern convincingly. If you cannot give a convincing case for the data being parametric then treat them as if they are not.

There are other ways of showing that data may fit a pattern besides plotting the data but these often rely on software or the use of a statistical test with a null hypothesis that there is no difference between the data observed and the required mathematical distribution.

Having discussed parametric data, we will now consider other sorts of data. Any investigation that involves other sorts of data is called non-parametric. Generally, categorical and ordinal data or any mix of parametric and non-parametric data gives a situation that is non-parametric. It is critical to identify whether to use parametric or non-parametric techniques. In general you should attempt to use parametric tests whenever possible as they give much more useful results, providing stronger evidence. On the other hand, non-parametric tests are much more robust and there are fewer factors that can upset the validity of the findings. The choice of test

depends how much evidence you have to support your choice. If sufficient evidence exists in favour of a parametric test then this is the one you should choose.

## Interpreting results

By applying a test to data a 'test statistic' is produced. There are many different kinds of test statistic each relating to a particular test, or tests. This result in itself is meaningless as it tells you nothing about the probabilities of 'accidentally' observing the data; it is a means to an end. The test statistic is used to generate a probability, or p-value which is of much more interest. The p-value generated gives evidence in favour of rejecting the null hypothesis. The lower the p-value, the less likely it is that the data observed occurred by chance and, more importantly, the more likely it is that you have observed something 'really happening'. In mathematical language, a low p-value provides evidence to reject the null hypothesis in favour of the alternative hypothesis. If the p-value is high we cannot get rid of the null hypothesis so we favour it instead. Remember that this process is not intuitive and may not seem to make common sense so do not think about it too hard!

There are two schools of thought about how this favouring process should work. One says that a predetermined limit should be applied to the p-value and if the value equals or falls below a fixed limit then the alternative hypothesis is 'true'. If the p-value is above the predetermined value then the null hypothesis is 'true'. This is called *fixed level testing*. The other way of using the result is to present it to the reader and let them make their own mind up, pointing out how significant the findings are. Not surprisingly this is called *significance testing*. A fairly standard way of interpreting the significance of p-values is on the verbal scale shown in Table 15.1.

## The process for a typical statistical test

Now we can draw all of the points above together and an example of the resulting statistical package, will be examined. As you read through this section, keep in mind the sections that come before; it is at this point that the relevance of each section becomes apparent.

The experimental hypothesis will be that for men born in the last 70 years, adults of later generations are taller than those of earlier ones.

**Table 15.1 Interpretation of p-values for significance testing**

| P-value | Interpretation |
|---------|----------------|
| Equal to or less than 0.01 | Strong evidence to reject null hypothesis |
| Greater than 0.01 and equal to or below 0.05 | Moderate evidence to reject null hypothesis |
| Greater than 0.05 and equal to or below 0.10 | Weak evidence to reject null hypothesis |
| Greater than 0.10 | Little evidence to reject null hypothesis |

The data will be height measurements on an interval scale. The data will be taken by randomly selecting unrelated adult male individuals from the population and placing them into one of two groups: below 40 years of age and over 40 years age. We will not concern ourselves with how this is achieved but assume that it is.

The initial null hypothesis is that there is no difference between the two groups (an older and a younger group), giving an alternative that there is a difference. As you are looking to see if there is an increase in height the process will involve one tail.

It has been mentioned earlier when discussing the normal distribution that this kind of measurement would be expected to be normally distributed in any particular group. Because the data could confidently be expected to fit a theoretical mathematical distribution, the normal distribution, then you can use a parametric test which relates to this. If we suspected that the data did not follow this kind of pattern you would have to choose a non-parametric test.

For this example you can use a commonly encountered family of tests called t-tests. More particularly an unrelated or unmatched t-test can be used. This test is sensitive to a number of assumptions, as follows:

- the data are randomly collected
- the data are independent
- the data sets are normally distributed with a similar spread about their mean values.

Notice that the way that the experimental hypothesis has been set up and the way that the collection of the data has been specified makes this t-test the ideal choice. It is always worth thinking about how you may test your data before deciding on a final experimental hypothesis.

The first step would be to calculate the test statistic or 't' statistic. How exactly this is arrived at is not important at this stage – if you are interested a more advanced book on statistics will tell you this. What is of interest is that the calculation involves the use of the *means* and *variances* of the two groups. The process is based on summary statistics which reflect properties of each group of measurements. Also the particular summary statistics involved are closely related to the theoretical distribution that the groups fit. The test statistic links properties of the groups to the chosen theoretical model (the normal distribution). If software is used to do the test then the test statistic will probably be included in the output.

If you are doing the test manually this statistic is now taken to a set of tables and converted into a p-value. If you are using software then the p-value will be given in the output with the test statistic. At this point it would be wise to check that the p-value has been generated for a one tail test; do not assume that software can read your mind – always check that the requirements of the test have been satisfied.

The p-value now needs to be interpreted. If you have chosen a fixed level approach then you now need to compare the p-value obtained against your chosen value. A widely accepted p-value is 0.05, representing a 1 in 20 chance that the results could have occurred accidentally. At this point, if a fixed level approach is used and the p-value obtained is equal to or falls below 0.05, then the result leads to the rejection of the null hypothesis and you conclude that younger males are (on average) taller than older ones. If significance level testing is being used and the p-value is just below 0.05, then you have 'moderate evidence' to reject the null hypothesis (see Table 15.1) and 'moderate evidence' in favour of the experimental hypothesis. The p-value chosen here is not the only possible choice. If you wanted to be really tough about making conclusions with a fixed value test then you could always lower the p-value at which the result becomes significant. A glance at Table 15.1 gives you an idea of how much this affects the credibility of your findings.

The steps taken for a non-parametric test are no different, but because there is no direct link between the data and a mathematical distribution the process is not quite as obvious. Non-parametric tests work because the test statistic calculated in the process relates to a theoretical distribution as opposed to the data themselves.

## Key points

- A correct choice of a statistical test is determined by the kind of information or data that has been collected.
- Tests can broadly be separated into two classes: parametric and non-parametric.
- A low p-value gives evidence to support the acceptance of the alternative hypothesis, that observations are not occurring by random chance.
- P-values can be interpreted using a rigid 'fixed level' approach or a more flexible 'significance' approach.
- The general process is similar for all tests.

# Common statistical tests

This section will look at some of the commonly used tests. The hypothesis for each test is included and it is very important that you have a clear idea of what each test actually does and how it allows you to draw conclusions.

Different tests are required depending upon the number of sets of data to be compared. The tests are considered to involve one, two or three or more sets of data. This is indicated for each test and examples are given to clarify how they are applied.

## The t-test (or Student's t-test) : compares two groups of data

The different names for this test reflect the origin of the test. It was created by a 19th-century statistician working for Guinness breweries in Ireland. As the owner of the brewery did not want his competitors to know that such 'underhand' industrial methods were being employed to control the quality of his product, and at the time it was quite a radical change of method, the statistician's name had to be kept secret. Because of this the test was published under the pseudonym 'Student'. It is called the t-test because it uses a mathematically determined distribution called the 't' distribution in order to generate its results.

The t-test can be used to compare two groups of measurements where the particular observations are on a continuous interval scale. An example of this would be an ionizing radiation dose. The doses recorded are on a continuous scale, down to the level of accuracy of the readout that has regular intervals, the units of the readout associated with it. An underlying assumption is that for each group the *mean* is a representative summary statistic. In the case where the data are obviously skewed the mean is not representative and this clearly rules out the use of this test. All t-tests have the underlying assumption that the groups of data have a *normal distribution*. This direct reliance on a mathematical distribution makes this a *parametric test*.

There are variations of this test. An *independent* or *unmatched* t-test allows comparison of two groups of data where the measurements in each group cannot have affected each other in any way.

*Example*: Using the example of ionizing radiation dose, this test could be used to compare patient doses associated with two different diagnostic or therapeutic radiographic techniques. A good example might be to compare the affects of different beam orientations on the dose to the thyroid gland during chest radiography. It is important to realize that it could only compare two orientations at a time and no measurement can affect any of the others for this test to work.

The null hypothesis of this test is that the means of both groups are the same. A low p- value indicates evidence that this is not the case and that the means (and hence the two groups) are different.

Another version of the t-test is the dependent, matched or single sample test. In this case the test is used to examine the possibility that a single group comes from a larger population which has a particular mean associated with it *or* to examine matched measurements of a group.

*Example*: This test could be used to examine changes in group of patients following a treatment of some kind. Observations could be taken of a particular continuous interval variable such as white cell count (WCC). If an antibiotic was being tested to assess its effectiveness as a treatment it could be administered to patients with a particular infection. Looking at WCC score for each patient before and after the administration of the antibiotic would provide a single data set comprising the difference in counts for each patient.

The null hypothesis would be that was no difference between the mean scores before and after the administration. A low p-value would give evidence to suggest that the treatment did create a difference.

In both cases notice that the choice of tails for the test is important. If a two-tailed test is used in either case then all that can be said is that there is a difference between two groups/circumstances. For a thyroid dose study or for an investigation of the efficacy of a drug, this is not enough to be useful. For cases like these one-tailed tests are necessary because they would tell us whether to change the way things are done. If one technique produces a lower dose or an antibiotic reduces the WCC then effective changes have been identified, but to do this we need to know if a reduction has occurred. In terms of null hypotheses this equates to whether one mean is greater or less than another, not just if there is a difference between them.

Generally it is also important that the spread of data in both sets is not too dissimilar. There are versions of the t-test that are specifically designed to cope with large difference in variance or standard deviation. Unless your test states this to be the case a useful rule of thumb is to make sure that the variances of the two data sets are within a factor of three of each other (i.e. neither one is three times bigger or smaller than the other).

## Mann–Whitney 'U' test: compares two groups of data

This test draws its name from the originators of the test and is much less interesting from a historical perspective.

The Mann–Whitney U test uses a calculation to produce a result called the 'U' test statistic which is then used to generate associated p-values. There is no directly underlying mathematical distribution involved and so this is a *non-parametric* test. Indirectly the distribution of 'U' is related to a normal distribution whose mean and variance are related to the size of the samples used and a mathematical pattern known as the uniform distribution. It is a highly versatile test that can be used to compare two *independent* sets of observations. The observations can be continuous or discrete and so it can be used on laboratory style measurements and whole numbers such as the ones that come from surveys or counting exercises. When it is not possible to perform a t-test this test is frequently chosen.

*Example*: If the recovery time following radiotherapy treatment was to be compared for different treatments, interval data could be collected for each treatment. If examination of one or both sets of data revealed a skew in the data then the Mann–Whitney test could be used to compare the treatments.

The null hypothesis would be that the two groups of recovery times belong to a single underlying set (population) of recovery times. A low p-value would give evidence to suggest that the two data sets do not belong with each other and that they are therefore different.

*Example*: The patients attending two different radiotherapy departments are given a series of 'satisfaction' questions to answer and their responses scored. The comparison of the two sets of patients could be made using this test.

The null hypothesis would be that the responses of the two groups are the same as the responses of a single larger group. A low p-value would give evidence to suggest that the satisfaction levels of patients at the two sites are different.

Notice that this test looks for differences, which is fine when addressing two-tailed hypotheses. If it was important to determine if one department was better, in terms of satisfaction delivered, than the other then some other evidence would be required. In this case comparison of a simple bar chart would indicate if one site scored higher than the other. There is nothing wrong with addressing one-tailed hypotheses in this way.

## Chi-square ($\chi^2$) test

The chi-square test, or Pearson's chi-square test to give it its full name, can be used to look at contingency tables. A contingency table is constructed of a number of boxes each of which is mutually independent, i.e. when an observation is made it can only belong to one box. An example of this would be the sorts of tables that are used to record data in *cohort studies* (see Chapter 9). In this case data are in a table which looks at exposure to a condition and whether or not a particular outcome is observed. Exposure to habitual smoking, for example, with an outcome of lung cancer could be represented on a contingency table. Each person observed can only belong in a distinct category or 'contingency' which is constructed from the options exposure/non-exposure and lung cancer/no lung cancer.

Although there is a mathematical distribution involved (the chi squared distribution), the data used in this are discrete, and categorical or ordinal. This means that the test is considered to be *non-parametric*. It is not only useful for cohort studies but can be applied to any contingency table. There is, however, one condition to bear in mind here. When looking at a table, each box or cell belongs on a particular row or column. Each cell has an 'expectation value' associated with it. This is calculated by multiplying the total number of observations for its row by the total number of observations for its column and dividing this by the total number of all observations in the table. If the *expectation value for any cell is lower than five then the test cannot be reliably used*. The reason for this is mathematical and requires an understanding of conditional probability which goes beyond the purpose of this book and so will not be elaborated on here. In these circumstances a similar test called Fisher's exact test should be used. This test can deal with all expected values for a cell. A particularly useful aspect of this test is that it can deal with ordinal or categorical data from questionnaires.

*Example*: As part of an audit in an X-ray department patients are asked to comment on their satisfaction with the courtesy of the staff. The question asks for a yes/no response. The answers for males and females are counted separately and placed in a contingency table with a view to investigating whether there is gender equality regarding the way which the staff behaves (Table 15.2). The auditors check that all of the cells have an expectation value of five or more using the subtotals and grand total, and find that all cells have at least this value.

The null hypothesis is that there is no association between gender and satisfaction. A low p-value suggests evidence that this is not the case and that males and females are being treated differently.

Note that this test only comes in a two-tailed form and so we cannot determine whether males or females are getting preferential treatment. Other evidence would be needed to confirm this.

This test can be used to investigate the response from Likert scales but the data need modifying before they will fit into a suitable table. The problem is that attitudinal scales are not discrete enough to prevent overlaps between cells. Using the example of patient satisfaction, if a Likert scale was used there would be degrees of satisfaction or dissatisfaction and a patient's response at any one time would be determined by their mood. A recent bad experience in another department could affect the response, e.g. a long wait in clinic before being sent for an X-ray examination. Because of this responses are not reliable in this case. The data from the scale would possibly need to be simplified into three options in this case, for example: satisfied, no preference or dissatisfied. This reduces the subtlety of the data and still has the problem that extreme recent experiences could adversely affect the data. It would be unacceptable to choose a simplification that would ignore some of the responses.

A final point that needs to be made is that the results of this test depend on the number of degrees of freedom involved. Again, the basis of this is beyond the remit of this book, but the number of degrees of freedom is very easy to determine.

(Number of rows in the table − 1)×
(Number of columns in the table − 1)
= degrees of freedom

## Goodness of fit (chi-square goodness of fit): can be used to compare two groups of data or one group with a theoretical distribution

The chi-square distribution can also be used to look at what is called 'goodness of fit'. This is the process of investigating how similar or dissimilar two distribution patterns are to each other. It can be used to investigate patterns in two sets of collected data and can also be used to compare collected data with a theoretical pattern. The examples below indicate how each works.

*Example*: A researcher wants to compare the work patterns of two radiotherapy departments and collects data about the kinds of therapies that they conduct. The patterns can be plotted in a bar chart for visual assessment but to find if the work patterns are significantly different (in a statistical sense) the researcher could conduct a goodness of

| Table 15.2 A contingency table for patient satisfaction | | | |
|---|---|---|---|
| Satisfaction | Males | Females | Totals |
| Yes | Satisfied males | Satisfied females | Subtotal – satisfied patients |
| No | Dissatisfied males | Dissatisfied females | Subtotal – dissatisfied patients |
| Totals | Subtotal – total males | Subtotal – total females | Grand total of all patients |

fit test comparing the categories of therapy against themselves, across the sites.

The null hypothesis will be that the patterns of work are not different. A low p-value indicates evidence that they may be different from each other.

In this case the patterns are not necessarily mathematical; they are generated by the frequency that observations fall into certain categories. The test could also be used for data that could be displayed in frequency histograms. Any patterns of matched categories or intervals can be used. The important point is that the data must be in a discrete form and the categories or intervals in the data must correspond to each other and be independent.

*Example*: In order to compare the waiting times for two diagnostic X-ray rooms data are collected and placed into groups or 'bins', e.g. waiting times are binned into 5 minute intervals: 0–5 min; 5 min. 1 s to 10 min; 10 min 1 s to 15 min . . . . A goodness of fit test could be performed to determine any differences between waiting times.

The null hypothesis is that there is no difference between the two rooms. A low p-value provides evidence that the waiting time for each room is different.

As with the Pearson chi-square test this is two tailed and further evidence would be required to discover which room had the shorter waiting times.

From the examples above it can be seen that this test can be used for all types of discrete numerical data, i.e. involving counting, and this makes it extremely flexible.

The same process is followed in order to establish whether a collection of data follows a mathematical pattern, although in this case the data must be interval data as all mathematical distributions are based on numerical scales. This test should only be used when the mathematical model is also discrete. Predictions can be made from discrete mathematical distributions and identifying this property in a set of observations can be extremely useful.

*Example*: A researcher wants to discover whether a set of observations follows a uniform distribution. This would mean that the responses in all of the categories are the same. A clinical department might, for example, wish to determine whether the rate at which patients arrive is uniform throughout the working day. Graphical representation might indicate that this is not the case and a goodness of fit test could then be performed to determine whether the pattern seen graphically was statistically significant.

The null hypothesis would be that patients are arriving at a uniform rate. A low p-value would provide evidence that there was a lack of uniformity and indicate if there was an underlying significance in the pattern. This could then be used to inform staffing levels based on the pattern.

## Analysis of variance (ANOVA): compares three or more groups of data

Analysis of variance is a technique that uses the spread (or variance) of each set of data. If the spread of the data sets covers similar ranges of values then it is likely that there is no difference between the sets of data. If the spread of any of the data sets are different then ANOVA will identify this.

With the notable exception that ANOVA is for three or more groups, this test is similar to the t-test. The test is used for interval data (e.g. dose measurements on a continuous scale) and there is an assumption that the data sets are *normally distributed*. This means that ANOVA is considered to be a *parametric test*.

A point of particular interest to notice here is that the test uses variance, not the mean of the samples as a t-test does. A potential problem here is that variance in a group of measurements comes from two sources. It can occur as a result of the process being measured (which is what the ANOVA test is looking for), but it can also occur because of errors of measurement (due to the measurement process and random variation). If measurement error provides too much contribution to the overall variance then the ANOVA test can give unreliable results. In other words the major contributor to a group's variance should be members of a group being measured, *not* the way that they are measured. A second related point is that variance in a group of measurements is also related to the number of measurements for independent random variables. This means that sample sizes are an important issue for ANOVA.

*Example*: A researcher is investigating the radiation doses given to different groups of patients undergoing different radiotherapy treatment regimens. There are three different regimens and separate (independent) groups are used. Provided that the sets of data for each group could be shown to be normally distributed then an ANOVA test could help to identify whether the different techniques deliver the same doses. If the variances in the groups are similar to the variances in measurement due to the dosimetry used then there are potential problems. Also it is important to note the number of patients in each group.

For this case the null hypothesis would be that all groups are receiving the same radiation dose. A low p-value would provide evidence that there was a significant difference across the groups.

There are some important points to notice about this example:

- The case above is a relatively straightforward one that involves only one variable, ionizing radiation dose.
- The subjects in each group are independent of each other.
- The result of the test only allows a difference across all of the groups to be identified, it does not allow the researcher to indentify which of the groups are different from each other.

The number of variables which the test can handle is referred to by the number of 'ways' that the test runs. A one way test looks at one variable (as is this case if measuring radiation dose), a two way test looks at two variables, a three way test looks at three variables, and so on. This book will only consider one way analysis, the simplest case. A further way of simplifying matters is to keep the size of each group of patients the same. This obviously minimizes the effects of variance differences which are produced by differing group size.

As with the t-test it is also possible to look at related or dependent groups with ANOVA. In the case of our example above this equates to using the same patients for each set of measurements.

The ability to detect a difference but not be able to identify a sense to the differences, i.e. how the groups are different from each other, make this a two-tailed test. It is also important to realize that this test on its own does not allow a researcher to examine specific relationships between groups, only the overall pattern of all of the groups together. If the example above used three groups, A, B and C, then a significant result would only say there is a difference between all of the groups. Groups A and B could be identical but the test could not tell that group C was causing the difference.

In order to investigate the situation further it is necessary to use a 'post hoc' test. In this case (a one way ANOVA for independent groups) a test called the Scheffé test can be used to look for relative differences between groups. It is called a post hoc test because it is carried out *after* ANOVA. This test uses both the mean scores of the groups and the results of the ANOVA, and to use it two conditions must be met:

- The results from ANOVA must be significant.
- It cannot be performed on its own, but only following ANOVA.

The results of the test are based on multiple null hypotheses that there are no significant differences between pairs of groups in the study. A low p-value for any pairing of groups provides evidence that there is a significant difference between the two groups. A simple comparison for the two mean scores then provides evidence of the sense of relationship.

*Example* – continuing from above: ANOVA provides evidence that there is a significant difference between treatment regimens A, B and C. A post hoc Sheffé test is conducted using the ANOVA results and the means of the measurements on groups A, B and C. The Sheffé test reveals that there is a significant difference between group A and the others with no significant difference between groups B and C. At this stage the process is still two tailed, providing evidence for difference but not saying whether Group A's dose is higher or lower than the others. Direct comparison of the group means gives an indication of this sense allowing a one-tailed result to be obtained.

## Kruskal–Wallis test: compares three or more groups of data

This test can be applied to three or more groups of data and uses an extension of the logic which lies behind the Mann–Whitney 'U' test. As with the Mann–Whitney 'U' test, the method is useful for ordinal data, or interval data that are not normally distributed (or where insufficient evidence exists to assume normality). The test is considered to be *non-parametric* and is used to investigate differences between groups.

*Example*: The researcher investigating patient dose as a result of different radiotherapy regimens has reason to believe that the data sets do not follow a normal distribution. In this case a Kruskal–Wallis test will enable a comparison of the groups as a whole.

As with ANOVA the process is two tailed and does not allow comparison of individual pairs of groups. In order to compare pairs of groups a post hoc test called Dunn's test would need to be applied (in an analogous way to the Scheffé test for ANOVA), but the process would still be two tailed. In this case the comparison between median scores would provide further information (remember that the median is a better summary statistic than the mean for asymmetrically distributed data).

*General note on the use of post hoc testing*: If post hoc testing is used it is considered dishonest to then retrospectively pretend that direct comparisons between pairs of data sets were performed and 'forget' to mention that this route was suggested by a post hoc test. It could be particularly tempting to modify the point of a piece of research based on the findings of this kind of testing and make it appear as if something is happening when in fact it was not the original intention. The hypothesis that generates the research should come first – you should not start off with a hypothesis and then modify or re-engineer it as a result of your findings. Retrospective alteration means that the data are used to find the hypothesis and this is not the basis of scientific investigation.

## Key points

- Inferential testing involves drawing evidence from observations which can then be used to infer ideas that go beyond the observations themselves.

- Inferential statistical tests perform the same function but vary depending on what kinds of observations have been made.
- Fixed level testing requires the assumption of a fixed p-value which is then used as a basis for accepting or rejecting a null hypothesis. Rejection of the null hypothesis leads to acceptance of the alternative hypothesis.
- Significance testing is more flexible and seeks to find the probability of the observations occurring and then using this as evidence to support the experimental (research hypothesis).
- Parametric tests provide stronger evidence.
- Non parametric tests are more robust and generally require fewer assumptions.

Figures 15.7 and 15.8 indicate how the process can work for some of the common tests described.

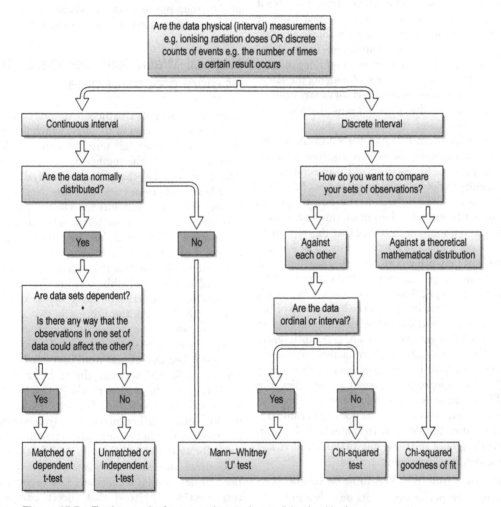

**Figure 15.7** • Testing results from experiments (a possible algorithm).

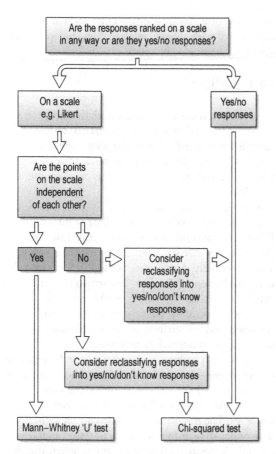

**Figure 15.8** • Testing results from questionnaires (a possible algorithm).

Note: not all of the conditions for the use of the tests are covered here and this should be used as a general guide. Small sample sizes could be problematic and this should be discussed with a statistician.

Note: agree/disagree responses can be treated in the same way as yes/no responses. The stages where the data are reclassified is a way of making dependent classes into independent classes. Remember that attitudinal scales have to be treated with caution. The combination of several responses into a score can be tested with the Mann–Whitney 'U' test.

## Getting it wrong

By now it is (hopefully) apparent that the whole process is driven by probability. By being careful you will *probably* be able to gain some insight into the circumstances leading to the data you have collected and into the workings of the world at large, but

*possibly*, owing to the influence of random chance, you might get it wrong. Not only can the testing process lead to flawed conclusions, but you should also consider the possibility that the way that you collect your data is flawed in some way. The sources of error were discussed in Chapter 1 and these can influence your data. The examples used in this section were based on the assumption that the data collection was flawless; however, in the real world it is very easy to introduce errors while collecting data. The errors of interest to this chapter are those introduced at the interpretation stage of a statistical test and there are two ways to get it wrong.

It is possible to reject the null hypothesis (i.e. to say the alternative is likely), when in fact it should not be. For fixed level testing this is less likely to happen if the p-value chosen for the level is higher rather than lower. The problem with raising the level is that the validity of your conclusion will be lowered, so some sort of compromise is necessary, which for most researchers occurs at $P = 0.05$. This type of error is referred to as a *type 1 error*.

It is also possible to fail to reject the null hypothesis (i.e. say that the alternative is unlikely), when in fact it is not the case. The effects of this kind of error can be overcome by using large samples repeating the research exercise in a variety of circumstances (a luxury which you may not have). This is referred to as a *type II error*. The ability of a test to resist this is called its *power*. Power calculations are mentioned in Chapter 10 so it is not necessary to revisit them in depth; however, we need to say that the power of a test is a measure of the probability that a type II error will be avoided. The power of a test can be calculated manually or more probably arrived at using software. With many software packages it is possible to select an appropriate power and then work backwards to decide how big a sample should be to make your findings significant.

Remember that all testing of data will be prone to these errors and there is no way to know when they happen or predict their occurrence.

## Summary

• Conducting a hypothesis test follows a well defined procedure which is common to all tests; data are used to generate a test statistic, the test statistic is used to produce a p-value, the p-value is then interpreted to accept or reject the null hypothesis and this is then interpreted in light of the original research hypothesis.

- The selection of hypotheses has a great influence on the success of the process and the exact wording of an experimental hypothesis can be influenced by the anticipated use of a particular test.
- Parametric tests should be favoured over non-parametric tests when it is practical to do so.
- The process of testing is subject to errors not only from the original data used but also from faulty interpretation of the results due to the influence of random chance. These errors are inherent in the process of testing because a fundamental condition for their use is the random acquisition of data.

So far we have been concerned with describing key aspects of sets of data and using these to answer questions related to research topics. These have related to the same quantity or variable being measured for different groups, e.g. the heights of adult males in different age groups. But what can we do when we have the opposite arrangement, which is when we have one group and different variables? This will be discussed in the following section.

# Correlation and regression

Both correlation and linear regression are alternative methods of examining the relationship between variables. The purpose of the two tests is distinct; which test you choose depends on the aim of the research, whether you are looking to describe a relationship (correlation) or you are using the data for modelling

or prediction (regression). This section is only concerned with linear relationships between two variables, known as bivariate.

## Correlation

A correlation is used to measure both the direction and magnitude of a relationship between two variables. The variables are usually from the same individuals or matched cases. The test is quite descriptive. If a relationship exists between variables this does not infer any causality.

Correlation can only be used for data where the numbers can be ordered, i.e. ordinal or interval data. If both the variables are measured on an interval scale the summary statistic used, assuming that each variable is normally distributed, is the Pearson's correlation coefficient (r). The Spearman's correlation coefficient (rho, ρ), which is the non parametric equivalent, is used when one of the variables is measured on an ordinal scale or the data do not approximate a normal distribution.

The tests produce a correlation coefficient that ranges from −1 to +1. The closer the correlation is to either −1 or +1, the stronger the correlation. Zero represents no relationship between the two variables. The direction of the correlation, either positive or negative, informs us how the two variables are related. A positive correlation exists when the two variables move in the same direction; a negative correlation is one where the two variables move in

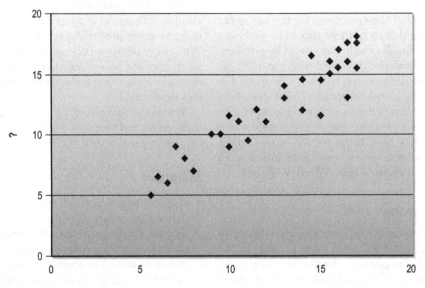

**Figure 15.9** • Strong positive correlation.

opposite directions. If we increased the repetition time in an MRI scan for a given number of slices and this was plotted together with the overall scan time we would see a negative correlation. As repetition time increases overall scan time decreases.

The best way to visualize the direction and magnitude of a correlation is to produce a scatter plot. Figures 15.9, 15.10 and 15.11 illustrate three different scatter plots demonstrating a strong positive relationship, a weak negative relationship and no

relationship between the two variables in question. The plots give you an idea of the strength of relationship but no exact figure.

## Obtaining a correlation coefficient

The first step is to look at the data and decide whether a Pearson's or Spearman's correlation is appropriate. To perform a Pearson's correlation the variables both have to be interval data, and they

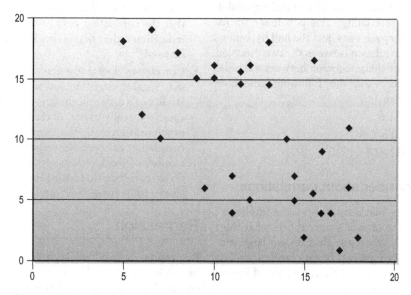

**Figure 15.10** • Weak correlation – negative relationship.

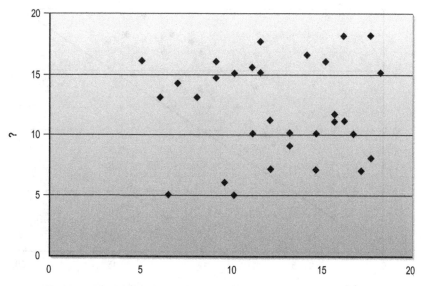

**Figure 15.11** • No correlation.

both have to approximate a normal distribution. The easiest way to check the assumption of normality is to perform a QQ plot or residuals plot. A QQ plot, Q standing for *quantile*, graphically compares the distribution of a given variable to the normal distribution. The normal distribution is represented by a straight diagonal line. The closer the points for the variable to this line, the greater the indication that the data are normal. Once this plot has been performed the appropriate test can be undertaken.

The output from a correlation analysis should provide you with a correlation coefficient and a probability value. If the probability value is below 0.05 (or pre-specified value) you can reject the null hypothesis that there is no correlation between the two variables.

The strength of the association between variables can be classified using the following guidelines provided by Cohen:[1]

- large: r = 0.5–1.0
- medium: r = 0.3–0.5
- small: r = ≤0.1–0.3

## Points to consider about correlations

- Do not assume that a smaller p-value implies a greater strength of association; this is what the r value explains. When sample sizes are large it is relatively easy to get significant correlations, but they may be weak associations that are of little if any practical significance.

- A good correlation does not necessarily mean good agreement. Figure 15.12 illustrates a scatter plot with a correlation of 0.963, P<0.001, a significant, very large association. A line has been added showing where the x and y values are equal, but of the 31 data points on the graph there is only one point on the line, so is there good agreement?

- Using a correlation on a rating scale is controversial. The numbers in the scales often do not have a true meaning and so are more ordinal in nature and in this case a correlation should not be used. However, if you are clear in the write-up that the correlation only provides a general indication rather than a specific value then it may be used.

- Correlation does not mean causation, although it may suggest causation and so may need further studies of a different design to investigate to see if causation really exists. A classic example of this problem is given by the significant and strong correlation between ice cream sales and the number of shark attacks on swimmers. From this do we conclude that eating more ice cream causes sharks to increase their attacks on swimmers?

## Regression

Regression is used to examine the relationship between variables. Unlike correlation, regression can explore non-linear relationships although only

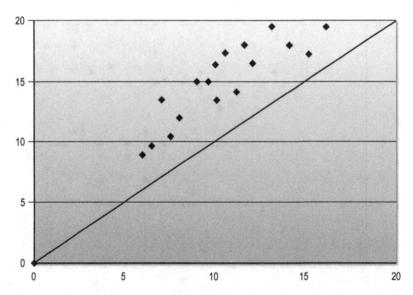

**Figure 15.12** • Graph showing difference between correlation and agreement.

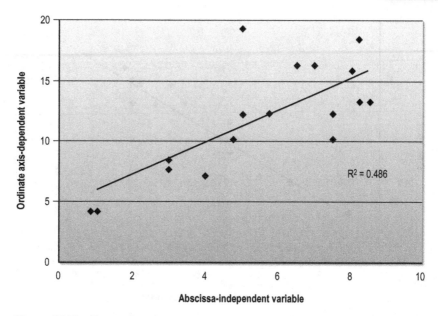

**Figure 15.13** • Regression plot.

linear regression will be discussed here. Unlike correlation, regression implies a direction of influence, of one variable on the other. Another difference is that both the dependent (observed or outcome) and independent variable (predictor) must be identified. When drawing a scatter plot of data for a regression the dependent variable is always placed on the ordinate ($y$ axis) and the independent variable on the abscissa ($x$ axis). In addition a line will be fitted to the data. There are a number of methods of fitting a straight line, but a common method is the use of the least square regression (LSR). This is a straight line that minimizes the sum of the squares of the distances between the line and the data points (Figure 15.13). The fit of the line to the points is explained by the value $r^2$, which is a value between 0.0 and 1.0, which has no units. An $r^2$ value of 0 indicates that knowing $x$ does not help you predict $y$. There is no linear relationship between $x$ and $y$, and the regression line is a horizontal line going through the mean of all $y$ values. When $r^2$ equals 1.0, all points lie exactly on a straight line and knowing $x$ allows you predict $y$ perfectly.

The resulting line, called the regression line, is characterized by the formula $y = a + bx$ where $y$ and $x$ relate to the dependent and independent variables, $a$ is the intercept and $b$ the slope of the line.

Figure 15.14 shows the regression line and is based on fictional data looking at the amount of time a student spends online using course resources and their exam result. The line has the formula $y = 8x + 9$, or exam score $= 8 \times$ online time $+ 9$. So for each hour on line the student's mark increased by 9%. We would expect a student who was online for 2.5 hours to get a score of 29% (exam score $= 8 \times 2.5 + 9$).

As with other tests it is possible to give a confidence interval for the regression line. This can be plotted on the scatter plot and gives curved lines above and below the regression line. And the area contained within these lines is the area that has a 95% chance of containing the true regression line. A second set of curved lines (95% prediction interval) can be added to the graph that gives an area in which you expect 95% of all data points to fall. The area within these lines is larger than the 95% confidence interval and would represent our confidence in predicting a single value on the regression line.

## Aspects to consider about regression

- Regression uses interpolation (the construction of new data points within the range of known data points) to make predictions of values. Do not use it for extrapolation (the construction new data points outside of known data points), as the predictions may be less reliable, as indicated by the dotted line in Figure 15.14.

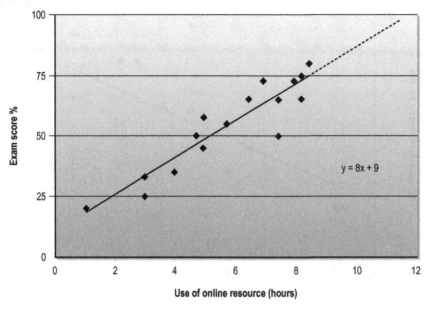

**Figure 15.14** • Regression line – formula and extrapolation.

• Regression is sensitive to outliers, particularly in certain locations, as is correlation; the model's ability to predict what is happening is seriously affected by outliers. The data should be checked very carefully for outliers. If we look at Figure 15.15 we can see some data points on the left and a regression line (light grey). If an outlier is added (purple circle) the regression line changes (solid purple line) and extends. The information between the outlier and the data point closest to it is based almost entirely on the outlier and even though we would be interpolating the data the confidence we have in the regression line being accurate must be suspect. Also the outlier has a large impact on the slope of the regression line.

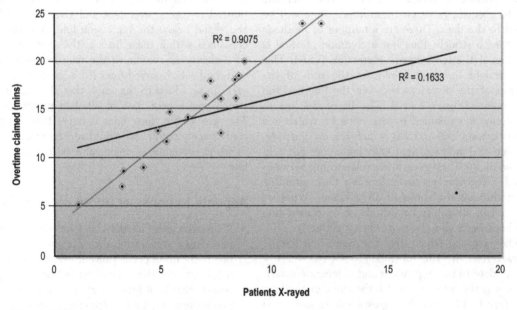

**Figure 15.15** • Effect of outliers on regression.

## The nature of proof and causation

Having displayed and/or analysed your data, a big question that needs to be addressed is 'what does it all mean'. It is not enough to present your findings – you must interpret them, use them to inform your research question, and ultimately draw some conclusions from what you have done.

In previous sections you have looked at some aspects of relationships in your data. Using *hypothesis testing* it is possible to look for *associations* or *lack of association* between groups. Useful conclusions can be drawn regarding how similar or dissimilar characteristics of groups are, for example the t-test looks at how similar or dissimilar the *means* of sets of data are. Correlations can give information about how two sets of variables can change in respect to each other, i.e. as observations of one variable increase, there is a similar tendency for a change to be seen with another variable, and this can be used to make predictions using regression modelling. An example might be the association seen between mental states such as depression and the use of some recreational drugs.

In all of these methods there is a serious pitfall which needs to be avoided. It is the assumption that one thing necessarily causes another or that anything has been proven. It may be the case that changes in one variable *cause* changes in another; however, it requires more than one piece of research to produce good evidence of this. The association between drug use and depression could be observed because depressives are more prone to seeking some form of escape.

Some criteria for providing evidence for causation are:

- How strongly one variable is associated with another, e.g. are smokers generally far more likely to die of lung tumours than non-smokers?

- How much the scale of association changes as one variable increases, e.g. do smokers who smoke more have a greater chance of dying from a lung tumour than smokers who smoke less?

- How well are the observations repeated when studies are done with different groups in different circumstances, e.g. does the association of death from a lung tumour and smoking change if you look at wealthy people as compared to poor people or if you look at groups from different countries?

### Key points

- When considering proof it is necessary to rely on repeatability and inference from other related research to suggest that proof has been obtained, e.g. ionizing radiation is taken to cause cellular damage because no experiment has ever found otherwise and slightly different styles of experiments will confirm the same result.

- One study on its own does not give enough evidence.

- Any bias in your data will mean that your evidence becomes progressively weaker as more bias is introduced.

- It is not only important to understand how fragile an argument for causation is when you are presenting one but it is also very important to recognize inappropriate claims of causation made by others.

- The safest course of action is to present the evidence and comment on its strengths and weaknesses.

- Allow the readers to form their own opinions guided by your observations rather than telling them what to conclude.

## References

[1] Cohen J. Statistical Power Analysis For The Behavioral Sciences. 2nd ed. New Jersey: Lawrence Erlbaum; 1988.

## Further reading

Altman DG. Practical Statistics for Medical Research. London: Chapman and Hall; 1990.

Campbell MJ. Statistics at Square Two. 2nd ed. Oxford: Wiley Blackwell; 2006.

Campbell MJ. Statistics at Square One. 11th ed. Oxford: Wiley Blackwell; 2009.

Miles J, Shevlin M. Applying Regression and Correlation: a Guide for Students and Researchers. London: Sage; 2001.

# 16

# Qualitative analysis

Peter Williams   Barbara Wilford   Susan Cutler

This chapter discusses the main qualitative research methods encompassed within this research paradigm, and some of the advantages and disadvantages of a range of data collection tools. We also discuss the data analysis process, the writing up of results and how to present your findings. We have included some examples of each qualitative approach that could be applicable to both diagnostic and therapeutic practice.

The principle qualitative approaches explored in this chapter have been divided into subchapters as follows:

1. Interviews (individual, focus group, structured/open). This approach tends to use language data (written or oral). The aim of these studies is to find answers to the questions that ask, how, what or why. This approach seeks to understand more about a phenomenon rather than measure it.
2. Questionnaires. This is a means of collecting data from a large number of people. Participants provide a written or an oral, if administered face to face, response which is either by selecting a predefined answer or by using their own words. Although qualitative responses will be considered in this chapter, it must be remembered that questionnaires are also used to generate quantitative data.
3. Observations. The researcher studies the phenomenon in question, with or without any intervention. It gives the opportunity to collect live data from live situations and to look at what is taking place in situ.
4. Case studies. This is when a specific instance or situation is used to illustrate a general

phenomenon. The focus could be on an individual, a family or a group. It is normal to use a multi-method approach to collect the data here.
5. Action research. This is where the researchers and participants work together to explore concerns and reflect on ways to change situations to achieve a positive outcome.
6. Content analysis. This is the systematic analysis or observations obtained from records, documents and field notes.
7. Critical review or systematic review. This approach aims to rigorously analyse primary research by evaluating high quality studies and synthesizing the findings.

First, then, what is meant by the term 'qualitative research'? It is an approach that seeks to *understand* human behaviour (i.e. what its essential *qualities* are) and, in our context, health behaviour and understanding of human health. Over recent years qualitative methods of data gathering and analysis have gained popularity among healthcare professionals as we seek to question traditional approaches to the delivery of health care. Qualitative research uses a number of different methods to collect the data which generates narrative or non-numerical information; it tends to use 'language data', which can be written or oral. In contrast, quantitative data collection focuses on collecting numerical data and then employs statistical analysis to test hypotheses. It should be remembered that similar ways of collecting data can be employed in both qualitative and quantitative methodologies. Also qualitative studies can employ frequency counts and language data can be used in quantitative studies. The overall aims of the study determine the methodical approach taken. A qualitative approach is utilized when you are asking questions that want to know, 'how' and 'why' rather than 'how often' or 'how many' where a quantitative approach may be more appropriate. It does try and gain insight into the individual's view of their own world. It is important that the researcher does not make any value judgements about the data collected. The focus is on the meaning and experiences of individuals or groups, to analyse how and why people form associations with other people, things and their immediate environment.

The key aspects of the qualitative approach are that:

- We are not trying to quantify or count things by gathering interview data (except where closed 'survey-like' questions are administered to a large sample of people).
- We are interested in *understanding* people and how they behave or think. We need to explore the ideas they hold in their minds as ideas are one of those things that we cannot observe.

This qualitative approach can be beneficial in the drive to expedite the service improvement agenda for the benefit of the patients, as it seeks to explore the patients' and practitioners' experiences of contemporary imaging and healthcare delivery.[1] The Society of Radiographers maintains that research will support change within diagnostic imaging, radiotherapy and oncology departments so ensuring practice- and patient-centred care become fully evidence based. In order to change and develop our practice for the benefit of the patient and client, we need to understand the environment in which we live and work and the patient's experiences and expectations. Any research we undertake must have a purpose; it would be unethical to undertake a study that did not attempt to explore phenomena relevant to the development of contemporary practice.

## Interviews

Any project which seeks to examine the attitudes, experiences or behaviour of people – in other words, social research – will almost inevitably involve data collection by some form of interview or survey. The interview might appear to be the easiest form of data collection – after all, who hasn't sat down and had a good chat with someone? And you only have to turn on your radio or television to hear an almost endless stream of interviews/conversations/ dialogues.

The first thing to say, however, is that an interview is NOT like a 'chat', despite the fact that the best interviewers make it appear so, and even though a research interview has been likened to a conversation. This distinction will become clearer later, but suffice to say here that, unlike a 'chat' or a 'normal conversation', in which you may expect a roughly equal contribution from the participants, a research interview should aim to be about 90:10 in favour of the interviewee – after all, it is their views we are interested in. By contrast, even the biggest pub bore would be hard-pushed to keep up that ratio, and if he did, his audience would soon be tiptoeing out of the back door.

So what is an interview, and why do we conduct them? Let us look at a couple of definitions:

- 'Rather than attempting to grasp quantities or measurements … interviewing is administered to develop a better understanding of how (people) interpret and experience some situation, process or event.'[2]
- 'Qualitative research [such as interviewing] attempts to understand meanings that people give to their deeds, experiences, or to other social phenomena'.[3]

Also, importantly, we are interested in individual experiences – stories, insights – things that you could not capture in questionnaire tick boxes. One of the present authors interviewed patients and medical staff at various GP practices where a touch-screen information kiosk had been installed. Interviewees not only had a wide variety of views, but ones which were totally unforeseen – and almost unforeseeable. One interviewee thought that the kiosk merely showed a plan of the surgery renovation; receptionists at a large hospital said that, as their kiosk was in a booth, it had been mistaken for a toilet cubicle. Given just these two responses, it is clear that a questionnaire could not have captured these perceptions, unless it approximated an interview format by using questions allowing for free-text answers.

One final point regarding the data accrued from interviews. People often worry about getting enough information to generalize or to make the research 'meaningful'. Here it might be useful to quote Henry Mintzberg, academic and author on business and management, who said: 'What is wrong with samples of one? Why should researchers have to apologise for them? Should Piaget apologise for studying his own children, a physicist for splitting only one atom?'[4] Similarly, television documentaries often contain individuals' descriptions of a particular event and quite often the recounted experience of four or five people gives a very rich picture, and offers an insight into what was going on beneath the surface.

As practitioners we deal with diverse and discrete client groups and their experiences of imaging or oncology may be considered for inclusion in this type of study. Interviewing of patient groups may be impractical for undergraduates owing to the complexities of the ethical approval process discussed in Chapter 6. But it is an avenue of exploration for qualified practitioners. Nevertheless this approach can be utilized in the university setting, with appropriate ethical approval, accessing the student body, either undergraduate or postgraduate, employees of the organization or the general public. For example you could explore the experiences of practitioners or students of working with hearing impaired patients or patients with learning disabilities. This has the potential to be extended to compare experiences with other health professional groups within the university setting, comparisons with students at different stages of their educational programme, different academic pathways, for example pre-registration undergraduate and postgraduate routes.

Using an open interviewing technique, possible questions could include:

- What is your definition of hearing impairment/ learning disability?
- Could you describe any experience you have had with a hearing impaired/learning disability patient?
- How did this make you feel?
- Do you think deafness awareness training would have helped?
- From your own experiences, in what way do you think the hearing impaired patient's visit to the medical imaging department could be improved?
- Are you in contact with or do you have experience of learning disabilities/hearing impairment outside the placement?
- How confident do you feel about dealing with people with learning disabilities/hearing impairment?

These questions are by no means exhaustive, but hopefully give you a feel of how questions could be phrased to enable the participant in the study to express their opinions and feelings about their experiences.

# Focus groups

Focus groups are unstructured interviews in which several participants discuss or explore together a specific set of issues. The focus group does not set out to change opinion or test knowledge, but like the interview, it seeks to explore the participants' experiences or attitudes. The role of the researcher is to facilitate and guide the debate and discussion by posing a series of questions that the participants explore. This approach can be used in its own right to explore issues, but is often used to complement questionnaire data or even as the preliminary tool for data collection from which a subsequent questionnaire is developed. The scope of the undergraduate dissertation possibly excludes utilizing this multi-method approach, due to the time constraints, but can be valuable in the clinical and post-registration context to explore in more depth issues relevant to practice.

The number of participants in a focus group varies, but the general rule is to include 6–12 people. Below this number there is the potential for little stimulus or for dominance of one of the participants. With too few participants, you also run the risk of the discussion and commentary from the participants being limited. Above this number you run the risk of having too many people talking at once and the essence of their debate is lost in the overall chaos of conversation. Also there is the opportunity for some of the participants to hide within the larger group and therefore not contribute. The group dynamics can be significant in the data collection as some do not interview well in groups and others may dominate. Sometimes the public setting of the focus group may inhibit the free flow of ideas or thoughts, which might be captured in a more intimate individual interview. Conversely the comment of one participant may provoke profound or animated debate among the others.

This type of interview usually takes from an hour to 90 minutes to conduct and can be quite demanding on the facilitator, who needs good social skills and interview technique. As a new researcher this can be quite a daunting aspect and it is worth trying to observe a skilled facilitator before commencing your data collection. Some of the key attributes required of the facilitator include:

- Alertness – attentive to the participants within the group; are there individuals who are dominating or others who are keeping quiet?
- Assertive – make demands of the participants to contribute to the discussion or allow others to speak, without being overbearing.

- Confidence – enough self-assurance to ensure that the focus group is appropriately conducted and relevant data are collected.
- Diplomacy – the ability to diffuse any potential confrontational situations.
- Empathy – the ability to understand and imagine the feelings of others.
- Encouraging – the flow of ideas from the participants without taking over.
- Interpersonal skills – the ability to establish a relationship with the participants.
- Listening – active listening is important in this context; the interviewer needs to be alert, reflect comments back to the group and seek clarification.

Before commencing the focus group, you will need to take into consideration the following three factors: the location of the interview, the physical environment and the group composition:

1. The location of the focus group should be such as to prevent the participants incurring any unnecessary expense.
2. The environment in which the interview takes place should be an adequate size so as not to inhibit any interaction and enable the participants to see each other, but not so large as to detract from the group dynamics or to prevent recording and observing effectively. It is advisable that the location is free from distracting elements such as noise, wall furniture and busy windows.
3. The participants: are they going to come from a disparate population or are they going to know each other or come from the same background, such as students in a cohort, practitioners from the same clinical department or practice area? Within the context of radiographic practice, whether therapeutic or diagnostic, the gender of the focus groups is unlikely to be representative of the population as a whole as the profession is still predominantly female. It is more important that the focus group participants do reflect the knowledge base or experiences required for the study.

One of the limitations of collecting data using focus groups is that only a limited number of questions can be addressed and are not usually explored in any detail. On the other hand the experiences of a larger number of participants can be captured and it is less time-consuming than individual interviews.

It is suggested that the focus group should be debriefed following the interview; this may include follow-up leaflets or phone numbers of relevant support groups if applicable. It is unusual for the transcription of focus group data to be sent to the participants, unlike interviews. Data produced from the focus group can be analysed in the same way as data generated from individual interviews. This is discussed later in the chapter.

Focus groups can be used to explore patients' experiences of health care. Particular reference, for example, could be made to different client groups such as the older patient, parent perceptions of their children's experiences, those with special needs. Conversely the practitioners, students, assistant practitioners, administrative staff perceptions could be expedited to give a contrasting perspective or to explore the context of the patients' or practitioners' experiences.

A study was undertaken to explore pre-registration students' experiences of using the virtual learning environment while on placement. A number of modules are delivered online to support their learning while undertaking clinical placements. To capture the diverse experience of as many students as possible a questionnaire was required (there were too many to interview individually). In order to develop the questionnaire for focus groups, one from each of the three cohorts studying at undergraduate level and one from the second year pre-registration Master's students, were undertaken. From these data a questionnaire was developed and subsequently distributed to the remaining student population.

## Recording your interview or focus group

Recording the data can be done in a number of ways: voice recording using a digital recorder, video recording or transcription of key points by the facilitator. The fear of relying on any recording equipment is, will it work? You could take the belt and braces approach and use two voice recorders. You could video record the interview or focus group, though participants may find video recording inhibiting and become self-conscious. It is useful to take notes during the session, but total reliance on this method means your focus is on scribing and not on the dynamics of the focus group, and as a consequence some comments may be missed and you may misinterpret meaning. It is important to ensure that the participants do not all talk at once so that data are not lost in the melee. When reviewing the recorded data it can be difficult to determine which participant is speaking on occasion. It should be remembered that this type of data can be 'messy' in comparison to that of an interview. In addition it can be time-consuming to transcribe and analyse the data.

## Advantages and disadvantages of interviews and focus groups

Many of the considerations for conducting an individual interview apply equally in the context of the focus group. The advantages and disadvantages of interviews and focus groups are highlighted below.

### Advantages

- *Participants' own words*: the interview/focus group offers unrivalled opportunity for interviewees to explain, reflect, and pontificate, using their own words and hence not being shoehorned into the words and the agenda of the interviewer.
- *Full and complete responses:* participants have the opportunity to expand on their answers, and often provide details not even considered by the interviewer.
- *Observational opportunities:* these are manifest when interviews take place in the subject's workplace or other location of interest to the researcher. It is amazing what important data can be gleaned from observing someone in action, fielding phone calls, having to break an interview to go and resolve some crisis, etc.
- *Non-verbal communication*: this can also be taken into account.
- *Clarification/follow-up questions:* these are possible, given the synchronous and dynamic nature of interviews.
- *Captive subjects:* as mentioned below, interviewees should be given the right to terminate the interview at any time. This happens only very rarely indeed, and usually simply because of work commitments or some unforeseen circumstance. Generally the interviewee is more or less captive. Hopefully, they will be interested enough in the topic to not

think in those terms themselves, but even if they do, they are often prisoners of their own politeness.
- *Known respondent:* unlike in a postal or online survey, you know who is responding – they are sitting right in front of you (unless they are not who they claim to be, which is pretty unlikely).

### Disadvantages

It all seems so fine and dandy up to here, but of course, as with every other research method, there are disadvantages too. Here are just some (and no doubt you will be able to find others if you think hard or cruise the Internet for long enough):

- *Conformity to expectations*: as you are right there with them, participants sometimes feel they have to say things that they feel you want them to say – people like to be nice, and to be cooperative. It is important, therefore, to stress that you are not judging them and also that you are not promoting anything. In our kiosk study we had to make it very clear we were not part of the company producing them.
- *Attempts to be rational*: in another manifestation of the desire to conform, people may try to be more logical than they really are. Having postulated that health information is very important in managing chronic illness, they may feel they cannot then say that, actually, they prefer to not think about it at all (so a good approach, instead of confronting them with questions about how much information they need for their health, would be to simply ask how they cope, and look out for where information crops up in their answer).
- *Reticence/shyness*: you may come across people who find the whole interview process intimidating, especially a 'research' interview. Unless you are good at putting them at their ease, you may find the time and expense yielding very little return. Of course, you as an interviewer may also be somewhat introverted. Before you decide on your project, to the extent to which you have a choice, consider carefully if it is one in which interviews are necessary.
- *Time/cost*: clearly, interviews are time-consuming and, if you have to travel around to undertake them, costly. As noted above, the prize is usually rich, fascinating and very worthwhile data. However, you do need to weigh up whether you

have the resources and, if so, whether the benefits that accrue are worth all the effort.

- *Data analysis difficult*: it is not easy to extract meaningful information from, sometimes, reams of transcripts or interview notes. More on this can be found below.
- *Unrepresentative samples*: sometimes, in carrying out qualitative research, there is a tendency towards finding and relying on a few key people or, alternatively, people who happen to have most time to speak to you. This can be an issue with undergraduate research when students often reciprocate participation in studies.
- *Poor articulation*: depending on the group(s) you decide to interview (individually or in a focus group), there may be a problem with participants being able to articulate their thoughts and opinions. In addition to possibly limiting the amount of data you accrue, there is a potential problem here of the articulate individual's views being over-represented, simply by their ability to express them.
- *Researcher bias*: you need to be aware that your own social background assumptions, attitudes and beliefs, and behaviour can affect the research process and should be acknowledged when writing up your project. It is important therefore to reflect on your own stance with regard to the research topic and acknowledge that your own personal experiences have the potential to lead to bias in the phrasing of your questions and interpretation of the data.
- *Participant overload*: one of the problems associated with pre-registration research is the potential sample size being limited to the number of students studying diagnostic or therapeutic radiography. There is a real risk that students become exhausted by participating in a number of studies. This also means that the results are contextualized to the population and may not be extrapolated to the wider population. As explored earlier with regard to researcher bias, there is the potential for participant bias in this context.

To obviate some of the problems, it is good to at least incorporate some of the following techniques to make your interview research more robust:

- *Purposive sampling*: focus on a specific population, so the participants have, as close as possible, the same or similar experiences of the phenomenon you are studying. This only works, of course, if you are not interested in a wide exploration.

- *Choose deviant case*: the exception proves the rule. If you can find someone who does not seem to conform, the data gathered will put the other research into perspective and will give you an overall richer picture.
- *Member check*: this refers to going back to the participants (if possible) or their peers and checking with them that this is what was said, and that the way you are interpreting it is correct.
- *Researcher 'reflexivity'*: this is simply acknowledging your own views and where you fit in. Reflecting on your analysis helps you to decide whether your own biases and pre-suppositions have 'contaminated' your data.

One other approach could be to use a process of:

- *Triangulation*: in other words, use another data gathering method and combine the results.

This approach is often used in the study of some aspects of human behaviour. A good idea is to combine interviews or focus groups with a questionnaire. Much survey research actually starts with a qualitative phase in order to tease out the main issues, around which a survey questionnaire can be constructed. However, each approach should stand on its own merit. Using just one method of data collection provides only a limited view of the complexities of human behaviour, so one method alone might introduce some bias. A multi-method approach that yields the same results can increase the confidence in those results.

## Preparing the interview

You will need, of course, ethical approval for your study, as described in Chapter 6, so this section assumes you have done this and the study has been approved. In terms specifically of interview preparation, the first thing you need to do is to go back to your original aims and objectives and determine the extent to which your interview will address and inform these. The aims of your interview will also determine the style with which it is undertaken. Briefly, there are three main factors involved: how specific a topic may be; the number and type of questions; and the order of questions. At one extreme is the interview in which there are very few, if any, pre-determined questions and the interview is led to a great extent by the interviewee; this is known as an 'unstructured' interview. This kind of interview is useful if the topic is vague or if you as a researcher have little prior knowledge of the field.

More common is the 'semi-structured' interview, where the researcher has a number of issues to cover and has a loose set of questions. Here the order of questions is not important, but the researcher tries to cover all the question areas, albeit not necessarily in a given order. There is also the 'structured' interview, where the questions are more specific, and asked in a predefined order. The structured interview is often undertaken on the telephone.

If possible, try to choose the interview location yourself. You really want to talk to your subjects in the environment of whatever it is you are studying. For example, if you are doing a study on some aspect of the work of radiographer or practitioner, it would be better to interview them actually at work, so you can see aspects of their work that they may (or may not) mention, and the contextual factors that may inform your study.

A very important part of your interview preparation will be to look at individual questions/areas/and themes. Questions can include those seeking:

- facts (e.g. age, gender, education, behaviour, experience)
- opinion/preference/attitude/feelings
- motivation or intention (e.g. likeliness, willingness).

You also need to decide whether or not to record your interview. Here you need to consider:

- the possible effect on the interviewee (will they be self-conscious, or as frank as they would be if it were not recorded?)
- listening/transcribing time afterwards, which may be prohibitive
- the reliability of machine/recording. Think what a disaster it would be if the interview did not record. It is always best to take notes as well, partly as a fall-back and partly as an orientation when playing the recording back or seeking a particular point.

## Conducting the interview

The guidance discussed below applies equally to individual interviews and focus group interviews.

A few basic rules for when you conduct the interview are:

- Thank your participants. Needless to say, this is the first thing you will need to do. Tell them how much you appreciate their time and effort in speaking to you, whoever they are, and make them feel important. This is especially advisable with people who may not ordinarily feel too important – frequent GP surgery attendees, for example. Second, set the scene. Explain the why/how/where and for whom of the study.
- Give an idea of the question areas, and more or less in what order they will be coming up (if there is a logical progression).
- Explain the ground rules. You will have to lay these out anyway in the information sheet they will have about the interview, but normally these will be that they can decline to answer any question, as they wish; they can terminate interview at any time; they can choose to remain anonymous if you decide to quote them in your dissertation or report, etc.
- Ask them if they have any questions before you start.

As you can see, the resemblance of an interview to a chat is already receding. Just to emphasize that, let us compare an interview with a pub chat.

Imagine, once you had got the 'hellos' and 'how are yous?' out of the way, then saying 'first, during this chat, I am going to ask you about how your day has been, with particular reference to that bloke in your office whom you wish to strangle; then we will briefly discuss the weather; and finally I'm going to lament the fact that my wife doesn't understand me and my teenage son is off the rails. I have a car problem I would like to discuss, but that will probably have to go on the agenda for next time'! I'm pretty sure your friend would exercise his or her right to terminate the meeting at any time – probably doing so immediately.

Back to the real interview. It is common to start with basic demographic questions to set the scene. It is also pretty standard to then continue with a general question and then funnel to the specific.

## Types of questions

Types of interview questions are:

### Open

- opening stages in a line of questioning
- invites opinion, general knowledge
- can cover areas where interviewer's own knowledge lacking
- no presumption about response.

## Closed

- elicits hard facts
- controls pace/direction of interview.

## Probing

- extracts more depth
- maintains a line of enquiry.

## Leading

- confirms interviewee's answer
- helps interviewee, by rephrasing answer
- brings a line of questioning to an end (summarizing).

# Analysing interview data

This is the part that worries people the most. How do you get meaningful data from the mass of interview transcripts or notes that you have? Although all of your interviewees will tell you individual and unique stories, each one of which will be valuable in its own right, your task will be to look for commonalities, themes and contrasts. Most important, of course, is to consider again your aims and objectives and to see how the interview data informs these.

There are several methods for sorting the raw notes and transcripts into meaningful research data. An approach which we favour is called 'framework analysis'.[5] This goes through a logical sequence which is relatively easy to follow. It consists of five stages:

- familiarization
- identifying a thematic framework
- indexing
- charting
- mapping and interpretation.

These are outlined below:

- *Familiarization*. This is the immersion in the raw data undertaken by listening to recordings, reading transcripts and notes, etc. so you can just get a feel for all the different ideas and themes that emerge.
- *Identifying a thematic framework*. Here you try to identify the key issues, concepts, and themes within the data. The best way to do this is to go through each interview with the aims and objectives of your study in mind, although issues raised by the respondents themselves which may not be central to your study aims might nevertheless inform the overall research. Write a

word or phrase beside each issue/concept elicited. By the end of this stage you will have a series of key words and phrases – and possibly questions – next to your main interview notes or transcripts.

- *Indexing/encoding*. This stage involves taking the comments, etc., grouping them into the themes identified, and coding them, possibly adding a few notes to the codes. By indexing the data like this, you are categorizing the original notes you made, and you may find you see the data in a new light.
- *Charting*. Here you take each index entry, lift it from its original place, and paste it into a new document which relates to one of the specific themes that have been itemized. Thus, all the text relating to a particular theme – such as 'changes in lifestyle' – will be in a single document. Before you do this, it would be a good idea to use some form of participant identification, so that you can trace back each comment to an individual. This is a good idea because it might be that all the participants who shared something in common, either demographically or in terms of job status or whatever, had similar views. This will only come out where each comment is attributable. There are a number of good suggestions about how to undertake the 'charting' process. One such suggestion is an approach which involves numbering each line of each transcript and printing transcripts relating to different kinds of interviewees on different coloured paper; e.g. green for nurses, blue for doctors and yellow for patients, etc. You can then write 'each question to be analysed', or each research aim, on large sheet of paper (preferably 'flip-chart' size) and you go through each page of coded transcript and relate the indexed entries to the research questions or aims, so that the interviewee comments that related to each point are all together. There may well be other data that do not fall naturally into the predefined categories suggested by the research aims or questions. This does not mean that they do not have any value. They will provide extra, perhaps contextual, data and may well suggest further areas for exploration in subsequent studies.
- *Mapping and interpretation*. Once you have 'charted' the data, you can really get something from it. The next, and final, stage uses the charts you have created to map the range and nature of phenomena, create typologies and find associations

between themes with a view to providing explanations for the findings. The process of mapping and interpretation – just as the 'charting' of the previous stage – is influenced by the original research objectives as well as by the themes that have emerged from the data themselves. During this stage the researcher reviews the notes, draws comparisons and matches similarities in the perceptions and experiences of participants, and resolves to explain these.

By the end of this stage you will have completed analysing the data and will be ready to either take the study forward onto a quantitative (e.g. survey) stage or make conclusions from your findings and write up your results, about which more below.

## An example of an interview with analysis

Below you will find an interview that has been transcribed. Pauses, silences, giggles, etc. have been removed, but in some instances verbatim transcription is essential as the pauses and hesitations enhance the data collected.

The five-stage process discussed above will be used as a guide for analysis of the following interview:

- Familiarization – once you have read, listened and transcribed the interview you can now start to analyse the data.
- Identifying a thematic framework – what we suggest is that you attempt to do this yourself first but you will need to consider the overall aims and specific questions while reading.

  Aim: to ascertain practitioners' perceptions of their role as a student mentor.

  The specific questions are:

  ○ What do practitioners perceive as challenges to the students' learning in the practice setting?
  ○ Do practitioners perceive there are any benefits of undertaking this role?
  ○ How do practitioners perceive the students learn in the practice setting?

- Indexing.
- Charting.
- Mapping and interpretation.

Here is an interview that you could practise on. Try this out yourself first. We have included some of our framework analysis later for you to look at and compare. Depending on who is interpreting the data, some

different themes can emerge; this does not mean that you are wrong, but that your analysis is different.

## Transcription of an interview with a practitioner about her role as a mentor

**Tell me about your experience of supporting learning in the clinical setting?**
Well I have been a mentor for 3 or 4 years now. I started by coming to the university for an induction procedure. I've gradually felt my way through it. I have a lot of experience so throughout the years I have had a lot to do with students training though not always on an official level. I've been a senior practitioner so I've always had some input into training but it is now more formalized with appraisal. I've just gradually got into it and do reports on the student's progress and I've done a few sessions where I have done some practical talks about basic views and the problems that they might encounter.

**What do you understand about the way adults learn?**
I think they learn quite a lot from their co-workers or other people, in actual fact I think the students learn from other students who are further on in the process but I think learn from observation really and from just being there whilst it's going on.

**Do you think that the learning needs of individuals can be met in the practice setting?**
Yes, yes I think so, it's just a normal thing that all students are different so that you match your teaching to what they are capable of taking in at the time. I think you have to play it by ear as some are capable of taking in things quicker than others. Some people are more confident and are prepared to go ahead and because they (the students) work with all of us (practitioners) and they get a bit of something different from every person that they work with. And here they get a good mixture of people to work with, so I think we can support individual needs. As mentors we often discuss students together so we can highlight strengths and weakness and put some support mechanisms in place to help students. The site coordinator is very good and helps us with ideas of how we can help the students.

**How do you use reflective practice to support the students' learning?**
Practice can be hectic, so quite often we can't take 'time out' to reflect immediately on what has happened.

It's often when we are relaxing, having a coffee when we actually have chance to discuss issues, but its more informal that way and we probably don't really think of it as reflection. But we do ask questions as we are going about practice, what about that patient who came from such and such a clinic, what did you make of the image, did you think it needed a lateral, why did you think that, for example. So you do it amongst yourselves, I've never actually sent anyone off to reflect.

### Do you think reflection is an important aspect of practice?
I do, but I think I'm not very good at documenting all these things, but when I think about it I've always reflected on my work. We discuss things about practice, such as barium studies with (names a colleague), you might not put a label on it as reflection, but I do reflect all the time.

### What is important about clinical education?
It's basically a practical occupation, you can theorize all you like, but until you've actually been there and done it I don't think you are ever quite as capable as you think you are until you have encountered the challenges of practice. Every patient is different and they all have different needs, so they (the students) might be taught about ageing but they don't really understand about the implications of that for taking an X-ray until they meet older people.

### What about professional socialization? How does the practice experience affect that?
I'm sure that is learning from example, the students need to find a good role model. I can say they get some good examples to follow and perhaps see some examples of things that aren't as they should be. When I was a student I wanted to be a professional and so tried to exemplify that and would take my lead from whoever I thought was worthy of that niche. But I think it takes a while to learn to work and fit in with a department, but by the time they qualify, they know what is acceptable and what is unacceptable, we tell them if we don't think they are acting properly.

### What do you think are the key goals of clinical education?
Well basically it's to have the confidence to make your own decisions and that comes from having a lot of experience of undertaking examinations. So they have a good base so that they know they can cope with any event that they encounter, well they can't do everything, but have the practical and thinking skills to work out what they need to do. It's about building up their knowledge so they have the confidence to make

decisions about referrals and how to examine the patient. You have to lead them through this process so they have the confidence in the end to do this on their own.

### How do you help to develop their clinical reasoning?
I think we have to start with the basics and ask them to think about what they are going to do before they do it. They then go and do it and afterwards think about what they have done, what they did correctly and what they did wrong. Why did they do what they did? What might they do next? Unfortunately it's time pressure really that means we don't always have the opportunity to discuss each case in depth as would be ideal, but over time we do iron out any issues over a period of time.

### What do you think your role is as a mentor in the management of clinical education?
I think it's about giving the students the chance to try things out but ensuring that they are doing things right the first time if possible. So sometimes it can be about saying that's not an appropriate examination for you to do at this stage of your training, or saying it's about time you were doing these types of examination now. It's about pushing them sometimes, but also about holding them back, maybe that's not the right term, ensuring they aren't attempting things they aren't currently capable of.

### How do you maximize their learning opportunities?
We do try and let them get on with what they are capable of. We do rotate them around the department so they get a chance to see and do lots of different things. Some do make more of their opportunities than others, in some ways I think all we can do is give them the chance to learn, to some extent they have to take some responsibility. Some of them will stand back and need to be encouraged all the time; others will ask 'can I do that?'

### What about the ethical issues relating to clinical education?
Well sometimes it can be difficult to manage the learning and the patient, the students often want to ask questions, which I might not want to answer in front of the patient. They sometimes might say or think that all old people are demented, but that's not right. I try to get them to think about what is right and wrong.

### How do you get the students to link theory with practice?
I get them to look at anatomy and pathology for example. But it can be difficult to get them to realize

that we apply theory all the time, but we don't talk in that way every day. But when I take an X-ray I do think about radiation protection all the time, but I might not say that I'm doing this or that as it helps to reduce the dose.

**How do you use assessment to promote learning?**
I think it's good, as its makes them learn things, but it does scare them. They have done things lots of times, but when you suddenly say, well this time I'm going to assess you, they can lose the plot. When I was a student people were watching me all the time and they could see I was progressing, I think it can be harder now as there is so much technology. I think it's good that they can make mistakes, and can learn from them. I think assessment is good it helps them realize what they need to know to do the job properly.

**What about feedback?**
I do it informally all the time; I fill in progress forms for the students, but (names colleague) she seems to do the more formal feedback, but I think they could do with more. But sometimes it's hard, you don't want to make them feel bad, but sometimes you have to be cruel to be kind as they can be hopeless sometimes.

**How important is CPD in learning and teaching to you?**
Well it's important as you want the students to have the best experience. So it's important you yourself are actually doing best practice yourself. I've always done it but haven't always recorded it, but need to now. I need to keep up to date with my practice, so that I can help and advise the students about what is now best practice, so in that way I'm using CPD to inform my teaching. But I haven't really done much about teaching as such; I've been on the training courses and update days, but not much else.

**Why did you decide to become a mentor?**
Well I think I have a responsibility to do it, but it's a big responsibility. I'm going to work with these people in the future, so I want to make sure they are moulded into the right sort of person. I think you volunteer for this role, which is better than 'pressed men'. But that doesn't mean you will be good at it.

**Is there anything else you would like to say?**
No I don't think so.

**Thank you for taking the time to participate in the interview.**
The data will now be categorized. An example of this can be found in Figure 16.1.

## Indexing and thematic framework

Included here is a copy of the interview which demonstrates the indexing process and from this we have developed the themes and codes. We started by reading through the interview and thinking about the questions. We then highlighted the issues and concepts (Fig. 16.1a). We have then written a word or phrase against each issue and concept. Look at all the words and phrases, including those highlighted in Fig. 16.1b (these will be referred to later in the analysis). How did these match to your indexing?

The next stage is when the original questions are reviewed and the indexed/encoded entries are related to the research questions.

## Mapping and interpretation

It is difficult with just the one interview in this example to undertake a full analysis and interpret the findings fully. Nevertheless we can see that some links and perceptions are emerging.

With regard to the question 'What do radiographers perceive as challenges to the students learning in the practice setting?'

The mentors indicate that assessment can be intimidating, but are also recognizing that they may not provide sufficient feedback. They recognize it is an active tool for learning. Observation is seen as an import aspect of clinical education.

You will need to look at all of the indexing/encoding and charting for all of your interviews and map responses to the relevant questions. You will also need to review the emerging themes. You need to be aware that it is not always black and white and there may be overlap of categories. The numbering helps you go back to the original location of the data to seek clarification if required.

## Key points

- Interviewing is probably the most common form of data gathering, but remember that an interview has to be well-prepared and takes considerable skill in conducting.
- The qualitative approach looks at the 'how' or 'why' rather than the 'how many', and has an emphasis on *understanding*.
- There are both advantages and disadvantages to choosing interviews and/or focus groups as data collection tools.

| Question and answer. Issues and concepts are highlighted | Words and phrases relating to each issue/concepts |
|---|---|
| **Tell me about your experience of supporting learning in the clinical setting?**<br>1. Well I have been a mentor for 3 or 4 years now. I started<br>2. by coming to the University for an induction procedure.<br>3. I've gradually felt my way though it. I have a lot of<br>4. experience so throughout the years I have had a lot to do<br>5. with students training though not always on an official<br>6. level. I've been a senior and superintendent radiographer<br>7. so I've always had some input into training but it is now<br>8. more formalised with appraisal. I've just gradually got into<br>9. it and do reports on the student's progress and I've done<br>10. a few sessions where I have done some practical talks<br>11. about basic views and the problems that they might<br>12. encounter. | 3. Gradual<br>4. Experience<br>5. Unofficial<br><br><br>8. Gradual  process<br><br>10. Teaching |
| **What do you understand about the way adults learn?**<br>13. I think they learn quite a lot from their co-workers or<br>14. other people, in actual fact I think the students learn from<br>15. other students who are further on in the process but I<br>16. think learn from observation really and from just being<br>17. there whilst it's going on. | 13. Co-workers<br>14. Each other<br>15. Observation<br><br>17. Being there |
| **Do you think that the learning needs of individuals can be met in the practice setting?**<br>18. Yes, yes I think so, it's just a normal thing that all<br>19. students are different so that you match your teaching to<br>20. what they are capable of taking in at the time. I think you<br>21. have to play it by ear as some are capable of taking in<br>22. things quicker than others. Some people are more<br>23. confident and are prepared to go ahead and because<br>24. they (the students) work with all of us (radiographers)<br>25. and they get a bit of something different from every<br>26. person that they work with. And here they get a good<br>27. mixture of people to work with, so I think we can support<br>28. individual needs. As mentors we often discuss students<br>29. together so we can highlight strengths and weakness<br>30. and put some support mechanisms in place to help<br>31. students. The site co-ordinator is very good and helps<br>32. us with ideas of how we can help the students. | 19. Different/Individualised<br><br>21. Pace of learning<br><br><br><br><br><br><br><br>28. Support individuals |
| **How do you use reflective practice to support the students learning?**<br>33. Practice can be hectic, so quite often we can't take "time<br>34. out" to reflect immediately on what has happened. Its<br>35. often when we are relaxing, having a coffee when we<br>36. actually have chance to discuss issues, but its more<br>37. informal that way and we probably don't really think of it<br>38. as reflection. But we do ask questions as we are going<br>39. about practice, what about that patient who came from<br>40. such and such a clinic, what did you make of the image,<br>41. did you think it needed a lateral, why did you think that,<br>42. for example. So you do it amongst yourselves, I've never<br>43. actually sent anyone off to reflect. | 33. Hectic<br><br>35. Informal discussion<br><br><br>38. Question practice |
| **Do you think reflection is an important aspect of practice?**<br>44. I do, but I think I'm not very good at documenting all<br>45. these things, but when I think about it I've always<br>46. reflected on my work. We discuss things about practice,<br>47. such as barium studies with (names a colleague) you<br>48. might not put a label on it as reflection, but I do reflect all<br>49. the time. | 44. Not formally recorded<br><br><br><br>48. Active reflection |
| **What is important about clinical education?**<br>50. Its basically a practical occupation, you can theorise all<br>51. you like, but until you've actually been there and done it I<br>52. don't think you are ever quite as capable as you think<br>53. you are until you have encountered the challenges of<br>54. practice. Every patient is different and they all have<br>55. different needs, so they (the students) might be taught<br>56. about ageing but they don't really understand about the<br>57. implications of that for taking an x-ray until they meet<br>58. older people. | 51. Practical<br>52. Challenges<br><br>54. Individual needs of patients |

**Figure 16.1 •** (a) An example of how interview data are categorized.

Continued

**What about professional socialisation? How does the practice experience affect that?**

| | |
|---|---|
| 59.I'm sure that is learning from example, the students need | |
| 60.to find a good role model. I can say they get some good | 60.Role model |
| 61.examples to follow and perhaps see some examples of | 61.Good examples |
| 62.things that aren't as they should be. When I was a | |
| 63.student I wanted to be a professional and so tried to | 63.Professional |
| 64.exemplify that and would take my lead from who ever I | 64.Exemplify |
| 65.though was worthy of that niche.  But I think it takes a | |
| 66.while to learn to work and fit in with a department, but by | 66.Learning to work |
| 67.the time they qualify, they know what is acceptable and | 67.Behaviours |
| 68.what is unacceptable, we tell them if we don't think they | |
| 69.are acting properly. | |

**What do you think are the key goals of clinical education?**

| | |
|---|---|
| 70.Well basically it's to have the confidence to make your | 70.Autonomy |
| 71.own decisions and that comes from having a lot of | |
| 72.experience of undertaking examinations. So they have a | |
| 73.good base so that they know they can cope with any | 73.Capability |
| 74.event that they encounter, well they can't do everything, | 74.Competence |
| 75.but have the practical and thinking skills to work out what | |
| 76.they need to do. It's about building up their knowledge so | |
| 77.they have the confidence to make decisions about | 77.Confidence |
| 78.referrals and how to examine the patient. You have to | |
| 79.lead them through this process so they have the | |
| 80.confidence in the end to do this on their own. | |

**How do you help to develop their clinical reasoning?**

| | |
|---|---|
| 81.I think we have to start with the basics and ask them to | 81.Thinking |
| 82.think about what they are going to do before they do it. | |
| 83.They then go and do it and afterwards think about what | 83.Reflection |
| 84.they have done, what they did correctly and what they | |
| 85.did wrong. Why did they do what they did? What might | |
| 86.they do next? Unfortunately its time pressure really that | 86.Time barriers |
| 87.means we don't always have the opportunity to discuss | |
| 88.each case in depth as would be ideal, but over time we | |
| 89.do iron out any issues over a period of time. | |

**What do you think your role is as a mentor in the management of clinical education?**

| | |
|---|---|
| 90.I think it's about giving the students the chance to try | 90. Providing opportunities |
| 91.things out but ensuring that they are doing things right | |
| 92.the first time of possible. So sometimes it can be about | 92.Encouraging them |
| 93.saying that's not an appropriate examination for you to | |
| 94.do at this stage of your training, or saying it's about time | |
| 95.you were doing these types of examination now. It's | |
| 96.about pushing them sometimes, but also about holding | |
| 97.them back, maybe that's not the right term, ensuring they | |
| 98.aren't attempting things they aren't currently capable of. | |

**How do you maximise their learning opportunities?**

| | |
|---|---|
| 99.We do try and let them get on with what they are capable | 99.Encourage |
| 100.of. We do rotate them around the department so they | 100.Provide opportunities |
| 101.get a chance to see and do lots of different things. | |
| 102.Some do make more of their opportunities than others, | |
| 103.in some ways I think all we can do is give them the | |
| 104.change to learn, to some extent they have to take some | 104.Learner responsibility |
| 105.responsibility. Some of them will stand back and need | |
| 106.to be encouraged all the time; other will ask "can I do that?" | |

**What about the ethical issues relating to clinical education?**

| | |
|---|---|
| 107.Well sometimes it can be difficult to manage the | 107.Difficult to manage |
| 108.learning and the patient, the students often want to ask | |
| 109.questions, which I might not want to answer in front of | 109.Appropriate responses |
| 110.the patient. They sometimes might say or think that all | |
| 111.old people are demented, but that's not right. I try to get | 112.Reduce prejudice |
| 112.them to think about what is right and wrong. | Right and wrong |

**Figure 16.1—Cont'd**

*Continued*

| | |
|---|---|
| **How do you get the students to link theory with practice?**<br>113.I get them to look at anatomy and pathology for<br>114.example. But it can be difficult to get them to realise<br>115.that we apply theory all the time, but we don't talk in<br>116.that way every day. But when I take an x-ray I do think<br>117.about radiation protection all the time, but I might not<br>118.say that I'm doing this or that as it helps to reduce the dose. | 115.Constant use of theory<br><br>117.Not explicit |
| **How do you use assessment to promote learning?**<br>119.I think its good, as its makes them learn things, but it<br>120.does scare them. They have done things lots of times,<br>121.but when you suddenly say, well this time I'm going to<br>122.assess you, they can loose the plot. When I was a<br>123.student people were watching me all the time and they<br>124.could see I was progressing, I think it can be harder<br>125.now as there is so much technology. I think it's good<br>126.that they can make mistakes, and can learn from them.<br>127.I think assessment is good it helps them realise what<br>128.they need to know to do the job properly. | 119.Active tool for learning<br>120.Intimidating<br><br><br><br>125.Reflect on errors |
| **What about feedback?**<br>129.I do it informally all the time; I fill in progress forms for<br>130.the students, but (names colleague) she seems to do<br>131.the more formal feedback, but I think they could do with<br>132.more. But sometimes it's hard, you don't want to make<br>133.them feel bad, but sometimes you have to be cruel to<br>134.be kind as they can be hopeless sometimes. | 129.Informally/Continuous<br><br>131.Written – formal<br>132.Insufficient  feedback<br>133.Consideration |
| **How important is CPD in leaning and teaching to you?**<br>135.Well it's important as you want the students to have the<br>136.best experience. So it's important to you yourself are<br>137.actually doing best practice yourself. I've always done it<br>138.but haven't always recorded it, but need to now. I need<br>139.to keep up to date with my practice, so that I can help<br>140.and advise the students about what is now best<br>141.practice, so in that way I'm using CPD to inform my<br>142.teaching. But I haven't really done much about teaching<br>143.as such; I've been on the training courses and up date<br>144.days, but not much else. | 135.Enhance learning experience<br><br><br>138.Best practice<br>139.Responsibility<br><br><br>142.Not teaching |
| **Why did you decide to become a mentor?**<br>145.Well I think I have a responsibility to do it, but it's a big<br>146.responsibility. I'm going to work with these people in the<br>147.future, so I want to make sure they are moulded into the<br>148.right sort of person. I think you to volunteer for this role,<br>149.which is better than "pressed men". But that doesn't<br>150.mean you will be good at it. | 145.Responsibility<br>146.Future practitioners<br><br>148.Volunteers<br>149.Quality of mentor |
| **Is there anything else you would like to say?**<br><br>151.No I don't think so<br><br>152.Thank you for taking the time to participate in the interview | |

**Figure 16.1—Cont'd**

*Continued*

| Thematic framework and indexing/encoding | |
|---|---|
| We read the interviews and immersed ourselves in the data. We looked at the issues and concepts that emerged from the indexing/encoding. And from these the initial themes were derived. You need to remember that these themes and encoding arise from one interview; more may emerge from other interviews. | |
| Themes | Charting |
| Mentor's role | |
| Reflective practice | |
| Clinical education | |
| Professionalism | |
| Assessment | |

| The next stage is **charting**, where the indexed/encoded items are related to the themes. | |
|---|---|
| Themes | Charting |
| Mentor's role | 3.Gradual<br>4.Experience<br>5.Unofficial<br>8.Gradual  process<br>10.Teaching<br>90.Providing opportunities<br>92.Encouraging them<br>99.Encourage<br>100.Provide opportunities<br>115.Constant use of theory<br>146.Future practitioners<br>148.Volunteers<br>149.Quality of mentor |
| Reflective practice | 35.Informal discussion<br>38.Question practice<br>44.Not formally recorded<br>48.Active reflection<br>81.Thinking<br>83.Reflection<br>86.Time barriers<br>104.Learner responsibility<br>107.Difficult to manage |
| Clinical education | 13.Co-workers<br>14.Each other<br>16.Observation<br>17.Being there<br>19.Different/Individualised<br>21.Pace of learning<br>28.Support individuals<br>33.Hectic<br>51.Practical<br>52.Challenges<br>54.Individual needs of patients<br>77.Confidence<br>117.Not explicit |

**Figure 16.1(b)**

Continued

| Professionalism | 60.Role model<br>60.Good examples<br>64.Exemplify<br>66.Learning to work<br>67.Behaviours<br>70.Autonomy<br>109.Appropriate responses<br>112.Reduce prejudice/Right and wrong<br>135.Enhance learning experience<br>138.Best practice<br>138.Responsibility<br>142.Not teaching<br>145.Responsibility |
|---|---|
| Assessment | 73.Capability<br>74.Competence<br>119.Active tool for learning<br>120.Intimidating<br>125.Reflect on errors<br>129.Informally/Continuous<br>131.Written – formal<br>132.Insufficient feedback<br>133.Consideration |

**Figure 16.1(b)—Cont'd**

- Interviews are used to explore deeper meanings of, for example, experiences, ideas or attitudes and are usually conducted on a one-to-one basis.
- Focus groups usually involve the participation of several persons in a discussion or exploration of a specific set of issues.
- Many methods can be combined to provide a rich picture of a particular phenomenon.

# Questionnaires

The questionnaire can be a useful tool to extract data from the wider population. The field of questionnaire design is vast and the aim here is to give some basic guidance on the development of a questionnaire that can be used in a qualitative research design. As this approach seeks to explore experiences and feelings as discussed earlier, the design of the questionnaire needs to be such as to capture the individual's perceptions. It is important to say that the structure of a questionnaire differs depending on whether the study is of a qualitative or a quantitative design. Under certain circumstances, both methods can be used to analyse the same questionnaire. Going back

to the example of the impact of a touch-screen health information system, questions could be asked on frequency of use, reasons for use, other information sources consulted, etc. Here one is seeking quantitative data, how many people use the system, how often, and for what purpose, as categorized in the survey, and responses need only be in the form of ticking a box. However, if one is interested in individual perceptions, ideas and attitudes, the questions will be framed differently, and the response options might include allowing free text.

Pay attention to questionnaire structure and style. Remember that respondents are subjects and not objects of research. Issues such as the informed consent of the participants and their right to withdraw have to be considered.

There is much debate about whether open or closed questions should be used for data collection. A problem with closed questions is that they have the potential to create false opinions, as limited options are open to the respondent. Closed questions are often perceived as easier to answer. The open-ended question gives the participant the opportunity to express their feelings and perceptions in their own words. But as a general principle the larger the sample size the more structured, closed and numerical the questionnaire is likely to be. Questionnaires, particularly those that are self-administered, are used for convenience and speed rather than in-depth analysis. They can be useful when exploring phenomena in a population that is distributed across a wide geographical area. This means that large population sizes are available and therefore expands the potential sample size to be included in the study.

An example of an open question may be:

- How do you feel about the care you received during your examination/treatment on your recent visit to the imaging/radiotherapy department?

Expressed in the closed format it could look like this:

- How do you rate the care you received prior to your examination/treatment on your recent visit to the imaging/radiotherapy department? Please circle one number

| | |
|---|---|
| Excellent | 1 |
| Very good | 2 |
| Good | 3 |
| Fair | 4 |
| Poor | 5 |

As we are looking primarily at language data the focus of this section will be on the use of semi-structured and open-ended questionnaires.

Open questions do generate more detailed responses from the participants, but as a consequence a great deal more effort is required to encode the responses. Open questions will take longer to complete and this should be taken into consideration when compiling the questionnaire. On the other hand it could be considered an economical approach in terms of the time spent distributing and collecting the data. This approach has the potential to capture honest personal comments from the respondent.

The wording and design of the questions does need careful consideration; this aspect cannot be rushed and is time-consuming. Otherwise you could potentially write:

- Double-barrelled questions – these are questions that essentially ask two questions at once, therefore the respondent could answer either part of the question. An example might be, 'Do you think the new appointment system is easy to use and what effect on waiting times do you think this will have?' It would be better to ask these questions separately as the answers given may elicit a positive answer to the first, but a negative answer to the second.

- Complex questions – such as 'Would you prefer to undertake a short programme of study, e.g. 3 or 4 sessions, that does not carry any award, which is delivered on a Wednesday evening each week, or a longer award bearing programme that is designed to be undertaken during the day rather than the evening?'

- Irritating questions or instructions – such as 'Have you ever attended a personal tutorial during your undergraduate programme', or 'Have you attended any continued professional development activities during your career?'

- Ambiguous questions – this is where the words are ambiguous, such as 'Do you regularly undertake self-managed study while you are on placement?' What do we mean by 'regularly'? Is this once a day, once a week, once during your placement?

- Biased and leading questions – these are questions which are worded in such a way as to suggest to the respondent that there is only one acceptable answer. An example might be: 'Do you prefer to plan your studies well in advance or to leave it until the week prior to submission?' If this was asked by your academic tutor, I think we can guess which response you might make!

The open questionnaire can be administered face to face or be self-administered. Clearly when undertaken face to face, this can be time-consuming and may limit the potential participants. However, it does give the researcher the opportunity to encourage the participants to expand on their responses. An example of this is given in the study (see previous section) involving the exploration of imaging practitioners' perceptions of their role as mentors. Initially interviews were carried out to get a feel of how imaging practitioners perceived themselves in that role. From this data an attitudinal questionnaire was developed. Open questions regarding aspects of the mentor role that participants found most challenging were asked as well. Questionnaires were used so that perceptions of a larger number of imaging practitioners could be captured.

Radiotherapy practitioners have a role as health educators, preparing their patients for treatment. A questionnaire could be used to explore practitioners' and patients' perceptions of that role using open questions.

When using or creating a questionnaire, reliability and validity of the tool should be considered:

- Reliability of a tool is the ability to reproduce the results.
- Validity is more concerned with the accuracy of the test used, and asks whether it measures what it is intended to measure.

For example, a questionnaire may be considered to be more reliable than interviews, as the respondent is anonymous and therefore may give more honest answers to the questions. When considering the validity and reliability of questionnaires in particular you must think about the sample size; a small sample may skew the results or be unrepresentative.

## Key points

- Questionnaires can be a useful way to collect large amounts of data from a large number of participants.
- Questionnaires are versatile and can be used in both qualitative and quantitative research designs.
- Questionnaire structure can incorporate open questions, closed questions or a combination of both.
- When using a questionnaire to collect data, pay attention to the criteria that may affect the validity and reliability of the study.
- Questionnaires are the most popular data collection tool used for cross-sectional surveys, for student research projects.

## Observation

Observation is often a preferred method or key component of case studies or action research. The method is often used to supplement other methods, such as interviewing, and also when the phenomenon we wish to study is not well known to us. Here, observation is inductive. We begin with specific or general observations; detect patterns and regularities; then formulate some tentative hypotheses; and finally end up developing some general conclusions or theories.

You may be surprised to know that the apparently simple act of looking at something can be done in a great many ways. Observational methods can be said to be a rough continuum from the extreme form of participant observation, where the researcher becomes one of the people he or she is observing, to being as invisible as possible as a 'non-participant' observer. The former research is favoured by sociologists and anthropologists. A 'classic' example is that of observers of a religious sect whose leader had prophesied that the world would end that year. They pretended to be followers for a considerable time. Unlike many such 'immersion' studies, however, they deliberately interfered with what they were observing by suggesting to cult members that their leader might be a fraud.[6] Observational research in which the observer tries to immerse himself or herself in a culture or environment is known as 'ethnographic'. It is not the only type of research for which observation may be used, however, as some of the examples below suggest.

By contrast, the extreme non-participant observation is where the observer is as unobtrusive as possible. One such example is that of a sociological study of infant schools, in which the researcher ignored children who came to him with their work, etc. to such an extent that eventually they learned to ignore him as much as he was apparently ignoring them.[7] Apart from being physically present and as discreet as possible, non-participant observation can be undertaken without the physical presence of the researcher (and here we generally part company with ethnography). For example, researchers can use:

- Recorded behaviour, e.g. using CCTV to record footage of people's use of a touch-screen health information system as one of a number of data gathering techniques to look at system usage.
- Human trace behaviour, which involves examining the things people leave behind as they go about their daily routines or undertake the activities researchers are interested in. A classic example of this was a study by Rathje[1], who examined household waste; however, be sure to consider all ethical implications of undertaking observational studies involving human participants.
- Computer log analysis, which entails observing computer usage through the transaction logs created by the system. As users in our health kiosk study were required to 'log-in' with these details, researchers were able to compare time 'online', pages accessed and navigational behaviour, and relate it to age and gender.

## Advantages and disadvantages of using observation

The advantages of using observational techniques include:

- capturing non-verbal behaviour, which may tell more than may be elicited from interviews
- subjects do not have to do anything, except 'act naturally'
- researchers do not have to ask questions and no interpretation is required by the subject
- good for preparing the ground for other fieldwork, by familiarization with a situation, process or environment
- good for triangulation, i.e. for combining with other methods
- phenomena are studied as they occur and there is no need for the participants to rely on memory
- a more intimate or informal relationship is permitted, where participant observation is involved.

The disadvantages of observation include the following:

- Observation could change what is being observed. This is as true of people as it is of subatomic particles, and has been given a name 'the Hawthorne effect'. This comes from a set of studies conducted in the 1920s and 1930s at the Western Electric Hawthorne Works in Chicago, by Harvard Business School Professor Elton Mayo, who was interested in productivity and work conditions at the works. Mayo found that the very act of being observed made the company employees work harder.[8] The experiments led to the term 'Hawthorne effect' being applied to research generally where researcher observation leads to a positive change in the behaviour of those observed. Although the effects have been questioned, it is a concept worth bearing in mind.
- The observer may pose an imagined threat. This may be particularly true in a work context, where people may be worried about their performance.
- It is hard to track many activities at once.
- Interpretation of observations is difficult.
- Observation is time-consuming.
- The researcher can feel a bit awkward. The term 'wallflower' springs to mind. This may seem a trivial point but the work will be your study, and

you will want to do your best. You may feel that you just would not be able to do this by feeling self-conscious or awkward.

## Collecting data

Having weighed up the pros and cons, and decided to go ahead with some form of observational process, you need to decide how to collect and record data. There are several techniques, which are often relevant to both participant and non-participant observation. The main ones, in addition to those not involving you as a direct observer, are:

- Protocol analysis log. Here participants describe what they are doing as you observe. This is common in looking at the usability or accessibility of information technology systems.
- Take field notes, but decide first on what you want to record. You can probably make notes that equate to approximately 500 words per hour. You may wish to record specific events, or to see what is going on generally. These can be described as:
  - ○ *event sampling*: an example might be to record communication activities between hospital staff
  - ○ *time sampling*: this is where you record what is happening at given times during an observational session. This was common in education at one time, where interactions in terms of frequency of 'teacher talk', 'pupil talk', 'silence' and 'confusion' among others were analysed.

## Recording tips

Much observational recording will be undertaken, by necessity, at the time of the observation. This is particularly true where specific instances, events or times are being recorded. Even where you just want to get an overall picture of an environment, without recording chronologically, you may like to follow these recommendations:

- Record during or straight after the event otherwise you will forget the details.
- Do not start a new observation session until you have recorded the last one.
- Recording can take as long as actual observation if you are meticulous.
- Include everything important, or which might be important.

## Analysing the data

As with interviewing, people get really worried about analysing observational data. 'What does it all mean?', one might ask. So, as also with interviews, consider the aims and objectives of your study, and how the observation fits in with those. Some tips are:

- Look for similarities and differences, and try to explain them. You may need to consult interview data if you have any, in this, or simply ask the people observed to explain certain actions.
- Watch for re-occurrences – why do the same things keep happening?
- Formulate 'rules', based on repeated occurrences, but look for exceptions.
- Try to explain the exceptions you find – do they mean your rule is wrong? If so, change it; or is the exceptional case really different in some way? If so, in what way, and how does it inform your study?
- To systematize observations it may be helpful to devise categories. If you did not do this for the actual observation, doing it afterwards is still valuable, in a way even more, as you will make the categories fit what you have observed not the other way round. With any luck patterns will emerge.
- If the observation is a preliminary 'staking out' of the field, consider what questions it raises that could be incorporated in any interview or survey you may be considering.

There is the potential to observe practitioners or students undertaking a specific radiographic examination or intervention to explore the variation in approaches to techniques or tasks. It might be useful to observe how practitioners use different approaches to a task, which may well produce a similar outcome. An example could be a task analysis of how a lumbar spine examination is undertaken, hand washing techniques, moving and handling of radiographic or therapeutic equipment, observing the tools applied when evaluating images on DR or PACs system. Task analysis is a range of techniques used by operators to describe and evaluate interaction between humans and machines and is a way of investigating participants' behaviour in a specific context.

Within the practice setting you could observe patients finding their way around the imaging and radiotherapy departments or their interaction with staff at the reception area. Again, remember the ethical implications of studies involving human participants.

## Key points

- Observational methods involve many approaches on a continuum from participant to non-participant; and the methods of data gathering, including 'event' and 'time' sampling.
- Observational research methods form a key component of case studies and action research.
- Observational research is often employed to supplement other research methods, e.g. interviews.
- Don't forget the 'Hawthorne effect' during observational studies.
- When analysing data, pay careful attention to the explanations drawn from the similarities and differences observed. In addition, participants can be asked to explain their actions.

## Case study

A case study is where a single instance is studied in depth, and can be considered as an approach rather than as a method, as several methods are employed in a case study. Examples may include where a patient, a group of specialist practitioners, a clique, a class, or an imaging department is studied as a unique case. A case study is used to explore and reflect what is happening in a unique situation and allow these specific situations to be explored in greater depth, which may not be captured using other data collection tools. One of the strengths of these studies is that they are drawn into the context of the case itself. Case studies aim to describe 'what it is like' to be in a particular situation and to give a rich description of the reality. Observation is a tool that is frequently used in the case study; it is discussed in greater depth in the preceding section.

A case study design is useful when:

- a randomized approach is not appropriate
- it is not possible to study a particular population as a group
- you need to evaluate intervention outcomes over a period of time
- pilot information is required.

Case studies are useful as a theory generating tools. When conducting a case study a number of factors need to be considered, such as negotiating access to people and how the data are to be collected. Data collection tools that could be employed in case studies include interviews, using open or semi-structured questions; observations or narrative accounts. In addition documents or diaries could be used to explore the uniqueness of a specific situation.

## Key points

- A case study can be considered an approach rather than a method.
- A case can be an individual or group of patients, practitioners, a class of students or an imaging department.
- Case studies are used to explore a 'happening' in a unique situation.
- Observations are frequently used as tools to collect data in case studies.

# Action research

The purpose of action research is to improve understanding of practices in a specific context with a view to making changes for the better and it is a reflective activity. Action research is designed to bridge the gap between research and clinical practice. It should bring about improvement, change and development to enable practitioners to have a better understanding of their practice.

There are three basic phases to action research:

1. Look – build up a picture of a situation and the context in which it occurs, thinking about what the practitioners, as well as the patients, are doing.
2. Think – this process requires you to interpret the situation and explain what is happening, reflecting on what the participants have been doing and look for any deficiencies or issues.
3. Act – whereby actions for change are identified and put into practice.

Action research is about looking at a local issue or problem and exploring that and making changes, as well as expanding knowledge. In addition, this research approach provides an opportunity for personal and professional development.

Methodologically it has a distinctive set of requirements. It should be:

- collaborative – the participants contribute to the overall project
- action oriented or participatory – intervention and change are a part of the process

- contextualized – it relates to a specific place, situation or circumstance
- reflective – through a process of planning, action, evaluation and critique

Action research relies on:

- communication of all group members
- time to reflect on the process and outcomes of the project
- verification of project – can it be replicated or reproduced?

It can be argued that the process of action research enhances the change process, a key agenda in the ever changing context of health care, but particularly in the fields of medical imaging and radiotherapy. It is an approach that enables the researcher actively to participate in development in their specific area or field and it is suited to small-scale projects. Action research generates change through reflection, communication, cooperation and collaboration and empowerment among participants.

The action research process consists of several stages:

- questioning existing practices and coming up with an idea
- collaborative decision making and planning
- action, implementing the changes with ongoing evaluation and monitoring
- critical reflection on the intervention and the process
- re-evaluation of original plan based on reflections, implementation of changes and continued monitoring
- reflection on the knowledge generated and the reshaped practice.

The actual methodological approach employed will depend upon the research question posed. As discussed earlier, triangulation is often employed to increase validity and to identify convergence and obverse patterns. But whatever data collection process is employed the validity and reliability of the chosen method should be considered. There are some potential problems associated with action research. These are the level of skill of the research facilitator and the culture of the organization in which the research is taking place.

A survey might elicit information from a patient group about waiting and changing facilities; the context in which this data is collected has to be taken into consideration. The data collected must be reflected on and discussed, a plan of action for any changes discussed and implemented. Follow-up focus groups, for example, could be employed to determine whether the interventions have affected change in clinical practice.

## Key points

- Action research is a reflective activity in which researchers aim to improve the understanding of their practice within a given context.
- The three basic phases involved in action research are look, think and act.
- Action research should be collaborative, action orientated, contextualized and reflective.
- Triangulation is often employed to increase validity and reliability of findings.

# Content analysis

Content analysis is used for studying the content of communication and documentary evidence. It is a careful, detailed and systematic examination of large amounts of data.[2] Content analysis is used to determine the presence of certain words or concepts within literature. The literature used can be from a variety of resources, books, journals, research articles, professional journals, departmental or hospital protocols, newspapers audio of video media material, etc. Any information, whether it is primary research or information which is in the public domain, can be used.

Content analysis can be qualitative or quantitative and usually involves inductive reasoning. This methodology can uncover underlying meanings within a text and enables the content to be quantified by the use of a set reproducible method of data extraction. Researchers quantify and analyse the presence, meanings and relationships of words and concepts within the literature. Categories and themes emerge from the data. These identify the focus of the research and the extracted data are assigned to these themes and categories as analysis of the data occurs.

Content analysis is generally categorized into two types:

*Conceptual analysis*, also known as thematic analysis, involves quantifying the existence and frequency of words of phrases in the literature being studied. The focus is examining the occurrence of selected terms within a text or texts. The terms may be implicit or explicit. While explicit terms are easy to identify, coding for implicit terms and

deciding their level of implication is much more complex, basing judgements on a more subjective system. The level of implication refers to how you have defined the words or phrases and must be kept constant throughout your analysis; using the example cited earlier about what is meant by 'regular', you need to define whether it means, for example, daily or weekly. To limit the subjectivity when coding such implicit terms specialized software packages can be utilized. These packages increase the reliability and validity of extracted data, adding rigor to the study and its findings. These packages are time consuming to use and are not usually used by students and entry level researchers because of this. Examples of such software packages are:

- ATLAS – software for text analysis and model building. It handles graphical, audio, and video data files and text.
- The General Inquirer – contains large content dictionaries (Lasswell Value Dictionary, Harvard Psycho-Sociological Dictionary) which are used in conjunction with text scanning software to determine patterns in the meaning of words.
- NUD*IST – allows authors to establish lexical and conceptual relations among words, to index text files, and to conduct pattern matching.

This is not an exhaustive list. Other packages include NVivo and Qualrus.

*Relational analysis*, also known as semantic analysis, involves searching for meaningful relationships present in a given text or set of texts. Relational analysis explores the relationships between the concepts identified.

The difficulty with content analysis is not locating relevant information but analysing the often vast amounts of available data. This makes the process very time-consuming and labour-intensive. Content analysis cannot easily investigate implied meanings and is not a useful methodology for assessing subtle meanings within the literature.

Patient information leaflets could be selected from a number of Trusts or from just one Trust. These are in the public domain, so you should not experience any difficulties accessing this information. Once you have collected your leaflets, you could randomly select a manageable number to review. These can then be scrutinized for the type, quality and level of language used within these texts. You could analyse the sentence length and count the number of syllables used, but you could also ask readers to rate the readability of the information provided.

You could search historical archives of professional material looking at the development of advanced practitioners or the development of non-traditional radiographic skills such as counselling, for example. This could be a specified timeframe, say the previous 5 or 10 years. Then you could look for articles, references or editorial comments relating to counselling skills and you could also look for training and educational programmes. You could explore whether definitions have altered and which areas of practice specific skills have focused upon, such as ultrasound, radiotherapy practice or mammography services.

## Key points

- Content analysis involves the study of the content of communication and/or documentary evidence.
- It can be both qualitative and quantitative and usually involves inductive reasoning.
- It can be categorized into conceptual analysis and relational analysis.
- Content analysis can be time- and labour-intensive.

# Critical reviews

Critical or systematic reviewing is a research methodology which aims to review primary research evidence with rigor. High quality reviews identify all relevant studies in a particular area of practice and assesses the studies, synthesize the findings in an unbiased way and present the results in a balanced and professional manner.

Evidence-based health care relies on systematic reviews ensuring that healthcare practitioners have a clear understanding of available research and ensuring that their practice is based on the best available evidence. Healthcare professionals are also turning towards current available research in order to aid in efficient clinical decision making. Critical reviews contribute to evidence-based practice by using explicit methods to select, critically appraise and summarize large quantities of information and literature, aiding the decision-making process.

## The search strategy

Carrying out a structured search is essential and of the utmost importance when undertaking a critical review because it helps to fully understand the topic in question. It enables awareness of existing research

in the same area and ensures the intended project has not been undertaken before. Even if the study has been done before there is often a need to review the latest available information and studies to ensure all evidence is current and this may necessitate undertaking a review that has been done previously. This is of particular importance if the new research will add knowledge to the literature already available. The Cochrane handbook for reviewers[9] recommends that a variety of sources should be systematically searched to reduce the risk of bias and broaden the search base. A critical review should include all available evidence.

The identification of the best evidence and selection of research literature requires the construction of an appropriate research question. A stepwise process named PICO has been developed to achieve this. PICO is an acronym for Population/Participants, Intervention, Comparison and Outcome. The research question should have elements of the population, investigation, comparative investigation and an outcome in its question. Formulating the question using these key components will assist in specifying the criteria used to select studies. The importance of developing a focused research question is crucial, ensuring it highlights the significance of the problem. Critical reviews in radiography often use the PICO system.

## Exclusion criteria

The method used for including relative literature is undertaken in three stages.

Stage 1 – is the inclusion of studies based on their title and abstract to decide whether they were relevant to the question posed.

Stage 2 – involves establishing if the studies met the inclusion and exclusion criteria.

Stage 3 – assesses the methodological quality of the study and extracts the data.

Ethical implications need to be considered and addressed when undertaking any systematic review or content analysis. Ethical release may be required from the ethics committee and the Higher Education Institution (HEI). An unbiased, objective approach should be followed, using published guidelines for critical reviews combined with good reflective judgement. This ensures the answers to the research question are based on available evidence rather than unsubstantiated claims that may potentially produce misleading results.

When comparing two imaging modalities in diagnosing a specific pathology, for example:

- Is magnetic resonance angiography (MRA) an alternative imaging modality to renal angiography in diagnosing renal artery stenosis (RAS)?
- Is ultrasound an alternative imaging modality to renal angiography in diagnosing RAS?
- Can CT colonoscopy replace the double contrast barium enema when screening for colorectal polyps or colorectal tumours?

## Writing up qualitative research

The manner in which your project should be structured and presented is explored in Chapter 17. But a number of considerations should be taken into account when writing up your study:

- Most importantly, you must refer to the original research question/aims and assess the extent to which your objectives have been reached.
- Try to be consistent with the data. In other words, do not try to make too much of one quote that seems to confirm what you already think at the expense of other data that do not.
- Treat all data 'fairly'. It is okay to say there was no apparent pattern in responses, and also to say that 'all the women in the sample thought X', as long as

you do not try to imply that this suggests any generality.

- It is always good to say that 'further research is needed to establish whether this represents a general trend'.
- Try to include appropriate quotes in your write-up, and also some individualized accounts/stories, etc.
- Your conclusion should include an assessment as to whether your research questions have been answered, what unforeseen results arose and, if possible, some recommendations for further research or practical action.

Undertaking qualitative research can be both fascinating and satisfying, and that information unearthed is often completely unexpected, and can be of immense interest and importance. Good luck if you go down this route.

## Key points

- The aim of a critical review is to rigorously evaluate primary research evidence.
- It is important that healthcare practice is based on the best available research evidence.
- A robust search strategy is essential when conducting a critical review (see also Chapter 3).
- Critical reviews in radiography often use the PICO system as a useful strategy.

## References

[1] Rathje W. Rubbish!: The Archaeology of Garbage. New York: Harper Collins; 1992.

[2] Curasi CF. A critical exploration of face-to-face interviewing vs. computer-mediated interviewing. Int J Market Research 2001;43 (4):361–75.

[3] Silverman D. Qualitative Research: Theory, Method, Practice. London: Sage; 1997.

[4] Mintzberg H. The Nature of Managerial Work. London: Harper and Row; 1973.

[5] Richie J, Spencer L. Qualitative data analysis for applied policy research. In: Bryman A, Burgess RG, editors. Analyzing Qualitative Data. London: Routledge; 1994. p. 173–94.

[6] Festinger L, Riecken H, Schachter S, et al. When prophesy fails. New York: Harper and Row; 1956.

[7] King R. All Things Bright and Beautiful: A Sociological Study of Infants' Classrooms. Wiley: Chichester; 1978.

[8] Mayo E. The Social Problems of an Industrial Civilization. London: Routledge and Kegan Paul; 1949.

[9] Higgins JPT, Green S, editors. Cochrane Handbook for Systematic Reviews of Interventions, Version 5.0.2 [updated September 2009]. Cochrane Collaboration. 2009. Available at: www.cochrane-handbook.org (accessed 1.10.2009).

# Section 6

## Writing up and disseminating

# Dissertations and projects: structure and presentation

# 17

Alan Castle

## CHAPTER POINTS

- The term 'project' refers to the process of research and data collection, while the dissertation is the written document designed to demonstrate your scholarly ability.
- Projects may take the form of a systematic review of literature (bringing together previous research and published work), clinical audit (measuring performance) or primary research (deriving new knowledge).
- Since there are many different types of project it is difficult to specify a single structure to suit every dissertation, but it should consist of a logical sequence of chapters to include a clear introduction, the main body of your argument and a conclusion.
- The purpose of your dissertation is to present the process, results and interpretation of findings in such a way that you get your message across clearly and effectively and in an appropriate academic style.

This chapter will provide detailed guidance on the structure and presentation of your final written document.

## Introduction

The purpose of a dissertation/project is threefold: to complete a higher education degree, to evidence your intellectual ability and to demonstrate that you can clearly and effectively communicate your findings. These three principles together shape the final structure and presentation of your thesis.[1]

There is often some confusion over the terminology used to describe the process of undertaking a project and writing a dissertation. You can consider a *project* as a process that involves a planned activity designed to achieve a particular aim. A *dissertation* is a written document discussing the background to, process of and findings, conclusions and recommendations resulting from, a project and is usually produced for an undergraduate or Masters degree. A *thesis* usually refers to a dissertation produced at Doctoral level. In this chapter I will use the term dissertation for simplicity and consistency.

Producing a dissertation is a major requirement of most higher education courses and is likely to be the largest single piece of work you will be asked to produce.[2] It involves undertaking some form of research, where you usually have the opportunity to pursue, in depth, some topic of your own choosing. Ultimately you will be expected to produce this extended documentation to demonstrate your ability to engage critically and analytically with appropriate literature, report on your own work, offer your own thoughts and interpretation on your findings, reflect on the research process and make an original contribution to knowledge. Essentially it is a document to demonstrate your thoroughness and ability to produce scholarly work.[3] As opposed to an essay, it requires more research in greater depth, more reading, more time, more independence, more planning and more writing. It is important therefore that you plan, manage and write it up effectively.

Getting started is often the biggest barrier.[4] Novice writers tend to be big procrastinators, finding many reasons not to get started, using delaying tactics such as having to make a cup of coffee, read more literature or collect more data.[5] However, writing requires you to make a conscious decision to start and then to discipline yourself to see the task through to the end, as the process is not complete until the findings have been written up.[6] Key tips to ensure good planning and management include setting deadlines, starting to write early, writing regularly and in stages and allowing time for revisions.

Whatever the nature of your project, a formally presented dissertation should be able to pass tests of readability (text clearly and quickly understood), organization (logical presentation so that a clear story unfolds) and referencing (to ensure claims made are based on evidence) and an appropriate and consistent style is adopted.[7]

Dissertations may vary in scope, but will probably take the form of a review of literature, clinical audit or primary research. A *systematic review of the literature* involves carrying out a systematic critical appraisal and synthesis of the current state of knowledge relating to the topic under investigation. Since all published literature is in the public domain no ethical issues arise. A *clinical audit* involves collecting data on current practice and comparing this data with some locally, nationally or internationally agreed standard in an attempt to find out *what we are doing* in an attempt to inform delivery of best care. You will normally need to obtain written department/hospital approval to collect such data. *Primary research* attempts to find out *what we should be doing* and to derive generalizable new knowledge. This involves collecting data, usually from staff or patients or using hospital equipment and resources, and you will normally need to obtain Research Ethics Committee Review approval to conduct a project of this nature.[8]

As the Latin word *dissertare* means to debate, a dissertation involves you being able to examine and discuss a topic from different points of view and advance an original opinion. You should be clear that the notion of original does not mean something that has never been done before, but rather something that you have done for yourself. Thus a dissertation will show that you are able to critically appraise relevant literature, apply principles of good project design and management and produce an academically rigorous document.

## Structure

There is no best way to structure your dissertation and educational institutions and funding bodies produce their own specific requirements about the format and length of the work. However, once you have got the structure right, the writing of the dissertation will be easier for you and the reading more

straightforward for an examiner. All dissertations should contain similar elements and below is a suggested approach to structure and organize your work. This generic structure is used in most academic writing, where the process is quantitative and linear, with the review of the literature preceding the collection of data. However, this may not be entirely suitable for qualitative projects where the literature and research may be more interconnected or where you are looking at several themes which would be better dealt with in separate chapters. Whatever the nature of your project, structure is important and possible ways to achieve a sensible and consistent structure should be discussed with your supervisor.

### Title page

This should be succinct, reflect the nature of the dissertation and contain enough information to attract relevant readers. Thus 'Women's attitudes to nuchal translucency screening' is better than 'Women's attitudes to undergoing the 11–14 week ultrasound scan to assess nuchal translucency where the risk of the fetus having Down syndrome is calculated',[9] as the first title contains enough key words (women's attitudes and nuchal translucency screening) to encourage further reading. Make sure the title has no spelling mistakes or typographical errors – first impressions are very important. In addition, this page should include the degree for which the dissertation is presented, the name (or number) of the student, the awarding institution, date submitted and word count (excluding reference list and appendices). Figure 17.1 shows a typical sample title page.

### Signed statement

You must declare that the dissertation is your own work. This page must therefore contain a signed declaration such as: 'I hereby declare that the text of this dissertation is substantially my own work.'

### Contents

This should be a list of the main chapters, subsections, figures/tables, reference list and appendices including page numbers. An example of a contents page for a project entitled 'A clinical audit to investigate the effects of simulator verification on the isocentric position of patients undergoing radiotherapy to the pelvic area'[10] is shown in Figure 17.2 (note that page numbers are usually indicated in Roman numerals before Chapter 1 and in Arabic numbers thereafter).

BSc (Hons) Diagnostic Radiography

Women's attitudes to nuchal translucency screening

by

Alan N Other

Submitted in accordance with the requirements of the
University of Hampshire

June 2009

Word Count: 10,356

**Figure 17.1** • Sample title page.

# Contents

**Figure 17.2** • Example of contents page.

## Abstract

The beginning of the dissertation should be especially clear and engaging for the reader if they are to be encouraged to explore further. The abstract should be a short summary telling the reader everything they can expect to find in the dissertation, including a statement of what the dissertation is about, some background to explain the focus, scope and rationale for the project (but should not contain any references), the project question, how the data were collected, the key findings and clear conclusions/recommendations. All this information should be contained within about 300 words (for a 10 000 word dissertation). For example an abstract for a dissertation entitled 'A review of the literature to assess the effectiveness of intensity modulated radiotherapy (IMRT) in the treatment of localized prostate cancer'[11] may be structured as illustrated in Box 17.1 (253 words).

## Acknowledgements

Where appropriate, acknowledgement should be made to the assistance given by individual supervisors and mentors or organizations that may have supported you, provided information or supplied equipment and materials.

## Glossary

This is a list of technical terms or abbreviations with definitions which can be included, if appropriate, in alphabetical order at the beginning of the dissertation. Examples are shown in Table 17.1.

## List of figures/tables

This can be used to guide the reader to specific illustrations in the text. For example, a project investigating whether computed tomography should become the primary imaging modality for trauma of the cervical spine might include the illustrations shown in Table 17.2. It is a good idea to number the illustrations according to the chapter in which they occur. Thus Figure 3.1 is in Chapter 3 (Methodology) and Table 4.1 is in Chapter 4 (Results).

# Chapter 1: Introduction

This is the scene-setting part of the dissertation and should explain enough background information so that the reader is clear about the nature of the project and why it is important for clinical practice. Definitions of any key concepts should be explained to help aid the understanding of, and context for, the study. You should assume the reader has some background

---

 Box 17.1

### Sample of an abstract

#### Aim

In the United Kingdom prostate cancer will affect 1 in 14 men during their lifetime. Successful treatment is greatly improved by early detection, but the most effective treatment is controversial and is dependent on the stage of the disease. The aim of this literature review was to assess the effectiveness of intensity modulated radiotherapy (IMRT) in the treatment of localized prostate cancer compared to three-dimensional conformal radiotherapy (CRT). Consequently the hypothesis suggested was that IMRT is more effective than CRT in the treatment of localized prostate cancer.

#### Methods

A literature review was conducted to collect information on the effectiveness of the two radiotherapy techniques. A total of 20 articles, including 10 prospective studies, 5 retrospective studies and 5 systematic reviews, were critically evaluated and summary tables generated for ease of data analysis.

#### Findings

The findings demonstrated that IMRT is more effective than CRT when the pelvic nodes are involved, as it was found to reduce toxicity to the surrounding critical organs. However, in the case of localized prostate cancer it was suggested that there was little or no significant clinical difference between IMRT and CRT.

#### Conclusions

Due to the findings of the studies reviewed producing equivocal results, the hypothesis was rejected as it was concluded that there was no definitive evidence to suggest that IMRT was more effective than CRT in the treatment of localized prostate cancer. However, since IMRT is still considered a relatively new radiotherapy technique, it is recommended that more research is needed before it becomes the treatment of choice.

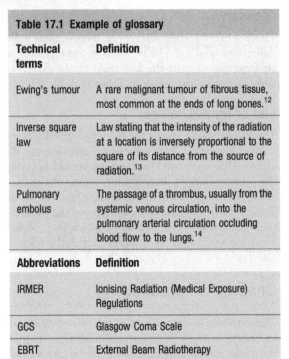

**Table 17.1  Example of glossary**

| Technical terms | Definition |
|---|---|
| Ewing's tumour | A rare malignant tumour of fibrous tissue, most common at the ends of long bones.[12] |
| Inverse square law | Law stating that the intensity of the radiation at a location is inversely proportional to the square of its distance from the source of radiation.[13] |
| Pulmonary embolus | The passage of a thrombus, usually from the systemic venous circulation, into the pulmonary arterial circulation occluding blood flow to the lungs.[14] |

| Abbreviations | Definition |
|---|---|
| IRMER | Ionising Radiation (Medical Exposure) Regulations |
| GCS | Glasgow Coma Scale |
| EBRT | External Beam Radiotherapy |

**Table 17.2  Example of list of figures/tables**

| Figure/table | Page number |
|---|---|
| Figure 3.1 Search strategy for bibliographic databases | 29 |
| Figure 3.2 Canadian C-Spine Rule | 32 |
| Table 4.1 Results of dosimetry studies | 42 |
| Table 4.2 Results of cost-effectiveness studies | 45 |

knowledge of your topic, but you need to bring them up to date and explain the current situation. For example, for a dissertation entitled 'A literature review to assess the comparative effectiveness of magnetic resonance imaging (MRI) and computed tomography (CT) in the diagnosis of acute stroke'[15] you could begin by outlining the etiology, epidemiology and pathology of the condition, followed by a summary of treatment options, a review of the role of imaging in diagnosis and the implications for practice.

Also included in this chapter should be a clear statement of the project question/hypothesis and clearly defined aim(s) and objectives. An example is outlined in Table 17.3.

## Chapter 2: Literature review

This is a review of published literature and should give the reader a clear understanding of the topic under discussion, key issues that arise, and the rationale for undertaking the project. You will be expected to demonstrate your ability to search for, and access, the breadth of literature informing the project and bring together past and present research and published work. The aim is to produce a distilled and *critical appraisal* of the relevant literature, showing how your project links to previous research and existing knowledge and how you intend to take this forward.

The purpose here is to *critically appraise* the literature you have read not simply collect references, describe them and make a list of what you have read. Critical thinking is a high level intellectual activity that requires you to assess and judge the value of knowledge and information.[17] This involves you looking at a piece of published work in an objective and structured way and asking such questions as:

* Is it an account of research or someone's views and opinions?
* How recent is the work and any other work discussed?
* What are the main points raised and are these supported in any way?
* Do you agree with the inferences and conclusions made?
* How does it fit with other work you have read in this area?
* What are its main strengths and weaknesses?

Thus you should be able to demonstrate that you can:

* make connections and see patterns in existing work
* organize your thoughts by being analytical, reflective and considered
* explore issues and identify reasons for any conflicting information
* take a new perspective on an issue
* assess whether practice should be changed.

For example, if you were undertaking a clinical audit to estimate how effective implementing the Ottawa Knee Rules in cases of acute trauma injuries is in reducing the number of radiographic examinations undertaken, your literature review might include the issues identified in Table 17.4.

Overall, the literature review is a piece of informative writing where you have the opportunity to 'tell a story' or 'paint a picture' about current knowledge

**Table 17.3 Example of project question, hypothesis, aim and objectives**

| | |
|---|---|
| • Project question | • Should CT or MRI be the imaging modality of choice for the primary and differential diagnosis of acute stroke? |
| • Hypothesis | • MRI is more sensitive at detecting and quantifying acute stroke artefacts than CT |
| • Aim ( a clear declaration about *what* you are going to do) | • To carry out a literature review to ascertain whether CT or MRI should be considered the gold standard for imaging of suspected acute stroke victims |
| • Objectives (a list of five or six specific statements which must be focused and precise and should be the bricks that build up your aim) | 1. Construct an effective search strategy for locating relevant studies undertaken within the last 5 years<br>2. Select and critically appraise 20 of the most relevant studies using the Critical Appraisal Skills Programme (CASP) assessment tool[16]<br>3. Conduct a meta-analysis of the quantitative results from these studies<br>4. Discuss the findings, draw appropriate conclusions and either accept or reject the hypothesis<br>5. Make recommendations for further practice and research |

**Table 17.4 Example of structure of literature review**

| Structure | Issues |
|---|---|
| Statement of question/hypothesis | The use of the Ottawa Knee Rule (OKR) will decrease the number of patients referred, following acute knee injuries, for radiographic examination without decreasing diagnostic sensitivity |
| Background/ rationale | • Extent of the problem<br>• Value of radiographic examination of the knee joint following acute injury<br>• Radiation dose<br>• Cost to health services<br>• Importance of undertaking project |
| Critical appraisal | • Range and value of clinical decision rules<br>• Derivation of OKR<br>• Application of OKR<br>• Comparison of effectiveness with other clinical decision rules |
| Summary | Your assessment of the effectiveness of OKR in reducing number of radiographic examinations based on the findings |

related to your topic. How the literature has shaped or informed the project is, consequently, an essential component of the dissertation.

# Chapter 3: Methodology

Chapter 3 is concerned with explaining *how* the question/hypothesis you posed in Chapter 1 was investigated and why you employed particular methods and techniques.[3] It requires sufficient detail for the reader to understand what you have done to collect and analyse the data.

The design of the project is a vital part of the dissertation for both a reader trying to judge the validity of the findings and for anyone interested in replicating the study. It is suggested that this chapter could be structured to include:

- a restatement of the aim of the project
- a discussion of the possible methodological approaches that you could have used to collect your data
- an explanation and justification for the approach you did use
- a description and validation of the ways in which the data collected were analysed

**Table 17.5 Example of areas included in methodology chapter**

| Aspect of methodology | Issues covered |
|---|---|
| Project design | Quantitative prospective study involving patients with lower back pain and sciatica who were referred for an MRI examination of the lumbar spine to determine whether they had intervertebral disc herniation (IVD) |
| Sampling method | A convenience sample of 50 patients was chosen and written permission obtained to carry out an MRI examination with the patient in the lateral position with their knee joints both flexed and extended |
| Measurements | Checklist devised to assess the resulting images in terms of degree of IVD (severity score) on a rating scale from no herniation (0), protrusion (1), extrusion (2) to sequestration (3) |
| Data collection procedures | Five radiologists recruited to blindly assess two sagittal plane images (knee joint flexion and extension) for each patient |
| Data quality | Content validity of the checklist assessed by three MRI radiographers and a pilot study undertaken with 10 patients prior to the commencement of the main project |
| Data analysis | • Spearman's rho correlation test used to measure the relationship between the severity scores for the flexed and extended positions<br>• Mann–Whitney 'U' test to compare the IVD mean severity scores for the flexed and extended positions |

- a discussion concerning any ethical issues and a statement that appropriate ethical/departmental approval was sought (written evidence that this has been obtained should appear in the appendices).

Details of any tools you used to collect data, for example measuring instruments, questionnaires, interview schedules, etc., should be included in the appendices. Table 17.5 illustrates an example of areas that should be covered in a methodology chapter from a project designed 'To compare the value of flexion and extension of the knee joints of patients during a magnetic resonance imaging (MRI) examination of their lumbar spine to investigate intervertebral disc herniation'.[18]

Thus, this chapter is important in allowing the reader to be clear about how you met the objectives identified in Chapter 1, what steps were followed in collecting the data, why you chose this approach and how you analysed the information obtained.

## Chapter 4: Results

Chapter 4 should provide an accurate and full summary of the data collected, possibly using illustrations (tables, figures, graphs and charts) to support the text. Quantitative data may include both descriptive statistics, for example, response rates, gender and age characteristics of the sample and inferential statistics (the results of any statistical tests). Generally, the text should be written after any illustrations so that it highlights significant aspects of the findings and not duplicate information, and placed in the dissertation as near to the relevant illustration as possible. All illustrations should be numbered consecutively, titled and appropriate legends supplied (units, axes for graphs, etc.) and referred to in the text.

Table 17.6 illustrates how the quantitative findings arising from the methodological approach outlined in Table 17.5 might be presented.

Qualitative results are usually presented as key themes that emerge from the data collected and may be supported by illustrations to demonstrate relationships between various components or sequences of events. Table 17.7 illustrates the findings that may be obtained from a project aimed at 'ascertaining the levels of awareness of diagnostic radiographers concerning issues of breast cancer in the United Kingdom'.[19]

Whatever the nature of the results, this chapter needs to be structured so that it takes the reader clearly through what was found.

## Chapter 5: Discussion

Here you should provide a broader and deeper interpretation of the findings and the possible implications they might have for practice. Simply reporting findings

**Table 17.6 Example of quantitative results**

| Type of results | Issues covered |
|---|---|
| Descriptive statistics | Fifty patients were recruited, but images for only 40 patients were obtained (80%) as 10 MRI examinations were not completed. Subsequently, two sagittal section images were obtained for each patient (80 images) and labelled 1A and 1B, 2A and 2B, etc. and each radiologist rated the images using the checklist. Pie charts and tables could be used to illustrate this data |
| Spearman rho correlation test | Data presented on a scatter plot graph to show the relationship between scores obtained for 1A and 1B, etc., for each of the five radiologists. Scores range from 0.998 to 0.935 suggesting that there is a high positive correlation between the radiologists' ratings for the flexion and extension images |
| Mann–Whitney 'U' test | The mean severity scores for the five radiologists could be demonstrated using a table, and the text could explain that, for example, the scores ranged from $P = 2.052$ to $P = 2.736$ and since they exceed the $P = 0.05$ level of significance it can be deduced that the mean scores for the flexion and extension images do not differ significantly |

**Table 17.7 Example of qualitative results**

| Type of results | Issues covered |
|---|---|
| Sample | A semi-structured interview was conducted with a sample of 10 diagnostic radiographers (five male and five female) aged between 25 and 40 years to ascertain their awareness of the risk factors associated with breast cancer in the UK |
| Awareness of the incidence of breast cancer | Most of the female respondents ($n=4$) and fewer of the male respondents ($n=2$) were able to accurately estimate the incidence of the disease. The other respondents ($n=4$) tended to overestimate the incidence by a factor greater than $\times 2$ |
| Awareness of risk factors for breast cancer | The majority of the respondents (female $= 3$ and male $= 3$) were aware of the key factors that both increased and decreased the risk of developing breast cancer. There was some confusion concerning the issue of menopause/menarche |
| Awareness of the ways of reducing the risk breast cancer | These were generally well known by most respondents ($n=8$), although one male respondent thought that a high fat diet decreased the risk and one female respondent thought that excessive exercise, particularly for women with large breasts, increased the risk |

**Key themes emerging:**

- Female respondents were more aware of the incidence of breast cancer than male respondents
- The relationship between menopause /menarche and the effects of oestrogen were seen as areas of confusion that need clarification
- There are some misconceptions concerning ways of reducing the risk of breast cancer

is not enough; you must give some meaning to what has been found. However, while qualitative results are by nature interpretative, usually the results and discussion are combined in one chapter. Conversely, as quantitative results consist of some form of statistical analysis, the interpretation of these findings is best undertaken in a separate discussion chapter. Whatever the nature of the project, the aim is to draw together the findings of the study and discuss these in light of what the project set out to achieve and in the context of previous studies. This involves more thinking than any other part of the process.

Any interpretation should be couched in tentative terms as the implications derived from the study are often speculative.[3] For example, the results of a project into 'Ascertaining the effectiveness of lead shielding to the thyroid gland during computed tomography of the head' may suggest that although risks are difficult to quantify for different scanning protocols, it would be beneficial to shield the thyroid gland because any radiation may be detrimental to health.[20]

In addition you should consider:

- whether the research question has been fully answered
- acceptance or rejection of the hypothesis
- any weaknesses or limitations in the project such as design constraints, sampling limitations, data analysis problems, etc.
- how problems encountered were overcome
- other approaches that might have been more appropriate with the benefit of hindsight.

Thus, this chapter should include an analytical interpretation of findings, a critical reflection of the process and to what extent your work has contributed to knowledge.

## Chapter 6: Conclusions

This chapter should be to the point and state clearly and succinctly what you have found. The conclusions should follow fairly obviously from the discussion, correspond to the original objectives, with no new material being introduced. However, only conclusions based on the findings should be made and you should avoid the temptation to drop in an opinion for which no evidence has been presented.

## Chapter 7: Recommendations

This chapter may not always be appropriate or may be included in the conclusions. Main recommendations include ways in which the findings of your project might improve practice or provide a stepping-stone for further research.

## References

This is a list of sources (books, journals, websites, documents, etc.) that you have referred to in the text of the dissertation. The list should be compiled exactly in accordance with the referencing system requirements of the institution (usually either the Harvard or Vancouver system). The Harvard system requires the references to appear in alphabetical order, whereas with the Vancouver system the references should be numbered and listed in the order in which they appear in the text.

## Bibliography

This is not an essential item, but may be a list of published work that you have consulted but not used in the text.

## Appendices

Again, this is not an essential component and should be kept to a minimum. You should include, for example, a copy of a questionnaire, interview schedule or data collection sheet used and copies of letters granting ethical approval for your project. Certainly you should not include numerous copies of journal articles or downloaded internet pages.

# Presentation

In addition to the general structure of a dissertation, the style of writing and presentation of material is important. Having spent so much time designing your project, reviewing literature and collecting data, it would seem illogical not to take care over the presentation of your dissertation. Therefore, your dissertation should be well organized and carefully presented, and you should adhere to the usual conventions which, although they may seem rather pedantic, are useful because they provide a standard form of presentation.

It is a piece of work you should be proud of, and one which will be of use to future students who want to inform themselves about the topic you have researched.

Remember, your dissertation is not an essay but a factual account of how and why a topic area was studied and what results were obtained.[3] It is essential to write simply and clearly, as the objective is to communicate your ideas and not to bury them in complex sentence construction or unnecessary jargon.

An excellent presentation makes the most of a good project and although the dissertation is judged largely on its academic content, some marks will also be given for good presentation. While each educational institution will have its own presentation requirements (so make sure you check details of specific requirements), the following points need to be considered if you are going to make your dissertation attractive to look at, easy to read and logical to follow.

## Box 17.2

**Example of 'house style'**

Chapter 3: Methodology

3.1. Introduction
3.2. Research Design
    *3.2.1. Research instruments*
    *3.2.2. Ethical considerations*

# Writing style

It is imperative that from the outset you develop a consistent 'house style' where your chapter and section headings all have the same numbering system, font type and size. Normally three levels of headings/section headings are sufficient, as shown in Box 17.2. Make sure that sentences are well punctuated and not over-long, paragraphs adequately developed and linking words or phrases used to guide the reader through the text.

Issues of correct spelling, punctuation and grammar are crucial if your final dissertation is going to be taken seriously. You have invested a lot of time and effort in the project and it is a pity that the impression or message resulting from your work may be diminished or lost because of poor attention to these details. Therefore, use a spell/grammar checker and make sure the meaning is clear and the language comprehensible. Paragraphs are best presented as fully justified (i.e. the left and right of each line of text line up) and make sure that contradictions, illogicalities and irrelevancies are avoided.

Take time to ensure silly mistakes are not made, for example paragraphs included twice, images indistinct, graphs poorly labelled, etc. and that everything is as neat and logical as possible. Where viable, all illustrations should be created using appropriate software tools, as hand-drawn images detract from the overall appearance of the dissertation.

Avoid the use of the first person singular, such as 'I developed a questionnaire', and write in the third person as 'a questionnaire was developed'. You should also write in the past tense, as ultimately your dissertation will be read as something that is completed and not as something that will be done. Thus, for example, you should write that 'the data were analysed using inferential statistics' rather than 'the data will be analysed using inferential statistics'.

It is usually a part of any university's equal opportunities policy to discourage the unnecessary use of gender related language. To overcome this problem it is easier to use the plural, e.g. 'practitioners should always ...', but if you need to use the singular try words like the patient, the student, the individual, the practitioner, etc.

Provide signposting by outlining the structure of the dissertation at the end of Chapter 1 and refer in the text to relevant points dealt with in other chapters/sections of the dissertation. It is a good idea to get into the habit of writing a brief summary at the end of each chapter (reflecting back on key issues) and a brief introduction at the beginning of each chapter (giving a flavour of what is to come).

All this is most easily achieved by making sure you write drafts of chapters well in advance of the hand-in deadline, read them through yourself, get others to read through your text and make appropriate revisions. Rigorous proofreading of your dissertation will allow it to be well crafted for its final version.

# Referencing

Referencing is an essential academic requirement as it demonstrates that extensive reading has taken place and that you properly acknowledge the work of others. Little or no referencing indicates insufficient reading to support the project or that you have copied ideas, data or facts from the source material. If you use text that is unreferenced (and generally work that is not your own is easy to spot), you may at worst be accused of plagiarism or at best poor academic practice. You should take particular care to make the references full and accurate, including the editors and publishers of books and volume numbers of journals in which articles appear. The Harvard system is often used in the social sciences and the Vancouver system in science and medicine.

The standard format for a journal article in the reference list is:

- Author, Initials. (year). Title of article. Title of journal, Volume number – if there is one (Issue number), start and end page numbers of article.
- *Example*: Law, RL, Slack, NF and Harvey, RF. (2008). An evaluation of a radiographer-led barium enema service in the diagnosis of colorectal cancer. *Radiography*, 14 (2), 105–110.

The standard format for a book in the reference list is:

- Author Initials (year). Title of book. Edition. Place of publication: Publisher.
- *Example*: Gunn C (2007). *Bones and Joints: a guide for students*. 5th Edition. Edinburgh: Churchill Livingstone.

For quotations in the text, an example of the same quotation, cited in the two different formats, is shown below.

Harvard system:

- 'A practitioner reporting sensitivity to colorectal cancer of 98% has been demonstrated' (Law, Slack and Harvey, 2008, p.109).
- Law, Slack and Harvey (2008) found that 'a practitioner reporting sensitivity to colorectal cancer of 98% has been demonstrated' (p.109).

Vancouver system:

- 'A 'practitioner reporting sensitivity to colorectal cancer of 98% has been demonstrated'.[21]
- It has been found that 'a practitioner reporting sensitivity to colorectal cancer of 98% has been demonstrated'.[21]

If the quotation is more than about 25 words, you should reduce the font size, indent and omit the quotation marks, as for example:

Harvard system:

> A practitioner reporting sensitivity to colorectal cancer of 98% has been demonstrated. The sensitivity achieved is probably as high as can reasonably be expected of any test, including more expensive techniques such as CT colonoscopy.
>
> (Law, Slack and Harvey, 2008, p.109).

Vancouver system:

> A practitioner reporting sensitivity to colorectal cancer of 98% has been demonstrated. The sensitivity achieved is probably as high as can reasonably be expected of any test, including more expensive techniques such as CT colonoscopy.[21]

However, there are many variations on these two themes, and details of how each system is actually adopted for use with a variety of material including books, journals, chapters in an edited book, internet websites, electronic material, student dissertations, newspapers, etc. should be checked with your educational institution.

Remember that presenting someone else's words, ideas or images as your own, without referencing them, is plagiarism. Therefore, if you incorporate material which is not your own without any adequate attempt to give appropriate credit, or you incorporate material as if it were your own when in fact it is wholly or substantially the work of another person, this is essentially cheating.

## Length

Make sure that you know the lower and upper word limits acceptable for your dissertation. The written project word limit typically excludes title page, abstract, list of contents, list of accompanying material, acknowledgements, glossary, references, bibliography and appendices.

Usually a word limit will be imposed, e.g. 10 000 words (+/− 10%), as it is believed that at this level the topic can be covered in sufficient depth and breadth in about 10 000 words providing it is well focused and structured. Thus, for example, if you write less than 9000 words, it is likely that you will not have dealt with the subject in sufficient depth or detail. Alternatively, if you find yourself writing significantly more than 11 000 words, it is possible that you have not sufficiently focused your ideas. While you may not be penalized for going under the stipulated word count (as it may be deemed that you have penalized yourself), going significantly over the word count (i.e. more than 10% in this case) may mean that penalties will be imposed. Diagrams, graphs, tables, etc. normally count as the word equivalence of the space they occupy.

## Pagination, margins and spacing

Number your pages consecutively throughout the dissertation, and locate them centrally at the bottom of the page, approximately 10 mm above the edge. Margins at the left hand edge should not be less than 40 mm (to allow for binding) and other margins not less than 20 mm. Double or 1.5 line spacing should be used for all text, although indented quotations should have single line spacing.

## Fonts

Arial and Times New Roman are the most common font styles as they are easy to read (avoid overelaborate font styles). Font size should be about 11, although the size of chapter headings may be larger and bold, while subsections may be italicized or underlined. Since you will be building up an argument, ensure you break up the text so that key issues can be readily identified by the reader. The important point is that once you have chosen the font style you should apply it consistently throughout the dissertation.

## Binding

You should use A4 size paper of good quality and of sufficient opacity for normal reading. Type or print on one side only and the dissertation should be professionally bound using either loose-leaf spiral binding or hard covers.

## References

[1] Glatthorn AA, Joyner RL. Writing the Winning Thesis or Dissertation: A Step-by-step Guide. 2nd ed. Newbury Park CA: Corwin Press; 2005.

[2] Levin P. Excellent Dissertations (Student-Friendly Guide Series). Maidenhead: Oxford University Press; 2005.

[3] Polit DF, Hungler BP. Nursing Research: Principles and Methods. 6th ed. Philadelphia: Lippincott, Williams and Wilkins; 2002.

[4] Bell J. Doing Your Research Project. 4th ed. Buckingham: Open University Press; 2005.

[5] Bogdan RC, Biklen SK. Qualitative Research for Education: An Introduction to Theories and Methods. 5th ed. New York: Pearson Education; 2006.

[6] Denscombe M. The Good Research Guide: For Small-scale Social Research Projects. 2nd ed. Buckingham: Open University Press; 2003.

[7] Edwards A, Talbot R. The Hard-pressed Researcher: A Research Handbook for the Caring Professions. 2nd ed. London: Prentice Hall; 1999.

[8] National Patient Safety Agency. National Research Ethics Service, Available at: http://www.nres.npsa.nhs.uk; (accessed 13 June 2008).

[9] Finney C. Women's attitudes to undergoing the 11–14 week ultrasound scan with nuchal translucency screening where the risk of the fetus having Down syndrome is calculated. Unpublished BSc (Hons) project, University of Portsmouth; 2008.

[10] Kember S. Is simulator verification necessary for pelvis patients? Unpublished BSc (Hons) project, University of Portsmouth; 2007.

[11] Lommerse P. A review of literature looking at the role of intensity modulated radiotherapy (IMRT) in the treatment of localised prostate cancer. Unpublished BSc (Hons) project, University of Portsmouth; 2008.

[12] Gunn C. Bones and Joints: A Guide for Students. 5th ed. Edinburgh: Elsevier Churchill Livingstone; 2007.

[13] Bushong SC. Radiologic Science for Technologists: Physics, Biology and Protection. 8th ed. St Louis: Elsevier Mosby; 2004.

[14] Renton P. Medical Imaging. Edinburgh: Elsevier Churchill Livingstone; 2004.

[15] Hawkes DJA. A comparative analysis of magnetic resonance imaging and computed tomography in the diagnosis of acute stroke.

Unpublished BSc. (Hons) project, University of Portsmouth; 2008.

[16] Public Health Resource Unit, England. Critical Appraisal Skills Programme (CASP). Available at: http://www.phru.nhs.uk/ Doc_Links/S.Reviews% 20Appraisal%20Tool.pdf (accessed 11 June 2008).

[17] Thomas G, Smoot G. Critical thinking: a vital work skill. Trust for Educational Leadership 1994;23:34–8.

[18] Mercieca L. Magnetic resonance imaging of the lumbar spine: knee flexion vs extension in patients with intervertebral disc herniation. Unpublished BSc (Hons) project 2008, University of Malta; 2008.

[19] Sparrow L. A research project investigating breast and prostate cancer awareness of the UK public. BSc (Hons) project, University of Portsmouth; 2008.

[20] Williams L, Adams C. Computed tomography of the head: an experimental study to investigate the effectiveness of lead shielding during three scanning protocols. Radiography 2006;12(2):143–52.

[21] Law RL, Slack NF, Harvey RF. An evaluation of a radiographer-led barium enema service in the diagnosis of colorectal cancer. Radiography 2008;14(2):105–10.

# Writing for publication and presenting at conferences

# 18

Richard Price

## CHAPTER POINTS

- Ensure that you consider the publication requirements of the journal you wish to write for.
- Prepare writing in manageable chunks.
- Read and reread your work. It is good practice to have another person read through your work as well.
- Prior preparation is key in successful presentations at conferences

This chapter will provide insight into preparing your work for publishing as well as preparing for conference presentations

## Introduction

The amount of research being undertaken by radiographers is increasing, which is not surprising given the age in which we live. In an age of rapidly developing technology which impacts on practice, the evidence base has to be continually revaluated if the best outcomes and service improvements are to be achieved. The duty of practitioners undertaking research is to communicate their findings to peers and beyond so that the best practices or important research data are shared for the common good.

The two most common methods of dissemination are via journal articles and conference presentations. Unless you are writing a feature for a magazine it is recommended that you submit your article to a journal that operates a peer review process. This is not to discourage anyone from writing a feature for a magazine, but if have undertaken research then it is in your interest to allow your work to be reviewed by peers.

Peer review is the process used to screen and select submitted articles for publication. Articles are 'refereed' by experts in the same field who offer advice to editors and authors on the standard of the work submitted. Peer review is not foolproof as there are instances where fraudulent research has beaten the system, but nevertheless the intention is that it should provide a robust scrutiny. Publications that have not been through peer review are likely to be regarded with some suspicion.

Writing an article for submission to a peer reviewed journal or proffering a paper to a conference of peers can seem daunting at the outset but very satisfying once the article has been published or the presentation has been given and the presenter is acknowledged with a round of applause. To maximize the likelihood of your work being accepted there are a number of points to take on board at the outset. It will become apparent that there is a lot more to getting an article published than just sitting down to write and as a potential author this is something you need to appreciate.

This chapter considers, firstly, the process of preparing an article for publication and secondly, a conference presentation.

## Writing for publication

Writing for publication may be a new venture for a health professional but the act of writing itself will not be. As a student you will surely have written essays or perhaps a dissertation. What you will have realized is that writing for a purpose is a disciplined activity and this is the same for an article which will be subjected to peer review.

Although this section will focus on preparing an article for submission to a peer reviewed journal there are other types of writing. For a practitioner this could include writing a book chapter, a technical report, or a feature in a professional magazine, but there is something that links all forms of writing – the need to communicate your ideas clearly and coherently to the readership. Authors will want readers to maintain their interest throughout the piece of work. Think of reading a novel and ask yourself, what do you want from it? You may say, I want to be introduced to the plot, the characters, the context and setting and be able to follow the story through to its conclusion. This, in principle, is no different from writing an article. You will have sections to explain the background, why and how the research was done, the consequences and implications, conclusions and recommendations. However, a scholarly article will normally be written in a more formal style while a novel or magazine feature is likely to be freer and less constrained in approach.

## Preparing the article

Before you put pen to paper or fingers to keyboard, be sure that you target a publication which is relevant to your area of work; refer to the 'instructions to authors' as these set out the journal's 'house' style. They will help you clarify your approach to presenting and formatting your article. The danger is if you do not present your work in the format required, at the very least you can expect to be asked to revise your article. Also do not expect that your article will be published immediately following submission. It could take several months before publication; the peer review process itself takes time to run its full course and will take longer if revisions are required. In the worst case your article may be rejected; it may be deemed unsuitable for publication in that particular journal or it is just flawed and not of the required standard. Even once an article has been accepted the editor will have to select the edition in which the article appears; this will be influenced by the frequency of publication and the number of other articles awaiting publication. It is fairly common practice for articles once accepted to be published electronically prior to appearing in a bound paper volume. Some journals now are only published electronically but many authors prefer to see their article appear as a hard copy; this may well be a matter for consideration when selecting a journal.

## Getting to grips with writing

Writing with confidence is something which all authors will aspire to, but do not worry too much about this as confidence will develop in time. Your first publication will certainly do wonders in this respect; it is that first step that is all important. There are steps that you can take to ensure your submission is both well written and well presented. The best approach in getting over your message is saying it simply. Write clear sentences with one thought; build paragraphs with a number of associated thoughts; make effective use of punctuation and match the style of writing to the readership. The latter you can determine by looking at back copies of your selected journal and turning to the instructions to authors.

There are some practical tips which are helpful:

- A common factor in any profession is the technical language or jargon that inevitably develops. While this may be alright in conversation with those by whom the terms are well understood that may not be the case with the written word. The best approach is to avoid jargon but if you do need to use it make sure you have explained its meaning.
- Abbreviations and acronyms can be used for terms that are repeated but make sure that the first time an acronym is used it is written in full with the abbreviation or acronym in parentheses, for example computed tomography (CT); source to skin distance (SSD).
- For some reason there is often a tendency to use upper case to begin common nouns e.g. 'The Radiographers and Radiologists both use Ultrasound in this Department'. This is incorrect and there is no justification for it. The words 'radiographers', 'radiologists', 'ultrasound' and 'department' are not proper nouns and must not be treated as such.
- Do not start a sentence with a number; for example, '12 respondents said yes' should be written as 'Twelve respondents said yes'.
- Avoid using shortened forms such as 'didn't' for 'did not'.
- Good English is very important in writing technical or scientific articles and the use of a spell check and someone to proofread your article before submission is advisable. The easier it is for the reviewer the easier it will be for you.
- Keep a clear focus on what you are writing, pay attention to detail, structure your sentences

carefully, do not raise questions which you do not address, do not jump from idea to idea and do not make assumptions.

- Selecting a title is important; it needs to capture what your article is about and be interesting enough to attract the attention of the reader. Take your time in deciding the title. A good approach is to have a working title which you can mull over while you are preparing your article.
- Bear in mind that you want to maintain the interest of your readers. Keep the article's purpose to the forefront of your mind, be clear on what you are trying to communicate, digress at your peril. The journal's instructions to authors will help authors maintain focus and will give guidance on the overall word length.

The journal will invariably require you to provide your work in a prescribed structure, e.g. an abstract, introduction, methodology, results, a discussion followed by conclusions, recommendations and references. Each of these will now be considered.

## Abstract

Although the abstract is likely to be read first it is the last section to write. It should summarize the article – i.e. what the objectives of the study were, how the study was undertaken, what results were obtained and their significance. It must make an impact because if it does not capture a reader's interest then the full article may not be read.

## Introduction

The introduction should explain the background to your study and provide the opportunity to discuss the results and conclusions of previously published work. The introduction has to include your aims and objectives plus any hypothesis.

## Methodology

This will provide all the details of your method including a description of statistical tests you may have used. It is essential that that what you did is explained clearly so there is no ambiguity. Ensure that your methodology can be duplicated by another researcher.

You must provide confirmation that the research complies with ethical principles and approval has been granted by an appropriate ethics committee if necessary.

## Results

There is no need to make any comment or interpret results in this section. You will have to decide what information to include but it is not advisable, nor is there any need, to present raw data. The approach should be to summarize data with text, tables or figures. Good advice is to only use a figure (e.g. graph) when the data lend themselves to a good visual representation. Also avoid using figures that show too many variables or trends at once, because they can be hard to understand.

## Discussion

This is where you have the opportunity to explain what the results mean or why they differ from what other studies have found. If necessary, note problems with the methodology and explain any anomalies in the data. You should interpret your results in the light of other published results, by adding additional information from sources you cited in the introductory section. Relate your discussion back to the aims and objectives and questions you raised in the introductory section but do not simply restate the objectives and do not introduce new material or facts. Avoid making statements that are too broad or general in nature which your results do not support.

## Conclusions/recommendations

The conclusion serves two purposes, one is to summarize the main points of your article and the other, to draw out your conclusions. Any recommendations should be set out along with future directions for ongoing research.

## Reference list

The reference list is extremely important for a number of reasons. It demonstrates that you have read around the topic, which can strengthen your work; it acknowledges the work of other authors, thus avoiding questions of plagiarism; and readers may wish to access the articles themselves. Make sure you provide accurate references for the publications cited. It is worth noting that although you may have looked at a number of articles and books as background reading, if you did not cite them do not list them in your reference list. There is no need to produce a full bibliography for an article, only the reference list.

How references are listed will depend upon the journal style. Medical publications tend to use a numerical or Vancouver system where citations are identified by a number in the text, usually in superscript. The citations are then listed numerically in the order they appeared in the text. An advantage of this system is that a number of references to the same article use the same number. Alternatively, a journal may use a Harvard style citation which cites author(s) and date in the text and lists them alphabetically. Education and social science journals tend to use the author date style. A numerical system can be tricky to manage where there are multiple references but with software programmes available for managing this aspect the task should not be difficult.

Examples of referencing articles using the Vancouver and Harvard systems are as follows:

1. Price RC, Le Masurier, SB. Longitudinal changes in extended roles in radiography: A new perspective. *Radiography* 2007: **13**, (1) 18–29

   Price RC, Le Masurier, SB. (2007) Longitudinal changes in extended roles in radiography: A new perspective. *Radiography* **13**, (1) 18–29

Within each system there are different conventions for referencing books, conference papers, correspondence, websites, etc. and you should refer to the journal's instructions to authors for detailed guidance. However, from the author's perspective there is no choice – you have to comply with the journal's style or you will be asked to revise your article.

## Submission

Before you submit make sure that your article has been spell-checked. It is advisable to ask a colleague to read the article; it is so easy to overlook a typo. What may seem complete sense to you may not be to another person.

Most journals have an electronic submission system and the instructions will tell you how to register as an author and how to submit. It is a fairly straightforward process. Typically the information required will include the name of the author designated as the corresponding author (if there are joint authors), e-mail address, full postal address, and telephone and fax numbers. You will also be asked to give four or five keywords for search purposes and sometimes a classification code, for example what type of article you are submitting, original research, review or case study. Make sure you submit any prints, tables and figures in the format requested, including instructions for colour reproduction, and if you are using any copyrighted material such as photographs or research tools make sure you have the owner's permission to do so.

Once your article has been submitted, peer reviewers will be invited to review it; the review process will take a number of weeks. Reviewers will report to the editor and make recommendations. There are three possible outcomes: rejection, major or minor revision or acceptance outright. A rejection means that the article may not be suitable for the journal but a matter you should have addressed before submission. Unfortunately, the article may be unsuitable because it is flawed, such as inconsistencies in your method, ethical issues not considered or conclusion not supported by your results. If you are asked to make a major revision then the article will be returned for you to make the necessary amendments. Once the amendments have been completed you will resubmit and your article will be sent once again to the reviewers and the process repeated until the article is suitable for publication. In the case of a minor revision you will be requested to make these and resubmit but the article may not be sent to reviewers a second time. If your article is accepted outright then that is a marvellous achievement and you can look forward to seeing the fruits of your labour in print.

## Presenting at a conference

There are usually two main options of presenting your work at a conference: in an oral presentation or by a poster. This section will consider the former.

You may be fortunate to attend a conference as an invited speaker. In this instance your work and reputation will have already made an impression. This being the case then it is unlikely your presentation will be peer reviewed; your work is accepted on trust, as you are already viewed as an expert. However, an invited speaker will be required to submit an abstract as the organizer will want to publish it in the pre-conference material. A conference theme or themes may be built around invited keynote speakers. Proffered papers will then follow on the same theme. Proffering a paper is a competitive process; an abstract will be subject to peer review and a decision taken on whether the work is suitable for presentation.

Preparing the abstract is the critical phase as if you fail to make an impression on the organizer you will not be required to present. As with submitting an article for publication, there are various phases to go through and 'rules' to observe which you must follow.

The first step is to identify the conference at which you believe it is most appropriate for you to present your work. The timings of major national and international conferences are well known in advance and dates for proffering papers are promoted widely. Most major conferences have a dedicated website which provides advanced programme information, themes and details for proffering papers including the submission date. For other conferences you will need to keep watch for advance notices in professional and other media outlets.

Once you have decided you want to proffer a paper there are four main phases: preparing an abstract, abstract submission, preparing the presentation, and finally the presentation itself.

## Preparing your abstract

As with the written article, the purpose of your presentation is to communicate ideas and research findings to a live conference audience. However, before you are in a position to do that, you have to convince a panel that your presentation is relevant to the conference theme and it is going to be of a good enough quality. You may have to achieve this in an abstract of as little as 100 words in some cases. Your abstract has to achieve maximum impact and with little room to manoeuvre it is imperative that your message is succinct but convincing enough to convey your ideas to the organizers.

The organizer should provide guidance on how to set out your abstract; for a scientific abstract, headings such as purpose, methodology, results and conclusion are appropriate. This is helpful as you do not have to worry about how to structure the abstract. If you are unsure on how to approach the abstract then it is worth looking at examples which can usually be found on some conference websites. Getting started can be the one of the hardest things.

Other abstracts may be based around a review, a case study or educational project. The headings and structure may differ but in essence you still have to make an impact. If there is no or little guidance, it is still preferable to have structured approach, as it will help keep focus and ensure you get your message over within the allowed word count.

If you are presenting research be clear about its purpose, provide brief details on the study and identify the problem to be resolved. Method can include how you carried out the work, where, when and with whom. Your results should be summarized, which

will lead directly to your conclusions, whether you solved the problem and consequently what your recommendations are. These will be the elements that the organizers will expect. You may wish to cite one or two key references which informed your research but this will depend upon how many words you are allowed. References should not be at the expense of getting your message over. Be careful if you cite yourself not to use the first person in the text as this will compromise your anonymity.

The writing style for the abstract should be disciplined as if preparing a research article for a peer reviewed journal.

## Submitting your abstract

Clearly, you must follow the rules for submission; do not exceed the word requirement and submit before the closing date or you may well be eliminated at the first hurdle. You can expect the organizer to be strict on this aspect. Late abstracts are unlikely to be considered, especially if there are more quality papers submitted than there are 'slots' available for presentation. If submission is online and the facility ceases to be available at the end on the given period, then there will be no way of making a late submission.

If the organizer requires the work to have a title make sure you provide one. If you are required to provide a number of key words associated with your presentation for promotional and abstracting purposes, make sure you supply them. Also ensure your contact details are given, especially your email address if this is the medium by which you will be contacted.

Online submission should be straightforward but unless you complete the required fields, submission will not be allowed. Once submitted it is usual to get an automatic email acknowledgement.

You should receive notification of the acceptance (or rejection) of your abstract in a timely fashion; if the organizers do not announce a notification date, you should contact them to find out when to expect a reply. If you do not receive notification by the specified date, follow it immediately. Your abstract may have fallen through the cracks, and it may not be too late for it to be reviewed.

## Preparing your presentation

Following acceptance it is time to work on your presentation. If it is a major conference you can expect detailed instructions about projection facilities, which you must keep safe. PowerPoint is used almost universally and most people who are contemplating presenting at a conference will have had some prior experience. If not, then using it for the first time at a conference will not be a good idea, so repeated practice beforehand, even if only to friends or colleagues, is a must.

In the earliest stage there are two elements to deal with: the first is what you are going to say and the second the number and content of your slides. There is normally an assumption that slides will be used and are important if you have results to display. Some of the most inspirational speakers get over their message without slides, but for a research presentation visual material is important. It is crucial that you have the correct balance between what you say and what you display. Too many slides will detract from the presentation, as will slides containing too much text.

You will know how much time you have for the presentation and there is no reason or excuse whatsoever for you to exceed your allocation. Remember others may have to follow and conference schedules run to tight deadlines.

The first step is to outline your key points. Your abstract will provide this and it is a good idea to structure your presentation around the headings used. So, if your abstract had headings purpose, method, results and conclusion you should plan your presentation around these – this is what the audience will expect. You will then need to allocate the time for each section. You may want to give more time to your results and the conclusion or if your methodology was particularly innovative or complex, then you may want allocate more time to that section. Do not allocate more time overall than you have been given. Once you have identified the key points you can start to think about the slides and make a first estimation of the number. As a guide, excluding the title slide, allow, on average, approximately 1 minute for each. Before you concentrate on the content of the slides good advice is to write out a draft of what you are going to say. On this occasion you do not have to write as you would for an academic paper. People do not normally speak in the manner in which an article is written and your oral presentation needs to be natural, lively and interesting. Remember you are not writing a paper for someone to read.

Once you have the essence of what you are going to say then start thinking about how the slides will enhance the message. Presentation of slides is important; if your institution has a corporate slide you should use it. Alternatively, you can use the slide master feature to create a template. If you do this, simplicity is a good rule to observe; you could use one of the already designed PowerPoint templates but some can be quite overbearing. Once you have your design template it is perfectly acceptable to vary the content format, for example a bulleted list, text only, graphic only, text and image are acceptable combinations. You need to be consistent with font type, size, colours and background. If your presentation is in a large auditorium slides may have to be seen from the back of the room as well as the front. A good contrast between background and text is essential; a dark text on a light background is preferable. Note that what looks good on a computer screen may appear less so when projected. Font sizes of 28 or 24 should be adequate for the main text although you may wish to use a larger font for titles. The font type and style will be the presenter's preference but *make it simple*, which will ease reading. The number of words on each slide should be limited to key phrases or headlines so you only include essential information. Punctuation should be limited, and do not put all words in upper case. Do not cram a slide full of text that no one will be able to read because there is not enough time or it is too small. There is nothing worse than a presenter saying: 'I am sorry but you will not be able to see that.' If a presenter knows that, why do it in the first place? Do not apologize for anything on your slides – if you have to do that you have not really thought about what you are doing.

If you are presenting data, think carefully what you want to show; there should be nothing too complicated or you may get bogged down; a graph is preferred to a table. Use a video clip if it will help you make a point but keep the time to a minimum.

Once you are happy with what you want to say and with the number and content of slides it is time to practise delivery. Practise on your own at first, making notes of any areas lacking continuity and noting the time taken. Practise speaking to the 'audience' and not to your slides, and the last thing you want to do is to read directly from them. If you have prepared a script, mark points where you should move slides forward. If you read from your script ensure you control the speed of delivery, including any pauses, and do not forget to look up at the audience from time to time. The more you know your script the more you can face the audience. (If you are provided with an autocue at the conference then delivery is easier and more natural.) If you know the conference will expect you to use a microphone try and practise with one beforehand.

Once you have sorted out any 'bugs' it is time to give your presentation to friends or colleagues. Ask them for constructive feedback on your delivery overall and specifically on voice projection, intonation, clarity of what you are saying and on the presentation and content of your slides. Listen to advice carefully and be prepared to make amendments.

Finally, it is as well to identify potential questions and think about how you are going to respond; your colleagues can help you with this aspect.

## Presenting your paper

By the time you arrive at the conference everything should be set. The organizer should be ready for you; your presentation will be rehearsed so what can go wrong? Well, you may like to take some precautions:

It is good to have means of a back-up presentation; at a large conference technical difficulties are less likely as technical help will be at hand.

It is worth checking to see which version of PowerPoint is recommended. Your presentation may be in the latest version but if the organizer's computer cannot handle it you have a problem. You can get around this by saving two versions, the second saved in an earlier version. Be aware that you may not be able to use all of the newer features in the older version but if you take your own laptop with you this can alleviate such problems. At smaller events you may wish to take transparencies and or handouts if the audience is not too large.

It will be your responsibility to ensure your presentation is loaded onto a computer prior to your presentation. Even if someone does this, double-check to make sure everything is okay. At a major conference there is likely to be a technician to help but at other events be prepared to set up yourself and taking a laptop as a back-up is advisable.

If you are part of a multi-speaker session, oral presentations will be allocated a strict time allowance and likely to be included will be an allowance for questions. This could take the form of a panel discussion involving all of the session speakers at the end of the session. This is preferable for overall time management. A weak chair could let questions run and run after one paper which puts unfair pressure on following speakers. All you can do is make sure that your presentation does not exceed the time allocation; it is discourteous and disrespectful to following speakers and can disrupt the schedule to do so.

It is likely that you will be anxious beforehand; this is natural. Try to relax and focus on the lessons you learned from your rehearsals. It is surprising that once you get started your nerves will probably disappear. Take a deep breath and focus on the delivery, do not talk too fast, move on your slides at the required point, keep to script and be natural. *You are in control*. It is surprising how quickly the time passes, and the round of applause will be a welcome sound.

What is the next step? What about converting your presentation into a formal article for a peer reviewed journal.

## And finally . . .

The achievements of seeing your work published in a peer reviewed journal or presenting at a conference are very rewarding. Both activities will be the result of hard work and commitment.

What at first may seem daunting exercises appear less so if tasks are broken down into more manageable parts. A structured and disciplined approach to writing has been considered which should assist authors in meeting their objectives. In particular, emphasis has been placed on submission processes both to a journal and to a conference. This means following a publisher's or conference organizer's instructions – these are ignored at the potential author's peril.

There is, of course, further reading you may find helpful and a selection is listed below. Happy writing!

## Further reading

Epstein D, Kenway J, Boden R. Writing for Publication. London: Sage Publications; 2005.

Kliewer MA. Writing it up: a step-by-step guide to publication for beginning investigators. Am J Roentgenol 2005;185(3):591.

Manning D, Hogg P. Writing for publication. Radiography 2006;12 (2):77–8.

Marshall G. Writing review articles. Radiography 2007;13(1):2–3.

# Applying for research funding

Gill Marshall    Leon Jonker

## CHAPTER POINTS

- Obtaining funds for research through a grant application is an essential activity to develop the evidence base of radiography practice. This will help promote radiography as an autonomous profession.

- A successful application is not written in a week or so; it takes up to a year to fully develop an idea and project plan.

- Apart from getting the science right, writing a grant proposal is a meticulous process. As mentioned in this chapter, there are common pitfalls associated with it. If these are avoided and the preparations for a grant proposal are done properly, then it will increase the chance of being successful in the selection process.

- Ensure you check all the items in Table 19.1. Having said that, with the current success rate of grant applications being 10–20%, it is much more likely that a grant application is rejected rather than accepted. If this happens, it is important to learn from the feedback.

- Most of the reasons for rejection can be addressed and worked on. For example, if there is criticism regarding the statistical aspects of the study then this can be reviewed. Even if the reviewers believe that the applicant does not have a strong enough track record, more senior peers can be contacted to propose collaborating.

Obtaining funds for conducting research is a challenge and the competition for grants and fellowships is fierce. Being able to write good quality grant proposals is an essential skill for a researcher in radiography since most high-quality research requires substantial funding. This chapter provides guidance for those interested in becoming involved in research and those already engaged in undertaking research. The research grant application process is covered in its entirety, from the initial idea to costing the project. An overview of common pitfalls to avoid is also given. The items covered here are generic and can therefore be applied to writing grant proposals for funding bodies in different countries. Ultimately, we anticipate that this overview will encourage people to apply for research funding and help to improve the chances of a successful application.

Research is an essential element of all professions and it is no different in radiography. Research facilitates the building of the profession's evidence base. As an emergent profession this is especially important in radiography because, for it to become an autonomous profession, practitioners must 'carve out a knowledge base that is dynamic and forward thinking'.[1] Furthermore, high impact studies in the field of radiography serve to raise the profile of the profession.[2]

Without exploring new ideas and development of novel treatments, techniques and applications, we would not have seen the amazing techniques in practice today, such as high resolution volumetric 3-D constructions and intensity-modulated radiotherapy. In the following sections of this chapter, the various tasks and activities that should take place in the several months it typically takes to get a good proposal together are laid out.

## From conception to grant proposal

The cornerstone of scientific research is having a novel idea or investigating an established area from a different perspective. Writing a grant proposal is

**Table 19.1 Checklist for grant applications (amended from[12])**

| Section of application | Item to check |
| --- | --- |
| Eligibility | • Check if you fit the requirements for eligibility<br>• Ensure the proposed study fits in with the funding body's priorities – especially when applying for a themed call for proposals<br>• Explain why the planned work is novel and necessary |
| Hypothesis and objective | • Check if the research has not already been done before; the need for the research should be justified<br>• Clearly define the hypothesis<br>• Place the proposed study in the context of the current knowledge on this topic |
| Methodology | • Explanation of the procedures involved for testing reliability and validity |
| Finances | • Justify the amount you are requesting<br>• Carefully calculate the total amount requested; double check all aspects of this, from number of hours for wages, to prices for equipment |
| Communication | • Public and patient involvement in preparation for the study and dissemination of the results is encouraged |
| Finishing touches | • Have you checked for grammar and spelling?<br>• Adhere to the guidelines: do not exceed the maximum number of words allowed<br>• Ask someone to proofread your application, particularly if some sections have to be intelligible for lay people |

an important piece of the jigsaw if you want to turn such ideas into practice. Research funding consists of grants, which are awarded in response to investigator-initiated projects, and contracts under which the research topic is proposed by the funding agency.[3] It may be necessary to submit the proposal to more than one agency in order to obtain sufficient funding to operate and support the infrastructure required for the research. There is much competition for research grants and so one cannot afford to make mistakes in a grant application, or the application is very likely to be rejected. Even so, many worthwhile projects will be rejected, particularly if the proposal is for qualitative research.[3,4] Only 10–20% of all grant proposals are generally accepted.[5] These guidelines apply for quantitative, qualitative and mixed methods proposals.[6] Applicants should choose topics that are of interest to them in order to maintain momentum. It is important to write a grant proposal that captures the uniqueness of your organization and shows the correct fit between your organization and the funding body.[7] Plenty of time should be allowed to minimize errors and optimize the quality of a grant proposal. Typically, up to 12 months will pass between generating the initial idea to the actual submission of a grant proposal. It is essential to document sufficient information to convince the

funders that the proposal is worth funding.[8] Bear in mind that grant writing should not be a lonely pursuit; there are many sources of help, for example books, videos, colleagues, consultants and the World Wide Web.[9] The writing is usually followed by an approximate 6 month wait for the outcome of the application. Although it can absorb a lot of the applicant's spare time, overall the development of a grant proposal should be enjoyable. It should also be seen as an opportunity for researchers to crystallize an idea and to critically appraise their research plans. This is an essential exercise, since it is likely to enhance the quality of the study. The scope of the proposed work can be evaluated and altered, and aspects including methodology and analysis can be thought through critically. At this stage potential follow-up studies will become apparent, which will effectively create continuity.

First and foremost, a propagated hypothesis should be tested against the current available data and knowledge in the area of interest using a comprehensive literature review. An additional simple yet effective method is to share your idea with colleagues and encourage constructive feedback. Typical questions to ask are: what am I trying to test/explain, what are the possible causes, what causes will I explore, and what are the possible mechanisms?[10]

This approach should be applied throughout the application process. At the literature review stage it will become clear whether an idea is simply a matter of building on current knowledge or if the idea goes against the grain of what others think. It is fair to say that a research grant of an evolutionary nature will stand a better chance than a plan involving a revolutionary hypothesis. However, a research proposal that promises very little in terms of added value will probably fail to impress. Advice on developing a research question and literature searching is given in Chapters 2 and 3.

Looking at current 'hot topics' in the field of radiography or researching themed calls for proposals will give an indication of what the experts in the field feel the priorities for research are. The Society and College of Radiographers in the UK recently published a list of research priority areas.[11] For diagnostic radiography this includes 'Sociological analysis of the profession of diagnostic radiography' and for therapeutic radiography, a focus area is 'Patient information'. If a project is tailored towards addressing these focus areas, it will further enhance the chances of success. Moreover, it also means a grant proposal will better fit the eligibility criteria.

## Added value of preliminary work and pilot data

The majority of, if not all organizations that fund research apply peer review for selecting the best grant applications. It is easier to convince reviewers of the merits of a proposed project if there is already some promising data accompanying the application. Obtaining preliminary or pilot data serves two purposes. Firstly, it will show that the hypothesis to be tested may be correct, or that the aims set can potentially be met. Secondly, by producing pilot data you can highlight to reviewers that you are capable of producing data. This indicates that, in addition, you can most likely handle larger, full-scale projects. It serves both as a teaser and a showcase piece. An important task is to explain the implications of the preliminary data to the aims of the proposed full project and to past work by peers in the field. One important thing to remember is that peer reviewers may have produced the data that your proposal is based on. Ignoring these people by not citing their articles and books may not go down well with them. A requirement of pilot data can lead to a 'Catch 22' situation if obtaining this data requires

funding. Sometimes, without financial backing no data can be generated, and without data, the chance of obtaining grant money is slim.

## Membership of the research team

To further increase the chance of being successful with a grant proposal, it is important to have the correct people on board. This certainly applies to less experienced researchers who wish to apply for funding. For professionals who want to become involved in research, or who want to start writing grants, it is best to join forces with scientists who have a track record in their chosen field. Having a senior co-author on an application will increase the faith reviewers have in your being able to deliver on what the grant proposal promises. Undoubtedly, a senior scientist will be able to give invaluable advice on how to write and develop a proposal. The temptation for junior researchers is often to try and do too much within the proposed time. A seasoned researcher will be able to evaluate if the planned work will fit in an allocated period, thereby avoiding a regular criticism by reviewers: a project being too ambitious.[12] Another sensible option is to link up with an established team of radiography researchers in a hospital, university or institute that provides good infrastructure and support.

While acknowledging the value of a more experienced peer, there are other people who can contribute to improving the quality of a study and therefore a grant proposal. Access to a statistician is imperative to decide the appropriate sample size for a study. This requirement applies for both qualitative and quantitative research, regardless of whether or not it involves human participation. Associated with this is the requirement to know the power of an experiment. For analysis of the generated data, it is also important to choose the correct type of statistical analysis.[13] It is even obligatory to obtain authorization from a statistician when applying for ethical approval at present, such is the importance of sound statistical appraisal of a project. An in-depth explanation of the application of statistical analysis in radiography studies is beyond the scope of this chapter but can be found in Chapter 15 of this book. If the proposed project observes a reduction in the length or number of treatments, or any other change that impacts on the costs involved in a service, there may be a requirement for the input of a health economist. Writing radiography grant proposals may be aided by consultation with a radiologist and/or physicist, depending on the precise nature of the bid. Co-investigators who complement your own background and training should be chosen.[14]

# Which grant and where to find it?

Once an idea has been thought through, the aims have been formalized, and possibly a team of people has been assembled, the next stage will be to identify a source of funding. Subsequently, we will cover the types of grants that are available and the different funding bodies that honour grants.

## Grant types

Grants come in different shapes and sizes, just like projects. Generally speaking, there are four different types of grants: research grants (money for one specific project), programme grants (large collaborative efforts that encompass a number of projects), studentships (to fund a research-based MSc or PhD degree) and fellowships (to fund career development). The latter two are awards made to a specific person. Naturally, variations on each type of grant exist. For example, certain grants promote collaboration between industry and the public sector and certain fellowships are intended specifically for, for example, clinicians. The type of grant for which one should apply depends entirely on the project and the applicant's circumstances. One area that the choice depends on is as follows: is the applicant employed as a radiography practitioner by a hospital or private organization, or by a university or other higher education institute? Employment status also impacts on what can be claimed in terms of salary.

For those wishing to establish themselves in research, career development grants are a good option. The grants are allocated to applicants who can demonstrate that they have the potential to become successful independent researchers; a track record is not an essential prerequisite. Apart from the need for a sound project proposal, other requirements have to be met to satisfy the reviewers. For the grant proposal, it must be evident that the candidate has a strong desire and commitment to work in research long term. The organization that the candidate works for also has to be committed to support and develop this person. It is therefore essential that

the infrastructure exists to provide that support, both through the presence of a mentor and adequate research facilities.[15] Even if the candidate shows promise and the research plan is of a high quality, his or her employer has to match this level of potential with sound back-up support.

## Funding bodies

There are several funding bodies that currently fund research for radiography and radiology. Although other countries also have charities and governmental research councils, for conciseness we will concentrate on the USA and UK only. In the UK, the Society and College of Radiographers offers research awards for smaller projects and it has an industry partnership scheme (see www.sor.org). This may be a good initial funding body for those researchers just starting out to apply to, since the funding is available specifically for professionals in the fields of radiography and radiotherapy. Larger grants are available from the National Institute for Health Research (NIHR) and from the more generic research councils, such as the Medical Research Council (MRC) and the Wellcome Trust. Depending on the topic of a project, other, more specific, organizations may be approached. For example, if a project looks into aspects of mammography then a charity such as Cancer Research UK may be an appropriate funding body to apply to. In the USA, the Radiological Society of North America provides support for professionals in radiography and radiotherapy (www.rsna.org). The main financial backer of research in the US is the National Institute of Health (NIH); they have a plethora of different grants available. For all funding bodies, the types of grants offered, and themed calls for proposals, are subject to change. Therefore, it warrants checking the websites for grant news on a regular basis. One website incorporates the calls for proposals and deadlines for applications: www.RDinfo.org.uk. It is a one-stop shop for virtually all there is to know about funding opportunities.

Once the decision has been made to apply for funding from a certain funding body it is useful to get in touch with this organization. People are employed by the funding bodies to provide guidance and information to (prospective) applicants. If in doubt about anything, or even when not in doubt, make sure to double-check your own eligibility or the appropriateness of your project with the programme or organization's administrator. There is nothing worse than going through the whole application process and finding out that the application cannot be considered. Different funding bodies use different software and formats for applications, which means that an application can often not simply be cut and pasted to fit another call for proposals.

# Writing a good grant application

A good grant application uses most of the elements discussed earlier in this book. It requires an understanding of what research is (Chapter 1), how to formulate a research question (Chapter 2), extensive literature evaluation (Chapter 4) and certainly appreciation of the ethical implications of the proposed research (Chapter 6). In addition, a research project should apply the most fitting methodology available. Data should be recorded and analysed by applying an appropriate statistical test if it is quantitative data, whereas qualitative data is usually analysed via themed analysis or quasi-statistics. These areas are covered in Chapters 15 and 16.

What we would like to stress is that writing a grant is time-consuming. Below, the main tasks and activities involved in developing an application are summarized from start to submission:

- Conceptualize the project and review the literature.
- If applicable, approach patients or the public about their involvement.
- Start work on, or collect, any pilot data (ensure compliance with governance and ethics).
- Identify potential collaborators or mentors.
- Further define the research question and methodology/analysis tools.
- Decide on the type of grant and funding body, contact the programme officer and review application forms and instructions.
- Outline and draft the proposal.
- If required, consult experts in statistics or other disciplines.
- Develop and finalize the budget.
- Review and draft second version of proposal.
- Critical appraisal by research team members, collaborators and lay persons.
- Final revisions and submission of grant application.

# Administrative elements of a grant application

A full research proposal is typically several pages long. Try to make life easy for the reviewer by strategically restating the key questions that the project will attempt to address. For a reviewer, who reviews numerous proposals in the space of days and who is not necessarily a specialist in your field, it is helpful to be gently reminded by the applicant how the proposal fulfils the key points in the proposed research. Likewise, each section of an application may benefit from a summary containing the key points. One also must be aware that, to a certain degree, when constructing a grant application, the candidate has to sell him- or herself to the reviewers and funding body. For applicants there is no harm in highlighting the fact that they have worked on a similar project in the past or attended a specialist course relevant to the proposed research project. The reviewer will most probably not know anything about the applicant's background; therefore, the reviewer has to be informed about any skills that may make the applicant qualified to deliver on the promised work.

Although it sounds obvious, the key is to adhere to the guidelines for submission. If the abstract can only be 200 words long, do not overstretch to 250 words because the application will be rejected. Stick to the instructions all the way through the grant application – from budget to bibliography. Following on, it is not compulsory to write to the nearest maximum word count – the grant application needs to be concise, clear and complete.[16]

Undertaking independent research with funding from a charity or research council also means getting to grips with calculating the costs of a project. Depending on the size and length of the project, this part of a grant proposal can vary from being manageable to requiring a specialist to do the sums. When writing a first grant it is vital to ask someone with previous experience to look at the finances. There are different costs incurred when carrying out a project and these costs need to be categorized. Directly incurred costs are the salaries for the people stated on the grant application, i.e. the people work specifically on the project and are therefore paid directly from the grant. Consumables purchased specifically for the project also fall under this category. Directly allocated costs are those costs inherent to conducting research in a department or an institute. These are, for example, charges for radiographic staff and overheads for research infrastructure such as the use of X-ray room time. Finally, there are indirect costs, which include costs for general back-up support staff such as library, human resources and finance staff.

There are certain things to bear in mind when preparing a budget for a grant proposal. Wages are calculated with inclusion of the on-costs the employer incurs – this means that pension and national insurance costs should be added to the gross wages. If a project runs for more than 1 year, one has to incorporate salary increases based on inflation or previous annual increments. For equipment and consumables costs it is important to find out if these figures should include (value added) tax or not. Ask for quotes from different companies when an expensive item is listed in the grant application to get an idea of the costs involved. It has to be noted that some grants do not allow asking for capital expenditure like equipment or machines. Finally, other costs associated with a research project must be considered. There are travel and registration costs associated with presenting research outcomes at a conference, and publishing a manuscript in a peer-reviewed journal. While on submission there is no charge for submission of the paper, it has usually incurred costs in its preparation. As with equipment, it is best to identify beforehand what conference the project will most likely be presented at; in this way, costs can be calculated more precisely. Sharing the outcomes of the project at conferences and in articles helps to gain a reputation based on the work carried out. Chapter 18 covers the processes involved in optimizing dissemination of data.

## Common shortcomings of grant applications

Grant applications can be rejected for various reasons. On the one hand, an application can be turned down because the candidate does not have a strong enough track record or the university, hospital or organization that the applicant works for is not renowned for hosting research. If this is the case, it will be fairly tricky for someone to turn this around in the space of a few months and re-submit an application. More common are content-related errors that make a reviewer decide to turn down a request for funding. In the past, funding bodies have been approached about why some grant applications are funded and others are not.[12,17] In their response

**Table 19.2 Common mistakes in grant applications**

| Percentage of grant applications in which the named issue was present[17] | |
| --- | --- |
| Study design issues, such as unclear design or too many measurements | 76% |
| Statistical issues including inadequate power calculations | 34% |
| General issues, e.g. issues with originality where it appears to be mentor's idea and not applicant's idea | 29% |
| Hypothesis problems, such as undefined aims or lack of novelty | 24% |
| Significance of the study and how it impacts on current knowledge | 18% |

it transpired that certain omissions, mistakes and deficits are more common than others. The major review issues, related to a National Kidney Foundation call for proposals, included those listed in Table 19.2.

More and more funding bodies demand input from patients or lay people in the design and dissemination of research project. User involvement during the development of a research bid can often have a positive effect on the design of a study.[18] Particularly in qualitative research involving patient questionnaires, lay people can highlight the use of too much jargon, acronyms and/or abbreviations. Similarly, discussions with patients may shed light on important ethical issues, such as how and when to approach patients for participation in a study. If we consider the research focus areas identified by the Society and College of Radiographers, it can be concluded that most topics could benefit from user involvement. As with the generation of pilot data for a research grant application, much user involvement work is unpaid.

What is important is to address any issues, not to try your luck with another funding body. This is especially so when dealing with niche subjects including radiography and radiology where there is a significant chance that the same reviewer may be approached again. If the perseverance and the efforts do pay off then this should certainly be celebrated. Obtaining a research grant is a prestigious feat and together with a positive outcome of the actual project work should lead to more successful grant applications and worthwhile collaborations.

# References

[1] Manning D, Hogg P. Writing for publication. Radiography 2006;2:77–8.

[2] Chung K, Shauver M. Fundamental principles of writing a successful grant proposal. J Hand Surg 2008;333(4):566–72.

[3] Woodward D, Clifton G. Developing a successful research grant application. Am J Hosp Pharm 1994;51(6):813–22.

[4] Carey M, Swanson J. Funding for qualitative research. Qual Health Res 2003;13(6):852–6.

[5] Frels L. Writing the grant proposal. AANA J 1993;61:32–5.

[6] Singh MD, Cameron C, Duff D. Writing proposals for research funds. Axone 2005;26(3):26–30.

[7] Sayer B. Writing organisation and funder profiles for a grant proposal. Nurse Author Ed 1999;9(2):7–9.

[8] McIntyre E, Reed RL, Kalucy E. Expressions of interest: writing for success. Aust Fam Physician 2006;35(4):255–6.

[9] Reif-Lehrer L. Applying for grant funds: there's help around the corner. Trends Cell Biol 2000;10:500–3.

[10] Gambling T, Brown P, Hogg P. This is not the end, nor is it the beginning—but it is the end of the beginning—getting to grips with the research process. Radiography 2003;9:161–7.

[11] SCoR. http://www.sor.org/public/pdf/research/research_priorities.pdf; 2007 (accessed 9 March 2009).

[12] Inouye SK, Fiellin DA. An evidence-based guide to writing grant proposals for clinical research. Ann Intern Med 2005;142:274–82.

[13] Ettarh R. Common descriptive and analytical statistics in investigative studies. Radiography 2004;10:299–302.

[14] Romm F. Practical grantsmanship: the application process in health care research. Fam Med 1991;23 (5):382–6.

[15] Gill TM, McDermott MM, Ibrahim SA, et al. Getting funded. J Gen Intern Med 2004;19:472–8.

[16] Bourne PE, Chapula LM. Ten simple rules for getting grants. PLOS Comput Biol 2006;2:e12.

[17] Agarwal R, Chertow GM, Mehta RL. Strategies for successful patient oriented research: why did I (not) get funded? Clin J Am Soc Nephrol 2006;1:340–3.

[18] Staniszewska S, Jones N, Newburn M, et al. User involvement in the development of a research bid: barriers, enablers and impact. Health Expect 2007;10:173–83.

# Good practice tips and pitfalls to avoid when writing up

# 20

Aarthi Ramlaul

## CHAPTER POINTS

- Choose a topic that you have a sustained interest in.
- Careful time management is imperative for successful planning and organization.
- Always maintain contact and clear communication with your research supervisor.
- Pay attention to analysis of information.
- Remember to present work using an academic writing style that has clarity, cohesion and good formatting.
- Read through written work to pick out and correct spelling and typographical errors.
- Reread your earlier work as you progress through your dissertation to ensure that there are no contradictions.
- Acknowledge the work of other authors by using references appropriately.
- Pay attention to the constraints of the word limit.
- Follow the guidelines and conventions of the institution to which you are submitting your work, e.g. word count equivalence of figures, binding and submission requirements, etc.
- Ensure that you have access to the resources you require in advance of your study.
- Lastly, answer the research question by evaluating your findings in light of your aim and objectives.

Albert Einstein said, 'If we knew what it is we were doing then it wouldn't be called research, would it?'

This chapter provides some tips to take account of during your research journey as well as a few pitfalls commonly encountered by students during the writing-up phase of the study.

## 1. Choose a topic that you are interested in

It is absolutely normal to feel worried and overwhelmed at the start of a research study. However, choosing a topic that you are really interested in will help keep you motivated and focused. Take some time at the beginning of the study to carefully read around the topic area and conduct broad literature searches to get a feel of what information is already available out there. Doing this at the beginning of the year of study would discourage you from changing your topic midway through the year. It is not necessarily a bad thing to change your topic provided you do so for the right reason, for example changing the focus of the research as more literature sources become available. It is not unusual to go through several ideas at a time. However, once you have settled on a topic area, try to stick to it and look at avenues to make it workable. Changing a topic later on means that you will have lost valuable time and this is what matters.

Choosing a topic can be a daunting experience as you may find that whatever it is you wanted to research has been done before; this may be coupled with the fact that institutions may encourage you to explore new territories to try and come up with original ideas and hypotheses. If at the beginning you do not have a topic in mind then do not worry as many institutions will give you guidance specific to a programme, especially if it is an undergraduate or postgraduate course that you are undertaking. They may be broad subjects, for example laboratory experiments involving aspects of dosimetry or evaluating students' experiences of a wide range of activities. In-house guidance would be provided for these. In addition, the Society of Radiographers regularly publish topics to research in radiography which are considered to be current priorities for the profession. You may also wish to consider radiography in light of the wider health team, thus contributing to developments in inter-professional practice. Attendance at seminars and conferences is a good way to learn about current topics in your field and will help generate some ideas which you can explore further. Looking at published work, such as the recommendations that authors have made in recent issues of peer reviewed journals, is also a good way to find topics.

## 2. Answer the research question

Another common pitfall is not answering the research question, or leaving it up to the reader to decide whether you have achieved this or not. This could happen by losing focus during the course of the study and not maintaining clear communication with your supervisor. The conclusion chapter of your dissertation (as mentioned in Chapter 17) is the chapter where you should pull together your findings and summarize them in light of your aim and objectives. The conclusions drawn from this summary should enable you to adequately answer your research question. It is possible that you may not have been able to answer all of your questions by the end of the study but be overt about this, as research is seldom perfect. You may need to make recommendations for further work. Recommendations for further work can then be picked up as a Masters level study and who knows, it may also lead to a Doctoral thesis.

## 3. Time management

Many of you may ask, 'What about time management?' Universities today have diverse student populations with a greater number of students having domestic responsibilities, part time employment and families to care for. Study therefore has to be carefully organized and well managed.

Time management is a valuable skill and an attribute to develop. Once you have it well established, it

becomes a transferable skill that can be applied in all situations. Time is something we often take for granted. It is said to be human nature to leave things to the last minute. However, while you may be able to write up a 1000 word essay in a few days, you will have difficulty applying this strategy to a 10 000 word research project. The importance of a carefully planned study that has been divided into small manageable chunks, mapped against a definitive time scale, cannot be overemphasized. Even a small-scale study involving just a few participants needs careful time management.

As you will have read in previous chapters, undertaking a piece of research requires a systematic approach. The merits of the completed study depend on your commitment to the steps within that process. A good practice measure would be to draw up a study plan or keep a research diary, with dates indicating practical time scales according to which you envisage moving your study along. This plan then becomes a working document and is monitored by the checking of completed tasks. Ticking off the completed tasks has the added therapeutic benefit of a 'feel good' factor that says, 'Well done!' at each stage throughout the process. It is important to reward yourself for these little accomplishments along the way and in so doing, help to keep you self-motivated and focused on your next target.

Keeping a well designed study plan also helps to identify additional time constraints, for example when applying for ethics approval from a relevant committee if your study requires this. Ethical approval is required for all projects that involve the use of human participants. These include academic or clinical staff, students, patients, the general public, and written or visual records that potentially allow identification of individuals. Remember that ethics, in a nutshell, is a critical reflection on morality. It is considered poor research practice to recruit participants in close contact with the researcher, such as good friends or members of the family. It is, however, considered acceptable practice as part of a course, in the interests of experience of the research process. Writing up an ethics application form and gathering supporting documentation can take several weeks depending on the nature of the study, so allow yourself ample time to get this done properly if going down this route. Pay attention also to the dates on which committees meet; and target a meeting early in the year to allow enough time for data collection. You (the researcher) must consider the ethical implications for the research participants (see Chapter 6 for more information on ethical considerations).

Keep the date by which your work must be handed in in view all the way through. Set aside ample time for putting your dissertation together, including organizing your appendices and printing and binding the final document.

## 4. Research supervision

All student projects (both undergraduate and postgraduate) are supervised by staff who are academic tutors, or clinical tutors, or both, depending on the research topics. The role of a research supervisor is to provide guidance and support throughout the research process. They form the first point of contact in all research project-related matters and will answer any query you may have in that regard. Once you have been allocated your supervisor, do not hesitate to contact him or her and arrange your first meeting. This first meeting is the most important of all those to come, as this meeting sets the ground rules for communication and establishes the manner in which supervision is to proceed. More importantly it gets the ball rolling. Your supervisor would normally expect you to have a proposal of your intended study at hand for discussion at this meeting. It is good practice to keep a log of meetings and a recording of the proceedings, again with target dates (see example

in Figure 20.1). These can then be used to inform and update your own personal planner, and to inform your supervisor of your progress.

All too often students meet with their supervisor at the beginning of the year, get advice and then do not get in touch until the very last minute when the hand-in date is looming. Do not let this happen to you. Be sure to schedule regular meetings with your supervisor for a steady drip-feed of guidance throughout the duration of the study. This will ensure that any problems or errors are picked up and dealt with efficiently and effectively and do not hinder the development of the final project. When you arrange to meet with your supervisor, ensure that it is at a mutually suitable time. It is the responsibility of the student to initiate and maintain contact with the supervisor. Although supervisors will act as mentors and motivators, they will not undertake the work for you. You have to be committed to follow their guidance and work to set targets within agreed timeframes. It is good practice to send in some work prior to the meeting. You could do this either electronically or drop off a hard copy. This will give your supervisor some time to read through and note points for discussion. The dissertation is unlike any other work you will have undertaken for your course as it provides a unique opportunity to actually work with your supervisor.

| Date | Summary of session | Details of target/s set | Duration of meeting | Mode of contact i.e. email, telephone ... | Target date | Date of next meeting | Signatures | |
|---|---|---|---|---|---|---|---|---|
| | | | | | | | Student | Supervisor |
| | | | | | | | | |
| | | | | | | | | |
| | | | | | | | | |
| | | | | | | | | |
| | | | | | | | | |
| | | | | | | | | |
| | | | | | | | | |
| | | | | | | | | |
| | | | | | | | | |

**Figure 20.1** • Supervision log sheet.

Make sure that you prepare for your meeting as well. Have a list of questions drawn up and take along some writing material to write down notes. Do not rely on your memory. You may prefer to record the proceedings of the meeting on an MP3 recorder. Ensure that this is agreed with your supervisor beforehand. Supervision guidance should be reflected on and used in a positive and constructive manner to improve your work. Using feedback positively should also 'snowball' into other aspects of your work so that you do not make the same mistakes over again. In this way you will begin to 'work smart' rather than work hard.

The research process has a certain degree of flexibility within it and the various stages are merely offered as guidelines to follow. These have been produced by experts in the field and are tried and tested recipes that have yielded successful outcomes. Find your own measure among them but be careful of deviating too much from the straight and narrow. It is good practice to read the guidelines after every little bit of literature searching or writing that you have completed. This helps you to keep focused on your aims and objectives.

Remember to use guidance from your supervisor, no matter how intelligent you deem yourself to be. Even experienced research students have the need for assistance. If stumbling blocks appear in the research process, do not be disheartened. Modify your work and carry on. Very little research is conducted exactly as it was envisaged.

# 5. Pay attention to analysis

It is good practice to get into the habit of evaluating your work as you go along and becoming your own severest critic. Think about how you would like to read a topic of that nature if written by someone else by putting yourself in the reader's position. It is harder to make yourself clear in written communication than it is during verbal communication. During verbal communication, you are easily able to 'fill in the blanks' as your conversation proceeds; however, written communication can be tricky in ensuring that every angle of the topic you are writing about has been adequately covered. Poor analysis of literature will impact on your review of literature and hence your discussion chapter(s) of your dissertation with the potential to rob you of a good mark. While on the topic of the discussion chapter, a common pitfall occurs when students introduce new information

towards the end of their dissertation. Remember that while it is good practice to keep on literature searching and constantly checking for updates on information and news that will be 'hot off the press', it is important that this information be analysed in your literature review first. You can then revisit this information in your discussion of findings later on.

Although students often carry out extensive literature searches and have seemingly exhaustive data extraction forms, one of the main areas in which students lose the most marks in their final write up is in analysis of literature, usually reflected in the literature review or discussion sections of their dissertations. These sections of your dissertation should be the areas that most clearly demonstrate your ability to evaluate and interpret the literature in relation to your original research topic and the findings of previous studies. Literature should be used in an integrative way to support an argument or justification but should also discuss material which offers a conflicting view. Look for gaps in your arguments and evidence to determine whether you have sufficient information to support your arguments. In this way, you are attempting to provide a well balanced view that can be built up into a discussion or an argument depending on the nature of the information. Remember to consider both theoretical (of concepts and theories) and empirical (of studies, e.g. randomized clinical trials) literature. The discussion chapter of your dissertation must link in with the literature review chapter, and although you are encouraged to develop your thoughts and present original ideas, be careful of introducing new literature in this chapter.

One of the reasons students often lose marks for analysis of literature is poor strategy in literature searching. A robust literature search strategy would help ensure that you have adequately covered your topic area's research base to include a good range and depth of material in your analysis. There is no fixed number of literature sources, such as journal articles, that is recommended for writing a dissertation; however, it is expected that you would conduct exhaustive searches in your field of study. Guidance on literature searching is given in Chapter 3 and on literature evaluation in Chapter 4.

To analyse literature, try breaking down the information into component ideas. Then look for literature that supports these ideas or criticizes them. Pull all those pieces of information together and then write up the information you gathered in an all-encompassing manner. This is known as synthesis of information – the building up of information using new ideas, concepts and theories, etc. from findings. Remember the quality of the online search engines used will determine the quality of information gathered. Google and Wikipedia are not considered to be credible sources of information for academic writing because what is published is unlikely to be peer reviewed.

In addition, when evaluating and interpreting your results be careful of over-interpretation of the findings, especially in qualitative studies. It is not uncommon for researchers to analyse their way through an emergent theme from their findings and then talk themselves completely out of the same theme. If in doubt or in need of clarification, it is good research practice to go back to the participants and have them verify the transcripts and discuss your dilemma with your supervisor. It is very easy to misinterpret or over-interpret transcripts. Being reflective and reflexive (see Chapter 5) throughout the process will help you acknowledge your own biases and opinions and will help in the accurate interpretation of research findings.

When drawing conclusions from your findings, remember to justify these from evidence. Recommendations made, for example for further study, should be feasible and contribute to advancing practice.

## 6. Writing style and presentation

Present your aims and objectives clearly. Do not spend paragraphs telling your readers what you are about to do. Simply be direct and get to the point quickly. Avoid 'flowery' talk or overt descriptions. Your work should be written simply but must be clear. Avoid the use of long, convoluted sentences and jargon. Do not try to impress your reader by using difficult or fancy words if you do not fully understand their meaning. If used inappropriately, they can hinder the clarity of communication that you are trying to establish. The manner in which you write should tell your reader that you understand your study thoroughly and have taken the necessary measures to make it of the highest quality.

Present your discussion points in a logical order, possibly using headings and subheadings. It may help to make a list of the points you are going to present. The quality of the writing is judged by the quality of evidence provided, therefore do not include unsubstantiated opinions unless you are stating observations.

An academic writing style should have a logical flow to the information provided and should be presented in an integrated fashion with literature. Be sure to state your rationale for the study clearly as this sets the scene and places your study into context.

The manner in which you present your information should be well organized. The main points of your work should be presented clearly. Pay attention to the overall structure of the dissertation and the chapters within it. Use paragraphs well to clearly present your ideas. Use different paragraphs for different ideas but be careful to link them in so that they provide a cohesive flow of information and draw the reader through your work. When you write, do not assume that the reader has any prior knowledge of the topic area. Consider the use of appendices to contain background information and then link this in with your writing. It is good practice to cover material from first principles, i.e. from basic to complex. Although this may seem elementary to mention, it is something that is often overlooked, especially by those who do not write very often.

While it is important to get your point across you need to bear in mind the nature and context of your writing. In this case it is a research project so you need to write using a style to suit that format. In the same way, writing this chapter is suited to a more conversational style so it would be acceptable for me to write this as though I was speaking to you. Your writing style has to match the medium within which you are trying to express yourself.

Writing in the first person as 'I' is not considered to be good academic practice, therefore writing in the third person is advised. However, if you are writing a reflective essay, for example; then writing as 'I' would be acceptable. Writing in the third person requires vigilance, as students tend to start off well and then by the sixth or seventh page of the dissertation, they have slipped into 'I' or 'my'. Pay attention to this as you do not want to lose valuable marks for avoidable mistakes like this one. It is good practice to give your work to someone else to read. Choose this person carefully as they should act as a critical friend who is willing and objective enough to give you constructive criticism. It is not advisable to ask a class mate to read your work, however well you get along with each other.

Presentation is not restricted to text. The manner in which you display your illustrations is also important. Try to choose the best fit for your data using the guidance given in previous chapters but do not present the same information in more than one way. The manner in which you present this should be appropriate, clearly labelled with descriptive titles and understandable without tedious amounts of explanatory text. If information does not appear clear, then the chances are that it really did not make sense to you anyway. You may either rework it to make it clear or leave it out entirely, provided it is not information critical to your study.

Pay attention to the use and presentation of abbreviations. Only use them if you have written the words out in full first. It is good practice to include a list of abbreviations as an appendix. This may be presented either alphabetically or in the order in which they appear in the text.

Be careful of the information you present as appendices. Students often put in lots of appendices but do not refer to these within the body of the text. If it is not important enough to be mentioned in your writing, then leave it out. Items that you choose to present as appendices should be laid out in the order in which they would be referred to within the text and clearly marked. It is good practice to present a list of all the appendices, sequentially numbered, attached to your dissertation.

## 7. Spelling and grammar

Grammar, syntax and punctuation are important as they enable the reader to make sense of what you are trying to say. Avoid the use of redundant words or phrases such as 'actually' or 'so to speak', etc.

Many people experience difficulty in spelling words accurately. The advent of technology, in particular the use of email and texting, means that the nature of communicating words is changing. Because people are often communicating via email and have to do this quickly, they tend to spell poorly out of haste rather than knowledge. But we can all overcome this by reading over our emails once quickly in order to make any changes to poor spelling before sending. In the same way, we can read through our work to make sure that we have got the grammar and spelling correct before submitting our written work. In this way, you will be paying attention to detail which is so important in academic writing.

Use the spelling and grammar checking software on your computer to help rid your work of spelling and typographical errors. However, you should check first that you have the software set to the correct version of English for the context, for example UK English or US English, as there are a number of variations in spelling.

The use of punctuation marks has become increasingly stylistic in today's writing. Only use as many as punctuation marks as you need for clarity. Do not overuse them as they tend to make writing look imprecise. Avoid also the use of emotive terms as this is a sure indicator of researcher bias and may invalidate findings.

## 8. Acknowledge the work of others and pay attention to the word count

It is good practice to keep just within the word count although plus/minus 5–10% is usually acceptable. If you exceed your word limit then penalties usually apply, depending on the criteria set out by the institution. Be careful when incorporating the use of diagrams, photos, images, graphs and tables. These usually contribute to the word count and should be considered in the final write up. A typical A4 page of writing, double line spaced, will yield approximately 270 words using an Arial font size of 12. If you include a diagram or table half the size of the A4 page, then you have used up approximately 135 words for your diagram. Acknowledgements, abstracts, references, bibliography and appendices do not usually contribute to the word count.

Avoid repetitive information and leave out all material that is irrelevant. If leaving out anything potentially valuable, you must indicate this briefly within the text and justify the exclusion, otherwise during the marking process your lecturer may comment on your omission by saying, for example, 'useful idea or argument developing, however, this could have been analysed in more depth'. While you cannot include every argument within the constraints of the word limit, choose the ones that you are going to present in light of your aims and objectives and write these well. Mention also the ones that the reader may not have thought about. The omission of any common ones, either because they are public knowledge or because they have ongoing attention, for example through the media, must be justified. Stating limitations and identifying constraints within your study enhances your work as a researcher rather than inhibits it. By so doing you are communicating in an open manner with your reader.

The average word limit for an undergraduate project is approximately 10 000 words and for a post-graduate dissertation, it is approximately 20 000 words.

Remember to acknowledge the work of others, both published and unpublished. Failure to do so is regarded as theft and is a very serious academic offence. Any piece of work and its content is regarded as the work of the author; therefore you must acknowledge all sources that are not your own in the correct fashion (see Chapter 17). Pay careful attention therefore when using a previous students' work as a source of inspiration.

If you are working in a group to collect data for your study, be careful of collusion. While plagiarism can be unintentional, collusion is always deliberate and can easily happen when working in a group with fellow students. Institutions may use plagiarism detection software, e.g. Turnitin, in cases where this is suspected and if found, students will have to comply with academic misconduct procedures. Some institutions require students to put their work through plagiarism detection software and submit an 'originality report' with their submission.

## 9. Use of equipment

If you are undertaking data collection using laboratory equipment, ensure that you have been trained to use the relevant equipment and that you allow yourself enough time to prepare the materials you will need. Some equipment needs to be calibrated or charged for defined periods of time. Ensure that this is written into your plan of study otherwise you will find yourself losing valuable time again. If you would like to conduct certain experiments that require specific equipment, for example thermoluminescence dosimetry (TLD) readers, ensure that you discuss this with your supervisor who would be able to advise whether the institution is able to provide this or not. Sometimes, it may become necessary to share resources with either a clinical site or another institution. Some institutions, if aware of your study needs in advance, will be willing to purchase the equipment for you and other students, so again, this requires strategic planning and decisiveness.

If you are to be conducting interviews or focus groups and plan to record the proceedings of the session for later transcription, you will need to ensure that the recording devices are fully charged or have fresh batteries. There is nothing more disconcerting than having your research participants turn up for your session and not being adequately prepared. Most qualitative studies require recordings and the more sophisticated the recording device is, the greater the chance that something that can go wrong with it, so be prepared. Have some writing material at hand to take notes if all else fails.

Do remember to thank the research participants who have given up their time to help you collect data.

Lastly, students are often encouraged to publish their project work and I would urge you to take up the challenge. Although the process can be lengthy and onerous, it is very rewarding for those who have persevered in contributing to the evidence base of the profession and advancing practice.

Radiography practice is changing at a fast pace and as practitioners we must keep up with the pace by evaluating our own and others' practices. This will ensure a commitment to continuing professional development and no doubt enhance quality in clinical practice, management and education.

# Glossary

**Aim of study** Purpose or goal of research plan.

**Analysis** The process by which sense and meaning are derived from the information gathered. It involves breaking down information to extract a deeper meaning from the key elements that make up the information, for example analysing literature for a review, or analysing findings from research results.

**Anonymity** Where the identities of participants are replaced by codes which the researchers use during the study. In this way, subjects cannot be identified by the reader, or sometimes by the investigators themselves.

**Attitude** Refers to beliefs, views or feelings about something specific, such as interprofessional learning. There is an emotional attachment which may be positive or negative.

**Baye's theorem** Known also as the 'inverse probability principle', which relates the probability of the occurrence of an event to the occurrence or non-occurrence of an associated event; or a theorem that updates the probability of an occurrence following new research findings or evidence.

**Bias** A subjective attitude or viewpoint which can cause distortion or deviation of research findings from its true value or meaning.

**Blind study** When researchers are unaware which participant is allocated to or belongs to which group, as during a RCT (*randomized controlled trial*).

**Clinically significant** Refers to a result that is large enough to be of practical importance to healthcare providers and patients, for example a new form of treatment or imaging technique. This has a direct effect on clinical practice and is not the same as being *statistically significant*.

**Coercion** Urging participants to participate in a study, by manipulation or intimidation, or by pressurizing or tricking them. Coercion forms an important ethical consideration during data collection.

**Collusion** Unauthorized collaboration; most commonly occurs during group work.

**Confidentiality** An important code of conduct whereby participants' identity and personal information is not made public knowledge.

**Confounding variables** A variable other than the independent variable that may have certain effects on your participants' behaviour. These need to be taken into account when drawing conclusions from your research findings.

**Contrast** To contrast is to draw comparisons or point to differences in data.

**Control group** The group that has not been exposed to the intervention being tested.

**Critical analysis** The development of argument when reviewing literature. It is an evaluation of the positives and negatives or the agreements and disagreements with the author's point of view and has been grounded in theory or justified using additional supporting evidence from literature.

**Delphi technique** This is a forecasting tool that does not require face to face participation. It is a useful way to get public opinion on issues or ideas for problem solving.

**Dose fractionation** Refers to exposing tissues to smaller (fractionated) doses of radiation resulting in less tissue death, rather than one large exposure, over a period of time.

**Dosimetry** The measurement of exposure to radiation from a radiation-emitting source.

**Effectiveness** Refers to how well an *intervention* works in practice, i.e. does it do what it says it is going to do?

**Efficacy** Refers to the measurement of how well an *intervention* works, i.e. does it produce the intended result?

**Empirical** Refers to research that has been based on evidence from observations or experiments.

**Epidemiology** The study of the health of whole communities and populations, not just of particular individuals.

**Ethics** A set of moral principles which researchers have to abide by in order to protect their participants and themselves.

**Evaluate** A thought-provoking process of asking and answering critical questions, collecting appropriate information, and then analysing and interpreting the information for a specific use and purpose.

**Evidence** Findings to support claims from research that would inform practice.

**Exclusion criteria** This refers to a specific set of conditions that participants may be subjected to in order to determine whether they are eligible to participate in a research study, for example a particular study might exclude persons under the age of 18 years.

**Experiment** A set of observations undertaken to solve a research question or problem in order to prove or disprove a hypothesis.

**Explore** To investigate or to examine.

**External validity** Refers to the extent to which research findings can be generalized or applied to other population groups.

**False negative** A false finding that a person does not have a particular condition, when in fact they do.

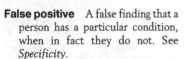

**False positive**  A false finding that a person has a particular condition, when in fact they do not. See *Specificity*.

**Feasibility**  Refers to the possibility, capability and practicability of, for example, a plan working.

**Generalizability**  See *External validity*.

**Gold standard**  A set of guidelines for a specific aspect of practice, such as a diagnostic test or protocol, that is regarded as definitive.

**Hypothesis**  A statement which is tested through research. This can be an experimental hypothesis (positive) whereby the researcher states, for example, that the public have good knowledge about the hazards of radiation; or it could be a null hypothesis (negative) which states, for example, that the public do not have good knowledge about the hazards of radiation.

**Inclusion criteria**  This refers to a specific set of conditions that participants must have in order to take part in a research study, for example females aged 18–30 years with a history of migraine headaches.

**Inductive reasoning**  Refers to making generalizations based on observations to support the conclusion of a study.

**Informed consent**  An agreement by participants to take part in the study after receiving a full explanation of the study procedure and any risks involved, etc. Consent may be given in an oral, written or implied format. The manner in which consent is gained from research participants is an important ethical consideration.

**Internal validity**  Refers to the manner in which the study was conducted free of bias, i.e. the extent to which the study actually did what it intended to do and the truthfulness of the results.

**Intervention**  Any measure put into place with the primary purpose of improving health or altering the course of disease, for example testing a new drug or therapy.

**Justify**  To support with evidence any assumptions, statements or assertions made.

**Negligence**  The behaviour or conduct of a reasonable person that fails to protect another person from foreseeable harm or risks, e.g. those associated with certain interventions.

**Objective**  To provide a balanced view taking into account the pros and cons of the issues involved.

**Placebo**  An inactive drug or intervention that is administered to 'blind' participants, for example in a randomized controlled trial where the effect of the actual drug or intervention is compared to the placebo. Participants sometimes feel a therapeutic, beneficial effect of receiving the 'treatment like' placebo and this effect is known as the *placebo effect*.

**Plagiarism**  Passing off other authors' work as your own and not acknowledging the work of others.

**Population**  All people who share certain specified characteristics, for example males aged 25–35years with a history of lower back pain. A sample of participants is usually then selected from this *population*.

**Probability**  The likelihood of an event occuring. Probability is measured numerically usually from 0 (never occurs) to 1 (always occurs).

**Qualitative**  Refers to methods whereby data collected is based on participants' experiences, attitudes and ideas; from these themes are drawn in order to extract deeper meaning and understanding of the specific issues.

**Quality**  Refers to the strength or appreciation of the study in relation to any methodological flaws and/or presence of bias.

**Quantitative**  Refers to methods whereby data collected is based on numbers; uses statistical analysis to draw meanings from which generalizations can be made.

**Randomization**  Refers to the process of randomly allocating participants to research groups, for example to the control group or experimental group of a *randomized controlled trial*.

**Randomized controlled trial (RCT)**  An experimental design which tests the effectiveness and efficacy of an intervention, e.g. therapy, health service or health technology. A sample of participants is randomly allocated into two or more groups so that the possible effects of the intervention can be compared with non-intervention under controlled conditions.

**Reflection**  A process whereby concrete experiences are reviewed in depth and analysed together with relevant theories to provide a plan of action to be implemented in practice.

**Reflexivity**  Refers to an acknowledgement or awareness of the involvement or influence that the researcher has in his or her own study, for example how the researcher's own values and experiences have influenced the study, and also how undertaking the study has impacted on the researcher.

**Reliability**  The extent to which the study is able to yield the same result if conducted under the same conditions or using the same measurements over again. The more consistent the result is, the greater the reliability of the result.

**Reproducibility**  The ability of the study to be done again (reproduced) in the same way, elsewhere.

**Sampling**  Method of drawing participants for your study from an identified population.

**Sensitivity**  This is the measure of 'positives' identified, i.e. a test's ability to correctly identify persons with disease.

**Specificity**  This is the measure of 'negatives' identified, i.e. a test's ability to correctly identify persons without disease.

**Statistically significant**  Refers to the probability that a result is not due to chance alone. The level of significance determines the degree of certainty or confidence with which we can rule out chance.

**Subjectivity**  Refers to the researcher's personal, introspective view.

**Synthesis**  'Building' of information using the key elements that has been 'broken down'(analysed) together with new found information (usually from literature searches). Where analysis is the breaking down of information; synthesis is the building up of information. Synthesis usually follows on after information has been analysed.

**Transactional analysis** Analysis of the emotion observed during communication in interpersonal relationships, where there are conflicting egos, for example in the doctor–patient relationship.

**True negative** A correct claim that a person does not have a particular condition.

**True positive** A correct claim that a person does have a particular condition. See *Sensitivity*.

**Validity** Refers to the extent to which the results or measurements are accurate, reliable and free from bias. See also *Reliability* and *Bias*.

# Index

Printed in the United States
By Bookmasters